Editors/Academic Advisory B

M000023460

Members of the Academic Advisory Board are instrumental in the final selection of article
Their review of articles for content, level, and appropriateness provides critical direction to
find their careful consideration well reflected in this volume.

ANNUAL EDITIONS: Nutrition 12/13
24th Edition

EDITOR

Amy Strickland, MBA, MS, RD
University of North Carolina–Greensboro

Editors/Academic Advisory Board continued

Preface

In publishing ANNUAL EDITIONS we recognize the enormous role played by the magazines, newspapers, and journals of the public press in providing current, first-rate educational information in a broad spectrum of interest areas. Many of these articles are appropriate for students, researchers, and professionals seeking accurate, current material to help bridge the gap between principles and theories and the real world. These articles, however, become more useful for study when those of lasting value are carefully collected, organized, indexed, and reproduced in a low-cost format, which provides easy and permanent access when the material is needed. That is the role played by ANNUAL EDITIONS.

Many of the articles in *Annual Editions: Nutrition 12/13* are based on the areas of concentration identified in the 2010 U.S. Dietary Guidelines. The Dietary Guidelines are published every five years by the U.S. federal government to address latest nutrition-related research findings and how they apply to the health of U.S. citizens. The 2010 Guidelines targeted obesity and other nutrition-related chronic diseases, food insecurity, physical activity, and the food environment in the United States. The majority of the articles in this edition address the challenges to improving the health of our country and many of the articles suggest possible solutions.

Annual Editions: Nutrition 12/13 is composed of eight units that review current knowledge and controversies in the area of nutrition. The first unit describes current trends in the field of nutrition with emphasis on the new guidelines for school meals and snacks, sports nutrition, and changes that are occurring in businesses that have historically provided "junk foods" to the U.S. markets.

This year a new unit has been added that focuses on childhood nutrition. The addition of Unit 2 is in response to the increased national emphasis on childhood nutrition and the "Let's Move" campaign. Articles on the importance of positive role models and family involvement in nutrition and health are the cornerstones of this unit.

Unit 3 includes five articles on the function and food sources of nutrients. Vitamin D, sodium, potassium, and fats are all emphasized in the 2010 Dietary Guidelines as nutrients of concern for Americans and are represented in articles in this section.

Units 4 through 6 include topics that focus on the relationship between nutrition and chronic diseases. Recent research findings on the role nutrients and diet play on diabetes, heart disease, hypertension, and obesity are emphasized.

Unit 7 covers food safety and technology, including information on the safety of imported foods and agriculture practices in other countries. Several articles in this section will discuss the use and prevalence of GM (genetically modified) foods.

Unit 8 focuses on hunger, nutrition, and sustainability of our food supply. Articles on the growing prevalence of nitrogen added to our environment, genetically altered grain crops, and sustainability efforts of the food industry make up this section.

Annual Editions: Nutrition is updated annually with the latest topics and controversies in the field as a way to keep students who study nutrition informed of the latest research findings, changes in policy, and trends in nutrition related topics. Keeping up with all of the nutrition research and policy changes is a challenging task, but thanks to books like the updated versions of *Annual Editions,* you can easily review the latest nutrition information taken from reputable sources.

Annual Editions: Nutrition 12/13 is to be used as a companion to a standard nutrition text so that it may update, expand, or emphasize certain topics that are covered in the text or present totally new topics not covered in a standard text. We hope that the reader will develop critical thinking and be empowered to ask questions and to seek answers from credible sources.

A *Topic Guide* assists students in finding other articles on a given subject within this edition, while a list of recommended *Internet References* guides them to the best sources of additional information on a topic.

There are two features in *Annual Editions* designed to assist students in their study and expand critical thinking. Located at the beginning of each unit, *Learning Outcomes* outline the key concepts that students should focus on as they are reading the material. *Critical Thinking* questions, located at the end of each article, allow students to test their understanding of the key concepts.

Your input is most valuable to improve this anthology, which we update yearly. We would appreciate your comments.

Amy Strickland
Editor

The Annual Editions Series

VOLUMES AVAILABLE

Adolescent Psychology

Aging

American Foreign Policy

American Government

Anthropology

Archaeology

Assessment and Evaluation

Business Ethics

Child Growth and Development

Comparative Politics

Criminal Justice

Developing World

Drugs, Society, and Behavior

Dying, Death, and Bereavement

Early Childhood Education

Economics

Educating Children with Exceptionalities

Education

Educational Psychology

Entrepreneurship

Environment

The Family

Gender

Geography

Global Issues

Health

Homeland Security

Human Development

Human Resources

Human Sexualities

International Business

Management

Marketing

Mass Media

Microbiology

Multicultural Education

Nursing

Nutrition

Physical Anthropology

Psychology

Race and Ethnic Relations

Social Problems

Sociology

State and Local Government

Sustainability

Technologies, Social Media, and Society

United States History, Volume 1

United States History, Volume 2

Urban Society

Violence and Terrorism

Western Civilization, Volume 1

World History, Volume 1

World History, Volume 2

World Politics

Contents

UNIT 1
Nutrition Trends

The concepts in bold italics are developed in the article. For further expansion, please refer to the Topic Guide.

UNIT 2
Childhood Nutrition

UNIT 3
Nutrients

The concepts in bold italics are developed in the article. For further expansion, please refer to the Topic Guide.

UNIT 4
Diet and Disease

The concepts in bold italics are developed in the article. For further expansion, please refer to the Topic Guide.

UNIT 5
Obesity and Weight Control

The concepts in bold italics are developed in the article. For further expansion, please refer to the Topic Guide.

UNIT 6
Health Claims

UNIT 7
Food Safety and Technology

The concepts in bold italics are developed in the article. For further expansion, please refer to the Topic Guide.

UNIT 8
Hunger, Nutrition, and Sustainability

The concepts in bold italics are developed in the article. For further expansion, please refer to the Topic Guide.

Correlation Guide

The *Annual Editions* series provides students with convenient, inexpensive access to current, carefully selected articles from the public press. **Annual Editions: Nutrition 12/13** is an easy-to-use reader that presents articles on important topics such as *nutrition trends, obesity and weight control, sustainability,* and many more. For more information on *Annual Editions* and other *McGraw-Hill Contemporary Learning Series* titles, visit www.mhhe.com/cls.

This convenient guide matches the units in **Annual Editions: Nutrition 12/13** with the corresponding chapters in four of our best-selling McGraw-Hill Nutrition textbooks by Schiff, Wardlaw/Smith, and Byrd-Bredbenner/Moe/Beshgetoor/Berning.

Annual Editions: Nutrition 12/13	Nutrition for Healthy Living, 3/e by Schiff	Contemporary Nutrition: A Functional Approach, 3/e by Wardlaw/Smith	Contemporary Nutrition, 9/e by Wardlaw/Smith	Wardlaw's Perspectives in Nutrition, 9/e by Byrd-Bredbenner/Moe, Beshgetoor/Berning
Unit 1: Nutrition Trends	**Chapter 1:** The Basics of Nutrition **Chapter 2:** Evaluating Nutrition Information **Chapter 3:** Planning Nutritious Diets	**Chapter 1:** What You Eat and Why **Chapter 2:** Guidelines for Designing a Healthy Diet	**Chapter 1:** What You Eat and Why **Chapter 2:** Guidelines for Designing a Healthy Diet	**Chapter 1:** The Science of Nutrition **Chapter 2:** Tools of a Healthy Diet **Chapter 3:** The Food Supply
Unit 2: Childhood Nutrition		**Chapter 18:** Nutrition from Infancy through Adolescence	**Chapter 15:** Nutrition from Infancy through Adolescence	**Chapter 17:** Nutrition during the Growing Years
Unit 3: Nutrients	**Chapter 5:** Carbohydrates **Chapter 6:** Fats and Other Lipids **Chapter 8:** Vitamins	**Chapter 4:** Carbohydrates **Chapter 5:** Lipids **Chapter 9:** Nutrients Involved with Fluid and Electrolyte Balance **Chapter 10:** Nutrients that Function as Antioxidants **Chapter 11:** Nutrients Involved in Bone Health **Chapter 12:** Nutrients Involved with Energy Metabolism and Blood Health	**Chapter 4:** Carbohydrates **Chapter 5:** Lipids **Chapter 8:** Vitamins	**Chapter 5:** Carbohydrates **Chapter 6:** Lipids
Unit 4: Diet and Disease	**Chapter 10:** Energy Balance and Weight Control **Chapter 13:** Nutrition for a Lifetime	**Chapter 7:** Energy Balance and Weight Maintenance **Chapter 17:** Pregnancy and Breastfeeding **Chapter 18:** Nutrition from Infancy through Adolescence **Chapter 19:** Nutrition during Adulthood	**Chapter 7:** Energy Balance and Weight Control **Chapter 15:** Nutrition from Infancy through Adolescence **Chapter 16:** Nutrition during Adulthood	**Chapter 2:** Tools of a Healthy Diet **Chapter 16:** Nutritional Aspects of Pregnancy and Breastfeeding **Chapter 17:** Nutrition during the Growing Years **Chapter 18:** Nutrition throughout Adulthood
Unit 5: Obesity and Weight Control	**Chapter 10:** Energy Balance and Weight Control	**Chapter 7:** Energy Balance and Weight Maintenance	**Chapter 7:** Energy Balance and Weight Control	**Chapter 10:** Energy Balance, Weight Control, and Eating Disorders
Unit 6: Health Claims	**Chapter 8:** Vitamins **Chapter 9:** Water and Minerals	**Chapter 10:** Nutrients that Function as Antioxidants **Chapter 11:** Nutrients Involved in Bone Health	**Chapter 8:** Vitamins **Chapter 9:** Water and Minerals	**Chapter 12:** Fat-Soluble Vitamins **Chapter 13:** Water-Soluble Vitamins **Chapter 14:** Water and Major Minerals **Chapter 15:** Trace Minerals
Unit 7: Food Safety/Technology	**Chapter 12:** Food Safety Concerns	**Chapter 16:** Food Safety	**Chapter 13:** Safety of Food and Water	**Chapter 3:** The Food Supply
Unit 8: Hunger, Nutrition, and Sustainability	**Chapter 13:** Nutrition for a Lifetime	**Chapter 15:** Undernutrition throughout the World	**Chapter 12:** Undernutrition Throughout the World	**Chapter 3:** The Food Supply

Topic Guide

This topic guide suggests how the selections in this book relate to the subjects covered in your course. You may want to use the topics listed on these pages to search the Web more easily.

On the following pages a number of websites have been gathered specifically for this book. They are arranged to reflect the units of this Annual Editions reader. You can link to these sites by going to www.mhhe.com/cls.

All the articles that relate to each topic are listed below the bold-faced term.

Internet References

The following Internet sites have been selected to support the articles found in this reader. These sites were available at the time of publication. However, because websites often change their structure and content, the information listed may no longer be available. We invite you to visit www.mhhe.com/cls for easy access to these sites.

Annual Editions: Nutrition 12/13

General Sources

American Dietetic Association
www.eatright.org

This consumer link to nutrition and health includes resources, news, marketplace, search for a dietician, government information, and a gateway to related sites. The site includes a tip of the day and special features.

The Blonz Guide to Nutrition
www.blonz.com

The categories in this valuable site report news in the fields of nutrition, food science, foods, fitness, and health. There is also a selection of search engines and links.

CSPI: Center for Science in the Public Interest
www.cspinet.org

CSPI is a nonprofit education and advocacy organization that is committed to improving the safety and nutritional quality of our food supply. CSPI publishes the *Nutrition Action Healthletter*, which has monthly information about food.

Food Guide Pyramid
www.mypyramid.gov

Visit this website and find out your daily needs for kilocalories and for protein intake.

Institute of Food Technologists
www.ift.org

This site of the Society for Food Science and Technology is full of important information and news about every aspect of the food products that come to market.

International Food Information Council Foundation (IFIC)
www.FoodInsight.org

IFIC's purpose is to be the link between science and communications by offering the latest scientific information on food safety, nutrition, and health in a form that is understandable and useful for opinion leaders and consumers to access.

My Plate
www.choosemyplate.gov

The USDA published My Plate to help simplify the message of eating a balanced diet. The site targets children, pregnant moms, and people who want to lose weight.

U.S. National Institutes of Health (NIH)
www.nih.gov

Consult this site for links to extensive health information and scientific resources. Comprised of 24 separate institutes, centers, and divisions, the NIH is one of eight health agencies of the Public Health Service, which, in turn, is part of the U.S. Department of Health and Human Services.

UNIT 1: Nutrition Trends

Food Science and Human Nutrition Extension
www.fshn.uiuc.edu

This extensive Illinois State University site links to latest news and reports, consumer publications, food safety information, and many other useful nutrition-related sites.

Healthy Hunger Free Kids Act of 2010
www.fns.usda.gov/cnd/governance/legislation/CNR_2010.htm

This piece of legislation, passed in December 2010, provides guidelines for breakfasts and lunches served in schools that receive federal funding as part of the breakfast and lunch program.

My Plate
www.choosemyplate.gov

The USDA published My Plate to help simplify the message of eating a balanced diet. The site targets children, pregnant moms, and people who want to lose weight.

American Society of Exercise Physiologists (ASEP)
www.asep.org

The goal of the ASEP is to promote health and physical fitness. This extensive site provides links to publications related to exercise and career opportunities in exercise physiology.

UNIT 2: Childhood Nutrition

Centers for Disease Control and Prevention— Obesity Trends
www.cdc.gov/obesity/data/trends.html

The CDC is the premier resource for statistics and latest research on diseases that impact U.S. citizens. This site is full of statistics on obesity among U.S. children and adults.

Centers for Disease Control and Prevention— Healthy Youth
www.cdc.gov/healthyyouth/obesity

The CDC is the premier resource for statistics and latest research on diseases that impact U.S. citizens. This site describes programs that are underway to help curtail the obesity epidemic.

U.S. Dept of Health and Human Services
http://aspe.hhs.gov/health/reports/child_obesity

This site describes the current research on how eating habits, lifestyle, socioeconomic status, parenteral influences, and marketing are impacting childhood obesity.

U.S. Dietary Guidelines
www.cnpp.usda.gov/DGAs2010-DGACReport.htm

A comprehensive view of the current state of nutrition and diet within the United States with recommendations for interventions, programs, and future research.

Internet References

UNIT 3: Nutrients

Dietary Supplement Fact Sheet: Vitamin D
http://ods.od.nih.gov/factsheets/vitamind.asp

The Office of Dietary Supplements fact sheet on vitamin D provides comprehensive information on the vitamin.

Food and Nutrition Information Center
www.nal.usda.gov/fnic

Use this site to find dietary and nutrition information provided by various USDA agencies and to find links to food and nutrition resources on the Internet.

NutritionalSupplements.com
www.nutritionalsupplements.com

This source provides unbiased information about nutritional supplements and prescription drugs, submitted by consumers with no vested interest in the products.

Office of Dietary Supplements: Health Information
http://ods.od.nih.gov/Health_Information/Health_Information.aspx

The Office of Dietary Supplements, a division of the National Institute of Health is the leading source on nutritional and botanical supplements. This website provides comprehensive information on the supplement industry.

U.S. National Library of Medicine
www.nlm.nih.gov

This site permits you to search databases and electronic information sources such as MEDLINE, learn about research projects, and keep up on nutrition-related news.

UNIT 4: Diet and Disease

American Cancer Society
www.cancer.org

Open this site and its various links to learn the concerns and lifestyle advice of the American Cancer Society. It provides information on alternative therapies, tobacco, other Web resources, and more.

American Diabetes Association
www.diabetes.org

The American Diabetes Association is the primary resource for type 1, type 2, and gestational diabetes.

American Heart Association (AHA)
www.americanheart.org

The AHA offers this site to provide the most comprehensive information on heart disease and stroke as well as late-breaking news. The site presents facts on warning signs, a reference guide, and explanations of diseases and treatments.

Medline Plus
www.nlm.nih.gov/medlineplus

This site provides health information from the National Library of Medicine and the National Institutes of Health.

National Eating Disorders Association
www.nationaleatingdisorders.org

This site offers information on the different types of eating disorders, programs, events, research, resources, insurance coverage, and a support line.

UNIT 5: Obesity and Weight Control

American Society of Exercise Physiologists (ASEP)
www.asep.org

The goal of the ASEP is to promote health and physical fitness. This extensive site provides links to publications related to exercise and career opportunities in exercise physiology.

Calorie Control Council
www.caloriecontrol.org

The Calorie Control Council's website offers information on cutting calories, achieving and maintaining healthy weight, and low-calorie, reduced-fat foods and beverages.

Centers for Disease Control and Prevention: Overweight & Obesity
www.cdc.gov/obesity

The Centers for Disease Control and Prevention is a component of the U.S. Department of Health and Human Services. It monitors and tracks the general health of Americans, conducts research, and implements health prevention strategies.

Shape Up America!
www.shapeup.org

At the Shape Up America! website you will find the latest information about safe weight management, healthy eating, and physical fitness. Links include Support Center, Cyberkitchen, Media Center, Fitness Center, and BMI Center.

UNIT 6: Health Claims

Federal Trade Commission (FTC): Diet, Health & Fitness
www.ftc.gov/bcp/menus/consumer/health.shtm

This site of the FTC on the Web offers consumer education rules and acts that include a wide range of subjects, from buying exercise equipment to virtual health "treatments."

Food and Drug Administration (FDA)
www.fda.gov/default.htm

The FDA presents this site that addresses products they regulate, current news and hot topics, safety alerts, product approvals, reference data, and general information and directions.

National Council against Health Fraud (NCAHF)
www.ncahf.org

The NCAHF does business as the National Council for Reliable Health Information. At its Web page it offers links to other related sites, including Dr. Terry Polevoy's "Healthwatcher Net."

Office of Dietary Supplements: Health Information
http://ods.od.nih.gov/Health_Information/Health_Information.aspx

The Office of Dietary Supplements, a division of the National Institute of Health, is the leading source on nutritional and botanical supplements. This website provides comprehensive information on the supplement industry.

QuackWatch
www.quackwatch.com

Quackwatch Inc., a nonprofit corporation, provides this guide to examine health fraud. Data for intelligent decision making on health topics are also presented.

Internet References

UNIT 7: Food Safety/Technology

American Council on Science and Health (ACSH)
www.acsh.org

The ACSH addresses issues that are related to food safety here. In addition, issues on nutrition and fitness, alcohol, diseases, environmental health, medical care, lifestyle, and tobacco may be accessed on this site.

Centers for Disease Control and Prevention (CDC)
www.cdc.gov

The CDC offers this home page, from which you can obtain information about travelers' health, data related to disease control and prevention, and general nutritional and health information, publications, and more.

FDA Center for Food Safety and Applied Nutrition
www.fda.gov/food/foodsafety/default.htm

It is possible to access everything from this website that you might want to know about food safety and what government agencies are doing to ensure it.

Food Safety Project (FSP)
www.extension.iastate.edu/foodsafety

This site from the Cooperative Extension Service at Iowa State University has a database designed to promote food safety education via the Internet.

Institute of Food Technologists
www.ift.org

This site of the Society for Food Science and Technology is full of important information and news about every aspect of the food products that come to market.

USDA Food Safety and Inspection Service (FSIS)
www.fsis.usda.gov

The FSIS, part of the U.S. Department of Agriculture, is the government agency "responsible for ensuring that the nation's commercial supply of meat, poultry, and egg products is safe, wholesome, and correctly labeled and packaged."

UNIT 8: World Hunger, Nutrition, and Sustainability

Food and Agriculture Organization of the United Nations (FAO)
www.fao.org

The FAO is the premier site for information on food production, consumption, deprivation, malnutrition, poverty, and food trade of countries around the globe. The FAO hunger map is a tool that is commonly used to demonstrate the areas of the world that suffer from malnutrition and food insecurity.

International Food Information Council Foundation (IFIC)
www.FoodInsight.org

IFIC's purpose is to be the link between science and communications by offering the latest scientific information on food safety, nutrition, and health in a form that is understandable and useful for opinion leaders and consumers to access.

Population Reference Bureau
www.prb.org

A key source for global population information, this is a good place to pursue data on nutrition problems worldwide.

U.S. Sustainable Agriculture Research and Education Program, University of California–Davis
www.sarep.ucdavis.edu/concept.htm

This UC-Davis sponsored site describes the main concepts of sustainable agriculture principles and practices.

World Health Organization (WHO)
www.who.int/en

This home page of the World Health Organization will provide you with links to a wealth of statistical and analytical information about health and nutrition around the world.

UNIT 1
Nutrition Trends

Unit Selections

Learning Outcomes

After reading this Unit, you will be able to:

- Evaluate the nutrition standards set by the Healthy, Hunger-Free Kids Act for meals served in the National School and Breakfast programs. Critique the breakfast and lunch standards.

- Describe the effects of the federal law passed in 2004 regarding vending in schools.

- Describe how PepsiCo is changing its business model to improve the nutrient density of its food and beverage items.

- Defend the requirement that chain restaurants must post nutrition information on their menus.

- Provide examples of how restaurants have eliminated trans fats from their menus.

- Explain how McDonald's in Europe has "cleaned up" its reputation.

- Assess why the definitions of meat products matter to food producers, marketers, and consumers. Identify the government agency that defines these terms.

- Define the nutritional strategies for athletes to optimize their physical and mental performance.

Student Website
www.mhhe.com/cls

Internet References

American Dietetic Association
www.eatright.org
American Society of Exercise Physiologists (ASEP)
www.asep.org
Food Science and Human Nutrition Extension
www.fshn.uiuc.edu
Healthy, Hunger-Free Kids Act of 2010
www.fns.usda.gov/cnd/governance/legislation/CNR_2010.htm
My Plate
www.choosemyplate.gov

The hottest trends in nutrition today revolve around reducing the incidence of obesity and chronic disease in the United States, improving the nutrient quality of school lunches, and holding the food industry and restaurants accountable for providing healthy foods to Americans.

Unit 1 addresses a few of these current trends in nutrition, including the new guidelines for healthy school meals and snacks, the recent paradigm shift in the operations of fast food restaurants, and the growing popularity of sports nutrition.

The recent passage of the Healthy, Hunger-Free Kids Act has prompted the USDA to modify the standards for the National School Lunch and Breakfast programs. The new standards for schools that participate in the federal program that supports free and reduced price breakfasts and lunches are addressed in Article 1, written by Nirvi Shah, "Ultimate Food Fight Erupts as Feds Recook School Lunch Rules." Schools who participate in the National School Lunch and Breakfast program have until next year to put the new guidelines in practice.

When the school food policies were tightened, thousands of vending companies fled the school vending market, leaving room for new concepts in healthy vending options. Nick Lieber focuses on some of the changes seen in the school vending market in Article 2, "Junk Food-Free Vending Machines Go to School."

An example of trends within the food industry to provide more healthy foods can be seen in the changes that are occurring at PepsiCo, covered in Article 3. PepsiCo, the parent company of soft drinks and snack foods, is working to improve its image and ensure that it is positioned to meet the demand for healthier snack foods and beverages. Indra Nooyi, the CEO of PepsiCo, is leading the company that traditionally has provided foods laden with added sugar, salt, and fats to a company that is leading the industry on research and development of healthier versions of snack foods and beverages.

McDonald's is taking strides to improve its image by offering healthier options in the United States and has changed its operations to more ethical and ecofriendly practices in Great Britain and Northern Ireland. McDonald's UK has made great strides to ensure no (genetically modified) foods are sold at its restaurants in Europe, discussed in Article 5.

Sports nutrition and nutrition to improve physical performance are popular topics among the general population and

© US Department of Agriculture

within the profession of dietetics. More Americans are increasing their activity level to meet or exceed the exercise recommendations published in the Dietary Guidelines. As a result, more people are exercising at the level of "athlete" rather than occasional exerciser. Article 6 addresses how to properly fuel and hydrate for optimal athletic conditioning.

Athletes need additional calories and nutrients to support training and optimal performance. As more Americans are choosing to increase their activity level to athletic and endurance conditioning, snacks may be the easiest way to meet the additional nutrient needs. Christine Rosenbloom offers practical advice on the best snacks for athletes in Article 7, "Snack Attack: Evaluating and Rating Snacks for Athletes."

The seven articles in Unit 1 focus on a variety of trends seen in nutrition and health environments. The selection of articles include topics that have been seen in popular media as well as trends observed within the profession of nutrition. These articles stretch across the topics commonly covered in general nutrition courses.

Ultimate Food Fight Erupts as Feds Recook School Lunch Rules

NIRVI SHAH

Across the country, school cafeteria managers, farm lobbyists, food companies, celebrity chefs, students, and parents have started the ultimate food fight.

The skirmish is over the U.S. Department of Agriculture's efforts, prompted by the recent passage of the Healthy, Hunger-Free Kids Act, to rewrite the rules about meals served through the National School Lunch and Breakfast programs. At stake is what will and won't be offered in the breakfasts and lunches schools serve millions of children every weekday.

"It's not your grandmother's school lunch anymore," Nancy Rice, the head of the School Nutrition Association, said at one of the advocacy group's gatherings last month.

The first rewrite of school-meal rules in 15 years, the proposed standards aim to cut sodium, boost the amount and types of fruits and vegetables students are offered, cut saturated fat, increase whole grains, and for the first time, limit calories. (The new proposed standards don't set limits on or address sugar, in part because sugar wasn't addressed in school meal requirements created by the Institute of Medicine. The USDA based its proposal largely on the Institute's recommendations.) The proposed rules, intended to simultaneously combat childhood obesity and malnutrition, have drawn thousands of emails, letters, and drawings that voice opinions about the proposed nutrition standards for school meals. And some of the interest has been high-profile, including school food activist Jamie Oliver, also known as "The Naked Chef," who has thrown his support behind the changes; the Berkeley, Calif.-based organic and natural foods company Annie's Homegrown, which created a website devoted to sending thank-you notes to the USDA for adding more vegetables to school meals; and the Washington-based National Potato Council, which also has a new website pushing for more potatoes to be allowed in school meals.

The proposed rules were published in January and comments are expected to roll in until the April 13 deadline. It may be next year before the rules are final, giving schools until at least the 2012–13 school year to put the new standards into practice. But stakeholders are asking for many concessions, saying some of the requirements would be impossible or have already proved so in school cafeterias.

"It is difficult to have one-size-fits-all," Agriculture Secretary Tom Vilsack told school nutrition directors in March. "I feel your pain. The trick is doing the balancing act . . . between what is appropriate . . . and fiscally responsible."

One of the biggest concerns is the expected cost to school districts: $6.8 billion over five years on food and labor. Some districts would have to buy new kitchen equipment, too.

The New Menu for Cafeterias

The nutrition standards for school meals would change dramatically under the new Healthy, Hunger-Free Kids Act. Among the proposed changes:

All Meals

- Milk: One-cup servings of unflavored milk must be 1 percent milk-fat or fat-free, and one-cup servings of flavored milk must be fat-free.
- At first, half of bread products served must be made with at least 51 percent whole grains. Two years after the USDA implements the nutrition regulations, all breads served must be at least 51 percent whole grain.

Breakfast

- Students must be offered one full cup of fruit at breakfast. Only half a cup could be juice, and that would have to be 100 percent fruit juice. Fruit could be replaced with vegetables.
- A meat or meat alternative, such as eggs, yogurt, or cheese, would have to be served every day. Tofu is not an approved meat alternative.
- The calorie range is 350 to 500 for elementary students, 400 to 550 for middle schoolers, and 450 to 600 for high schoolers.

- No starchy vegetables—potatoes, corn, peas, or lima beans—are allowed.
- Over the course of 10 years, schools must reduce sodium to 430 milligrams or less per breakfast for elementary students, 470 milligrams or less for middle schoolers, and 500 milligrams or less for high schoolers.

Lunch

- Elementary and middle students must be offered a one-half cup serving of fruit every day. High school students must be offered a cup every day.
- The calorie range is 550 to 650 in elementary school, 600 to 700 in the middle grades, and 750 to 850 in high school.
- Elementary and middle school students must be offered at least one ¾-cup serving of vegetables every day; one cup for high school students.
- Starchy vegetables must be limited to a one-cup serving a week.
- A one-half-cup serving of dark-green vegetables must be offered at least once a week.
- A one-half-cup serving of orange vegetables must be offered at least once a week.
- A one-half-cup serving of legumes—black beans, black-eyed peas, garbanzo beans, green peas, kidney beans, lentils, lima beans, soy beans, split peas, and white beans—must be served once a week.
- Over 10 years, schools must reduce sodium to 430 milligrams or less per lunch in elementary school, 470 milligrams or less in middle school, and 500 milligrams or less in high school.

The price tag was a main reason the American Association of School Administrators, the National School Boards Association, and the Council of the Great City Schools lobbied against the law. Because of the cost, the state of the economy, and the possibility that additional federal money per meal to meet the requirements may not materialize until after they go into effect, the Arlington, Va.-based AASA, in its comments, said districts need more time to put the final regulations into practice. The School Nutrition Association, a group of 55,000 school nutrition directors based in National Harbor, Md., also wants more time, in part because some foods required aren't available in some regions.

Adding more fresh fruits and vegetables this year to school meals in Norfolk, Va., cost about $500,000, said Helen Phillips, the school district's senior director of school nutrition and president-elect of the School Nutrition Association. But at least in her district, changes in anticipation of the federal regulations have been put in over time, allowing her to space out the added costs. For districts with less progressive menus, costs could shoot upward more quickly.

"The cost is big anyway," Ms. Phillips said. But compounding the change, "food costs are at an all time high."

But Margo G. Wootan, the director of nutrition policy at the Center for Science in the Public Interest in Washington, which lobbied for the law, finds neither the timeline nor the costs insurmountable.

"There are lots of school districts that are serving healthy meals under the current reimbursement rate," Ms. Wootan said, referring to how much school districts are paid by the USDA per meal.

The federal agency has suggested districts raise prices, if necessary, to offset costs, although school nutrition directors fear that could turn off some students.

Whole-Grain Everything

Aside from cost, there are concerns about nearly every part of the regulations. One proposed rule requires schools to switch all breads—tortillas, pizza crust, pancakes—to whole grains. At first, half of all bread products must be whole-grain rich, or made with at least 51 percent whole grains. Two years after the rules are final, all grains served would have to be whole-grain rich.

In the Sioux Falls, S.D., schools, Child Nutrition Supervisor Joni Davis said her 21,500-student district is halfway there.

"We've been talking to vendors, and they're listening," Ms. Davis said, although at first, they thought she was "a little bit crazy" for asking for whole-grain breading on chicken patties.

But the Anne Arundel County schools in Maryland abandoned a yearlong effort to switch to whole grains for some lunch items, said Jodi Risse, the supervisor of food and nutrition services in the 75,000-student district. While students didn't seem to notice the change in breakfast breads, they quickly learned to avoid pizza and egg rolls made with whole grains. "We couldn't tell as adults," Ms. Risse said, but for students, "over a few months we saw the consumption of egg rolls just go away. They probably don't eat it that way anywhere else." And there can be a tradeoff when adding whole grains: more sugar. For example, when the Schwan Food Co. of Marshall, Minn., reformulated the pizza it makes for schools to increase whole grains, it added sugar, a comparison of the printed nutrition facts for the two products shows. The USDA said it hopes that calorie requirements will keep sugar levels in check.

'Bok Choy? Watercress?'

In the Burlington, Vt., schools, Food Service Director Doug Davis said his 4,000-student district has easily incorporated orange and dark-green vegetables into menus, in part because of a farm-to-school program that emphasizes local produce.

Lunch Letters

In letters to the Agriculture Department, children thank the federal agency for the proposed nutrition rules:

"Those are the kinds of things that grow best for us," Mr. Davis said, so students are used to eating kale and butternut squash. The proposed rules require at least one half-cup serving each of dark-green and orange vegetables a week.

They include bok choy, broccoli, collard greens, dark green leafy lettuce, kale, mustard greens, romaine lettuce, spinach, turnip greens, and watercress, and acorn squash, butternut squash, carrots, pumpkin, and sweet potatoes.

Burlington students eat vegetables, including zucchini and carrots, in breakfast breads, too.

But back in Sioux Falls, Ms. Davis said her district hasn't been big on squash and pumpkin, and including dark-green vegetables, other than broccoli, may be tricky.

"Bok choy? Watercress? That's going to be different. Can you put broccoli on your menu every week as your dark green?" she said. "When we think of kids trying new vegetables, the first time they look at it. The second time they smell it. And the fourth, maybe, they eat it."

Besides the challenge of adding new items is the required serving size, said Bob Bloomer, a regional vice president for Chartwells-Thompson Hospitality of Charlotte, N.C., which provides meals for about 470 Chicago public schools. The proposed regulations would require a minimum of one cup of fruit at breakfast for all students, only half of which may be 100 percent fruit juice. For elementary and middle school students, another half cup of fruit and a ¾-cup serving of vegetables would be offered at lunch, when high schoolers get a full cup each of fruits and vegetables.

"A cup of vegetables? No high school student is going to take a cup of vegetables," Mr. Bloomer said. He and others worry much of the additional produce will end up in the garbage instead of students' stomachs.

Potato Pushback

While children must be served more veggies, the proposal also says cafeterias must reduce starchy items. Potatoes, corn, green peas, and fresh lima beans—those that weren't picked dry off the plant—would be limited to one cup total per week at lunch. Sweet potatoes aren't considered a starchy vegetable in the proposal.

"It doesn't make any sense at a time when you're telling kids to consume more vegetables," said John Keeling, the executive vice president and chief executive officer of the National Potato Council. He said the bad rap on french fries has tainted the popular, cheap tuber, which is high in fiber and potassium and low in calories.

Many schools serve "fries" that are actually baked in the oven, he said. His organization recommends allowing four half-cup servings of spuds a week, plus a serving of another starchy vegetable, and allowing potatoes at breakfast. The School Nutrition Association goes further: They asked for four half-cup servings of potatoes a week in elementary school, and no limits on the number of days those half-cup servings are offered in middle and high school per week—as long as kids can't take seconds and neither potatoes nor any other vegetable could be fried.

The recommendation isn't because cutting back on potatoes isn't impossible, said Ms. Phillips, of the SNA. In her menus in Norfolk, Va., there are weeks when potatoes aren't offered at all. But other districts may rely more heavily on potatoes. "It goes back to where districts are currently," she said, and "a concern . . . that we do have for children. Some of their favorite vegetables are starchy vegetables. To limit them to just that to one cup a week might discourage them from eating vegetables at all."

But Ms. Wootan of the Center for Science in the Public Interest, said the problem with potatoes isn't whether they are fried or roasted.

"It's just the variety," she said. "If kids were eating carrots as their only vegetable at every meal, that wouldn't be a good thing either."

Got (Fat-Free Chocolate) Milk?

The National Dairy Council worries that chocolate milk, long the dairy king among students, may be less inviting in fat-free form. Flavored milks that are anything but fat-free wouldn't be allowed under the new guidelines, although schools could serve unflavored milk with up to 1 percent milk-fat. "We want to make sure there are not unintended consequences," said Ann Marie Krautheim, senior vice president of nutrition affairs of the Council, based in Rosemont, Ill. In other words, if students dislike fat-free flavored milk, they might not drink milk at all.

But in Anne Arundel, students never noticed the switch to skim chocolate and strawberry milk this school year, Ms. Risse said. To make up for the missing fat, the milk has a little more sugar and flavoring, but the district's milk consumption is virtually unchanged. For some districts, however, including Norfolk and Burlington, fat-free flavored milk isn't available from the closest dairies, one reason the School Nutrition Association wants more time before the regulations take effect.

"We need to get the standards out there, let industry meet the standards, and then have time to bid those items," Ms. Phillips said.

Districts do have 10 years to cut back on sodium. While that's enough time for manufacturers to reformulate recipes and for districts to develop spice blends to compensate for the reduced salt, the sodium requirements are unrealistic, said the School Nutrition Association, adding that they are so low they're less than what a hospital might serve a patient on a low-sodium diet.

"School food will taste so dramatically different from what a child would eat at home and at a restaurant that participation will drop," Ms. Phillips said. The association endorses only the first two phases of sodium reduction, but not the final limits. She pointed out that a cup of milk has 120 milligrams of sodium naturally, or about 1/5 of what will be allowed.

In Chicago, the district has already cut sodium to the level required in the first phase of the reductions. Mr. Bloomer said he has been hounding food manufacturers to cut sodium further in processed foods they supply to the district. And district policy doesn't allow added salt on vegetables, to which a blend of spices is now added. Some kids haven't been impressed.

"No matter how good a fresh vegetable is, it needs a little bit of something," he said, which his district adds in the form of spices and herbs.

Whether it's no-salt-added vegetables, roasted butternut squash, or fat-free chocolate milk, by far the biggest challenge for school districts will be to convince kids to eat what will be offered after all the meticulous meal planning and calorie counting.

David Just, a professor at Cornell University in Ithaca, N.Y., and co-director of the school's Center for Behavioral Economics in Child Nutrition Programs, works on ways to get students to eat healthier at lunch through the placement of items, renaming foods, and other subtle measures.

"It isn't nutrition until it's eaten," he said.

Critical Thinking

1. Describe the nutrition standards set by the Healthy, Hunger-Free Kids Act for meals served in the National School and Breakfast programs.

2. Explain why sugar is not addressed in the Healthy, Hunger-Free Kids Act.

3. Critique the breakfast and lunch standards. What do you think will be the most challenging standards to meet?

4. How will these new standards impact food suppliers and food companies?

From *Edweek,* April, 2011. Copyright © 2011 by Editorial Projects in Education. Reprinted by permission.

Junk Food-Free Vending Machines Go to School

Nick Leiber

Jeff Lowell, an assistant principal at Interlake High School in Bellevue, Wash., normally dismisses the e-mails he gets from businesses trying to sell to his 1,500 students. He was intrigued, however, by the pitch he received in September from **Fresh Healthy Vending,** a San Diego franchise operaton that offers vending machines stocked with snacks and drinks it touts as alternatives to junk food. "Everybody [understands] what eating right does for you and how much it ends up affecting your ability to think," Lowell says. "We decided we wanted to try it."

Lowell signed a one-year contract allowing Fresh Healthy to park its machines near Interlake's gym in exchange for 15 percent of profits. In late November, Fresh Healthy installed three machines, featuring goodies such as Kashi granola bars and Stonyfield Farm fruit smoothies, next to older machines that sell Powerade and Dasani water—though no soda—through a long-standing agreement with **Coca-Cola Enterprises.** The top seller in the new machines so far: Pirate's Booty cheese puffs.

Fresh Healthy is one of more than a dozen small companies that aim to bring healthier fare to school vending machines. To do so they must navigate a tangle of rules created in the wake of 2004 federal law that required school districts to establish local policies aimed at improving student nutrition and reducing childhood obesity. Those rules prompted the bulk of the 10,500 U.S. vending machine companies to avoid schools. "There were fewer and fewer operators handling school accounts because it was a tough process to find products that met the patchwork of school guidelines," says Ned Monroe, senior vice-president for government affairs for the National Automatic Merchandising Assn. The trade group estimates that just 10 percent of its vending operator members sell in schools now, down from about 25 percent a decade ago.

1500—Schools with Fresh Healthy's vending machines

The hodgepodge of local policies will soon be replaced. Under a law that regulates schools participating in the federal school lunch program, which President Barack Obama signed on Dec. 13, the U.S. Agriculture Dept. now can impose nutritional standards on all snacks and refreshments sold in schools. The national guidelines will make it easier for vending companies to sell to many local districts. Producers are likely to be more willing to make foods suitable for vending machines if they know what requirements they must meet. "Food companies [are] trying to be ahead of the game and have products in the marketplace available to meet those standards as soon as they're published," says Diane Pratt-Heavner, a spokeswoman for the School Nutrition Assn., a trade group of food companies and school cafeteria managers.

Small vending machine operators that specialize in healthy snacks are confident the new law will boost their business. "I can't even tell you the response we're getting since this latest piece of legislation passed," says Fresh Healthy founder Jolly Backer, who launched the company in May to sell and supply franchises. He charges franchisees about $11,000 per machine, which they then manage, ordering from Fresh Healthy online and restocking once or twice a week. Fresh Healthy has machines in more than 2,000 locations, about three-quarters of them schools. "Our race is to get space," says Backer, 55. "A lot of schools would just as soon get rid of vending programs because they haven't found out about healthy options yet." He expects revenue at the 22-employee company to at least double this year, to more than $10 million.

Sean Kelly, the 27-year-old chief executive of **Human Healthy Vending** in Los Angeles, says the new law will help him expand from 300 machines to perhaps 1,500 by yearend. He hopes to convince schools that the vending machine business isn't "synonymous with scam" and that it sells more than junk food. Kelly expects revenue to triple this year to more than $9 million. "We see tons of opportunity," he says.

The biggest U.S. vending machine operators—**Canteen, Sodexo,** and **Aramark**—have started offering healthier food in recent years. Canteen has a fledgling operation of about 200 machines (out of a total of 300,000) selling vegan foods and local fare. Since 2003, 15 percent of the products in its company-owned machines have met Canteen's reduced fat and sugar criteria. In 2001, Sodexo introduced a similar program for 20 percent of its products. The company says it plans to increase healthy choices to 30 percent by April. Aramark followed suit in 2005 with a labeling program showing nutritional values for products in its machines.

The new entrants say they aren't worried about industry giants muscling in on their niche. "I don't get that concerned about it because of the uniqueness of what we do," says William H. Carpenter Jr., president of **Vend Natural** in Annapolis, Md., which counts USDA headquarters among the locations for its 535 healthy vending machines. He says the company's revenue, "well north of $10 million," is on track to increase by more than 25 percent this year. "The growth is just so huge," Carpenter says, "not only because of what's happening under the current Administration but just how people want to eat."

Critical Thinking

1. Describe the effects of the federal law passed in 2004 regarding vending in schools.

2. How did the 2004 school vending law impact the number of vending companies that sell to schools?

3. Evaluate whether the law passed on December 13, 2010 will impact vending in schools. Explain your reasoning.

4. Defend the statement regarding the December 2010 school vending law, "Producers are likely to be more willing to make foods suitable for vending machines if they know what requirements must be met."

From *Bloomberg BusinessWeek*, January 17–23, 2011. Copyright © Bloomberg 2011 by Bloomberg BusinessWeek. Reprinted by permission of Bloomberg LP via YGS Group.

Pepsi Brings in the Health Police

The snack food behemoth has hired a team of idealistic scientists to find alternatives to Doritos.

Nanette Byrnes

In February 2007, when Derek Yach, a former executive director of the World Health Organization and an expert on nutrition, took a new job with PepsiCo, his mother worried that he'd lost his mind. "You are aware they sell soda and chips, and these things cause you to get unhealthy and fat?" she asked him. Yach's former colleagues in public health circles murmured similar concerns.

Yes, he said, he knew what Pepsi made. But he wanted to help guide the $43 billion snack food multinational toward a more balanced product menu. The company describes its current portfolio of "healthy" fare as a $10 billion business—a figure CEO Indra Nooyi says she wants to see jump to $30 billion over the next decade.

The question is, will Yach, now senior vice-president for global health policy, really have the influence his boss has promised? If he does, will Pepsi's strategy prove profitable? Can its growing team of health advocates—who in times past might have seen Pepsi as the enemy—come up with an apple treat that tastes as good as a deep-fried Lay's potato chip?

Over the past two years, Pepsi has hired a dozen physicians and PhDs, many of whom built their reputations at the Mayo Clinic, WHO, and like-minded institutions. Some researched diabetes and heart disease, the sort of ailments that can result in part from eating too much of what Pepsi sells.

Yach and his comrades aren't subversives. The goal, says Mehmood Kahn, Pepsi's first-ever chief scientific officer, is to create healthy options while making the bad stuff less bad. "It's O.K. to have a slice of birthday cake on your birthday," says Kahn, formerly a practicing physician specializing in nutrition who did a stint at the Mayo Clinic. "Would you eat it every day of the week? That's a different question." At Pepsi, he and the other scientists "can say we can actually make an impact on what is available for consumers."

Flight From Junk Food

Khan hunts for benign ingredients that can go into multiple products. Last year, technological improvements to an all-natural zero-calorie sweetener derived from a plant called stevia allowed Pepsi to devise several fast-growing brands, including Trop50, a variation on its Tropicana orange juice that has half the calories of the breakfast standby. Introduced in March, Trop50 has become a $100 million brand. Two Trop50 line extensions are hitting the shelves: Pomegranate Blueberry and Pineapple Mango.

Chief Executive Nooyi says she has no choice but to move in healthier directions. For more than 15 years, consumers have gradually defected from the carbonated soft drinks that once comprised 90% of Pepsi's beverage business. Many switched to bottled water. Meanwhile, the cloud of criticism shadowing Pepsi's largest business, oil- and salt-laden Frito Lay snacks, grew steadily. The company acquired Quaker Oats and other wholesome brands but until recently didn't emphasize research. Nooyi, who took over in 2006, is changing that. She has increased the R&D budget 38% over three years, to $388 million in 2008.

"Society, people, and lifestyles have changed," Nooyi says. "The R&D needs for this new world are also different." Her goal of expanding healthy products to $30 billion in sales would require annual growth in those lines of more than 10%, twice the company's overall historical average.

Society, people, and lifestyles have changed. The R&D needs for this new world are also different.

Coming off a tough 2009, during which once high-flying brands such as Gatorade slipped, Pepsi hasn't convinced Wall Street that Nooyi's plans will pay off. The company trades at a significant discount to its rival, Coca-Cola. While securities analysts say that healthier foods look like a good long-term market, for now, the slowdown in the company's far larger traditional snack-and-soda portfolio cannot be ignored. "The consumer can move to baked chips, or pretzels, or Sun Chips, but they're not yet giving up their chips for an apple or carrot stick," says Bill Pecoriello, CEO of Consumer Edge Research, an independent stock-research firm in Stamford, Conn.

Pepsi built its empire on the manufacture and distribution of instantly recognizable products. It could get a bag of Lay's or a can of Mountain Dew to customers practically anywhere in the world. So far, healthier options have produced only modest hits, including TrueNorth nut snacks and SoBe Lifewater. "We're not building Pepsi again," Nooyi says. She aims to sell a wider variety of products to meet all kinds of consumer demands.

Pepsi's health push includes a controversial plan to sell new products to undernourished people in India and other developing countries. This isn't charity, notes Nooyi, herself a native of India. The goal is to make money. As one of its exploratory ventures, Pepsi is supporting a nonproflt operation in Nigeria that distributes a protein-rich peanut-based paste. Khan says that once the company has figured out what's needed most, Pepsi will shift to for-profit production of nutritionally beneficial processed foods.

One potential hazard of marketing in the developing world is that Pepsi could be accused of trading on misfortune and not serving the overall dietary needs of the poor—a criticism that has haunted sellers of infant formula. Kelly D. Brownell, director of the Yale University Rudd Center for Food Policy & Obesity, says Pepsi's developing-nations initiative deserves scrutiny. But Brownell, an industry critic, praises Pepsi for improvements in its mainstream products, such as removing bad fats from its chips. "They're the most progressive player in the industry," he says.

Critical Thinking

1. What are some of the changes that have been made to improve Pepsi's image as a soda and snack food company?

2. What three products have been developed as healthier versions of processed foods/beverages?

3. How much money is Pepsi expecting to earn from healthy products by the year 2020?

From *Bloomberg BusinessWeek,* January 25, 2010, pp. 50–51. Copyright © Bloomberg 2010 by Bloomberg BusinessWeek. Reprinted by permission of Bloomberg LP via YGS Group.

Calorie Posting in Chain Restaurants

Sarah H. Wright

Nutrition labeling on packaged food has been mandatory in the United States since the early 1990s, and printing tiny lists on cans and bags has long been accepted practice. Yet, in spite of this improvement in providing information, the share of Americans who are obese has continued to rise, increasing from 15.9 percent in 1995 to 26.6 percent in 2008.

The fraction of calories consumed in restaurants also has risen in recent years. In 2008, New York City extended nutrition labeling to chain restaurants, requiring them to post clearly the number of calories in every one of their foods and beverages. In March 2010, new federal health care legislation mandated calorie posting for chain restaurants nationwide beginning in 2011. Will these point-of-purchase postings have any public health effect? Could menus with "350 calories" printed beside "eight grain roll" drive a consumer to buy a banana (100 calories) instead?

In **Calorie Posting in Chain Restaurants** (NBER Working Paper No. 15648), study authors **Bryan Bollinger, Phillip Leslie,** and **Alan Sorensen** ask whether mandatory calorie posting influences consumers' purchase decisions. They use detailed data from Starbucks stores in New York City, where calories are posted; from Starbucks in Boston and Philadelphia, where calories are not posted; and from Starbucks stores throughout the nation. The researchers find that mandatory calorie posting influenced consumer behavior at Starbucks in New York City, causing average calories per transaction to drop by 6 percent (from 247 to 232 calories). They also find that these effects are long lasting: after the posting began, the calorie reduction persisted for at least 10 months (the duration of the sample period). There is also evidence of persistent learning effects: commuters who lowered their calories per transaction on weekdays in New York City also lowered them in transactions at Starbucks outside the city, where calories were not posted.

Mandatory calorie posting influenced consumer behavior at Starbucks in New York City, causing average calories per transaction to drop by 6 percent.

The researchers also find that almost all of the calorie-reduction effects in Starbucks are related to food—not beverage—purchases.

Following calorie posting, average food calories per transaction fell by 14 percent. The effect is larger for high-calorie consumers: individuals who averaged more than 250 calories per transaction reacted to calorie posting by decreasing calories per transaction by 26 percent—dramatically more than the 6 percent average reduction for all consumers.

Beverage consumption was largely unaffected by calorie posting. Consumers tended to underestimate the calories contained in Starbucks' food and bakery items, but they overestimated the calories contained in Starbucks beverages. According to the researchers, consumers who discovered by calorie posting that an Ice d Cafe Latte contains just 130 calories were pleasantly surprised—continued buying.

Noting that calorie reductions on the order of 6 percent at chain restaurants would yield only modest decreases in body weight, the researchers suggest that the direct effect of calorie posting on U.S. obesity may be small. The most meaningful effect of the calorie posting law may be its long-run impact on menu choices, as restaurants will have an economic incentive to offer low-calorie options. The new policy may also benefit public health as consumers grow accustomed to counting calories and choose or demand healthier foods.

The study also explores how calorie posting affected corporate profits. The authors find that it did not cause any significant change in Starbucks' overall revenue. At Starbucks stores located within 100 meters of a Dunkin Donuts store, revenue actually increased by 3 percent—suggesting that calorie posting may have caused some consumers to substitute away from Dunkin Donuts toward Starbucks.

Critical Thinking

1. What year will mandatory calorie posting be enforced for chain restaurants?
2. Describe how calorie posting affected consumer behavior of Starbucks customers.
3. Predict the long-term impact on restaurant's menu offerings considering the likely increased demand for lower calorie items.
4. Defend the requirement that chain restaurants must post nutrition information on their menus. In your response, consider the perspective of a restaurant owner, a politician, and a nutritionist.

From *NBER Digest*, May 2010, pp. 1–2. Copyright © 2010 by National Bureau of Economic Research. Reprinted by permission.

Behind the Brand: McDonald's

In the first of a major new series following on from the ground-breaking "Behind the Label," Peter Salisbury takes a look at one of the biggest brands in the world—McDonald's—and asks: Has the burger giant done enough to clean up its act?

PETER SALISBURY

Chances are that you have had a McDonald's meal in the past or if not, you certainly know a lot of people who have. It's the biggest fast food chain in the world, with 32,000 outlets in 117 countries. The clown-fronted burger outfit employs a staggering 1.7 million people, and in the first three months of 2011 alone it made $1.2 billion in profits on the back of revenues of $6.1 billion. The company has come in for huge amounts of criticism over the past 20 years, for the impact it has on the diets of people worldwide, its labour practices and the impact its business has had on the environment. From *Fast Food Nation* to *Supersize Me* by the way of the McLibel trials of the 1990s, plenty has been written and broadcast to tarnish the golden arches' shine.

Declining sales in the early 2000s, which saw franchises being shut for the first time in the company's history, caused a major rethink of the way McDonald's operates, and its recent rhetoric has been that of a firm with a newly discovered zeal for ethical end eco-friendly practices, garnering praise from champions as unlikely as Greenpeace and the Carbon Trust. But is this just marketing hype or has McDonald's had a genuine change of heart?

The answer is yes and no. First of all, because of the way the company is run, it's hard to generalise. Around 80 per cent of McDonald's outlets are run by franchisees who have to meet standards set by the company, but who can—and do— go above and beyond them. Further, McDonald's branches are run by country and regional offices, each of which is subject to domestic standards. The production of much of the raw products which go into McDonald's meals, from burger patties to sauces, is subcontracted to different suppliers, making it impossible to assess the company in terms of a single golden standard. Its sole global supplier (for soft drinks) is Coca-Cola.

The UK branch of the company has certainly made great strides since the 1990s, when it became embroiled in the 1997 McLibel court case, in which McDonald's Corporation and McDonald's Restaurants Limited sued Helen Steel and Dave Morris, a former gardener and a postman, for libel after they published a series of leaflets denouncing the company.

Exploitation

The judge overseeing the case decided that, although the pair could not prove some of their accusations—that McDonald's destroyed rainforests, caused starvation in the third world or disease and cancer in developed countries—it could be agreed that the company exploited children, falsely advertised their food as nutritious, indirectly sponsored cruelty to animals and paid their workers low wages: a major blow to the brand in an age of increasing consumer-consciousness.

Since then, the UK branch has committed to a number of initiatives to improve its image, running an aggressive marketing campaign at the same time to portray itself as an ethical employer which is both farmer and eco-friendly. It has also moved to become more transparent, putting ingredients lists for all of its products on its website and setting up another website, Make Up Your Own Mind, inviting customers to voice concerns and publishing accounts of critics' visits to its production sites.

All of this should be taken with a grain of salt however. It's not surprising that a multibillion-dollar corporation, which has been hurt in the past by concerns over its practices, will do its utmost to sell itself as a reformed character. And it's suspicious that any web search of the company brings up a hit list of sites almost exclusively maintained by the company.

Yet research conducted by the *Ecologist* shows that in many areas the company has improved its record of ethical and environmental awareness over the last decade. The company's burgers, for example, are now 100 per cent beef, and contain no preservatives or added flavors whatsoever. All of McDonald's UK's burgers are provided by Germany's Esca Food Solutions, which claims to maintain rigorous standards at its abattoirs and production plants, and which works closely with 16,000 independent farmers in the UK and Ireland to maintain high standards.

Since the early 2000s, McDonald's UK has maintained that none of its beef, bacon or chicken is fed genetically modified grain. Farmers working for McDonald's have independently confirmed to the *Ecologist* and Esca that they have a 'decent' working relationship with the company.

In 2007, Esca won the UK Food Manufacturing Excellence Awards for its burgers, and in 2010 McDonald's announced that it was launching a three-year study into reducing the carbon emissions caused by the cattle used in its burgers (cattle account for four per cent of the UK's emissions). Meanwhile, all of the fish used in Filet-O-Fish and Fish Finger meals in Europe are sourced from sustainable fisheries certified by the Marine Stewardship Council. Fries are largely sourced from McCain's, the world's biggest potato supplier, and McDonald's claims that the vast majority are produced in the UK, again by independent farmers. The fries are prepared in-store and are cooked in vegetable oil containing no hydrogenated fats. At the beginning of the potato-growing season, dextrose—a form of glucose—is added as a sweetener, and salt is added after cooking (the company claims to have reduced the amount of salt used by 23 per cent since 2008).

The bread for McDonald's buns and muffins is sourced from a single unnamed supplier based in Heywood, Manchester, and Banbury, Oxfordshire. McDonald's would not comment on where it sources the grain for the bakeries but says once more that it does not buy genetically modified crops. Meanwhile, the company has been working with its suppliers and franchise-holders to make sure that they are as energy efficient as possible. In 2010, the Carbon Trust awarded McDonald's its Carbon Trust Standard for reducing its overall carbon emissions by 4.5 per cent between 2007 and 2009. The company is currently experimenting with a series of energy initiatives based around turning its waste, from packaging—which is 80 per cent recycled—to vegetable oil into energy.

Certification

Since 2007, the company—which is one of the world's biggest coffee retailers—has committed to selling only Rainforest Alliance certified coffee. Although the certification body has certainly been responsible for improving conditions and practices in many farming operations worldwide, it has been the subject of controversy—most recently after an undercover investigation by the *Ecologist* revealed allegations of sexual harassment and poor conditions for some workers at its certified Kericho tea plantation in Kenya which supplies the PG Tips brand.

Certification issues aside, McDonald's has undoubtedly become considerably better at taking criticism. In 2006, Greenpeace activists stormed McDonald's restaurants across the world dressed in chicken suits in protest at the destruction of the Amazon rainforest, which they attributed to greedy soy producers—who in turn were selling their produce to chicken farms, of whom McDonald's was a major customer. They subsequently praised the fast food chain for leading a unified response among soy buyers, pressuring producers to adopt a 'zero destruction' approach to growing their crops. Despite praise from Greenpeace, the Carbon Trust and personalities such as Jamie Oliver who have praised the company for its ethical stance on meat and buying its produce locally, the firm is by no means perfect.

One of the biggest incongruencies in its newly discovered zeal for ethical practices comes from its seemingly differing approaches to the conditions chickens live in depending on whether they produce eggs or are used as meat in Chicken McNuggets and similar meals. The firm proudly trumpets that its UK branch only buys eggs from Lion-certified free-range producers, a laudable effort from a huge buyer of eggs, and that the meat in each nugget is 100 per cent chicken breast (the final product is around 65:35 meat and batter).

Factory Farming

Yet by the same token, the company buys most of its chicken from two suppliers, Sun Valley in the UK and Moy Park in Northern Ireland, who are in turn owned by the controversial American firm, Cargill, and Brazil's Marfrig. Sun Valley has been accused of using intensive chicken farming methods to produce their meat, which campaigners say can typically involve birds being cooped up in giant warehouses for much of their natural lives with barely any space to move. Sun Valley was embroiled in a scandal in 2008 when the activist group Compassion in World Farming secretly filmed poor conditions at its supplier Uphampton Farm near Leominster.

Furthermore, although McDonald's is happy to advertise the provenance of its beef, dairy products and eggs, it is more circumspect about chicken meat. This may be because up to 90 per cent of the meat it uses in the UK is sourced from Cargill and Marfrag facilities in Thailand and Brazil, where regulations in the farming sector are perhaps less stringent than in the UK.

Meanwhile, the fact remains that despite attempts in recent years to cultivate a more healthy image, McDonald's primary sales come from fast food in a time when there is increasing recognition that obesity has reached epidemic proportions in the UK and the US. Although the European, and in particular the UK, arm of the company have become increasingly ethically aware, the same cannot be said for the US arm, which uses livestock farmed using intensive methods and fed in some cases on GM crops. And by buying McDonald's in the UK, you are still buying from the same clown.

Critical Thinking

1. Identify a US city that has a population equals to the number of people employed by McDonald's worldwide.

2. Explain why McDonald's made the decision to "clean up" its reputation? When did this begin?

3. Justify the following statement: "It's impossible to assess the operations of McDonald's in terms of a single golden standard."

4. Explain why McDonald's restaurants in Europe do not sell foods containing genetically modified (GM) ingredients, whereas in the United States, McDonald's produces foods with GM ingredients.

Nutrition for Optimum Athletic Performance—The Right Fuel Can Be the Difference

ELLEN COLEMAN, MA, MPH, RD, CSSD

Three primary factors influence athletic performance: genetics, training, and nutrition. Athletes have no influence over their heredity, but they can control their training and diet.

Athletes are constantly looking for a competitive edge. Though the appropriate diet won't guarantee athletic success, a poor diet can undermine training efforts. In many events, especially among elite athletes, the margin between victory and defeat is very small. Attention to nutrition can make that critical difference.

The foods an athlete chooses will influence performance in both training and competition. Diet may actually have its biggest impact on training. A healthful diet supports regular, intensive training and decreases the risk of illness and/or injury. Appropriate food choices can also enhance adaptations to the training stimulus.

Several prestigious organizations have recently issued guidelines on nutrition and athletic performance after meticulously reviewing the literature. This article will provide sports nutrition recommendations and highlight key points from these documents:

- the new International Olympic Committee Medical Commission consensus statement on sports nutrition, released in October 2010[1]; and
- the American Dietetic Association, American College of Sports Medicine, and Dietitians of Canada's 2009 update on their position statement on nutrition and athletic performance.[2]

These documents emphasize that diet has a significant influence on athletic performance. Athletes should adopt specific nutritional strategies before, during, and after training and competition to optimize their physical and mental performance and promote health. The proper amount of food, the composition of the meal, and the timing of food intake can help athletes train and perform more effectively and reduce the risk of illness and injury.[1,2]

Energy Intake

Energy requirements depend on an athlete's periodized training load and competition program and vary from day to day and with the competition schedule. An appropriate diet will help athletes reach an optimum body size and composition to achieve greater success in their sport.[1,2]

Excessive energy intake relative to expenditure increases body fat, which may hinder performance. Inadequate energy intake relative to energy expenditure impairs performance and adaptations to training.[1,2] Insufficient energy consumption causes the body to use both fat and lean tissue for fuel. Loss of lean tissue decreases strength and endurance and may compromise immune, endocrine, and musculoskeletal function.[2]

Energy availability is defined as "dietary energy intake minus exercise energy expenditure." Low energy availability should be avoided as it may be harmful to brain, reproductive, metabolic, and immune function and bone health.[1,2] The well-documented "Female Athlete Triad," consisting of low energy availability (with or without disordered eating), amenorrhea, and osteoporosis (alone or in combination), is a major concern and poses significant health risks to young and adult female athletes.

When energy intake is restricted to reduce body weight and/or fat mass, it is important to select nutrient-rich foods to reduce the risk of developing nutrient deficiencies that will impair health and performance.[1]

Dieting in young athletes should be discouraged as this may hinder their growth and development.[1] Athletes at risk of disordered eating patterns and reproductive disorders should be promptly referred to a qualified health professional for evaluation and treatment.[1]

Although exercise performance is influenced by body weight and composition, these physical measures should not be seen as criteria for sports performance. Athletes may be pressured to lose weight and body fat to improve their power-to-weight ratio (eg, running, distance cycling, triathlon), achieve a desirable body composition for aesthetic sports (eg, gymnastics, figure skating, diving), or compete in a specific weight class (eg, wrestling, lightweight rowing, boxing) in spite of having an appropriate weight for health and performance. Scholastic athletic governing bodies have instituted weight-loss procedure guidelines that limit the rate of loss for collegiate and high school wrestlers, but the potential for abuse still exists in other sports. Losses of both muscle and fat mass due to extreme energy restriction may adversely influence an athlete's performance and health.[2]

Body fat percentages of athletes vary depending on an athlete's gender and sport. The estimated minimal level of body fat compatible with health is 5 percent for males and 12 percent for females. However, optimal body fat percentages for an athlete may be much higher than these minimum levels and should be established on an individual basis. An athlete's optimal competitive body weight and relative body fatness should be determined when an athlete is healthy and performs at his or her best.[2]

A diet that provides adequate energy from a wide range of regularly available foods can meet the carbohydrate, protein, and fat requirements of training and competition.[1] Athletes do not need a diet substantially different than that recommended in the 2010 Dietary Guidelines for Americans.[2]

Carbohydrate

During high-intensity training, particularly prolonged exercise, an athlete should consume enough carbohydrate to meet the energy needs of the training program as well as replenish carbohydrate stores (muscle and liver glycogen stores) during recovery between training sessions and competitive events. For competitions lasting one hour or longer, the athlete should emphasize carbohydrate-rich foods in the hours and days before the event.[1]

Carbohydrate recommendations for athletes range from 5 to 12 g/kg/day, as shown in Table 1. These are general recommendations and should be adjusted with consideration of an athlete's total energy needs, specific training needs, and feedback from his or her training performance.[3]

Guidelines for carbohydrate intake should not be provided in terms of percentage contributions to total dietary energy intake. These recommendations are neither user friendly nor strongly related to the muscle's absolute need for fuel.[3]

Protein

Protein metabolism is influenced by exercise type (endurance vs. strength), exercise intensity, carbohydrate availability, training state, energy balance, gender, and age.[1]

Table 1 Daily Carbohydrate Recommendations for Athletes

- 5 to 7 g of carbohydrate/kg/day: athletes engaging in moderate-intensity exercise for 60 to 90 minutes per day
- 7 to 12 g of carbohydrate/kg/day: athletes engaging in moderate- to high-intensity endurance exercise for one to three hours
- 10 to 12 g of carbohydrate/kg/day: athletes participating in extreme endurance exercise for four to six hours per day (eg, Tour de France)

Athletes should take in more protein than the 0.8 g/kg/day recommended for the general population. Endurance athletes should consume 1.2 to 1.4 g/kg/day and strength athletes about 1.2 to 1.7 g/kg/day. The increase in contractile proteins allows a weightlifter to achieve a greater absolute power output, whereas an increased mitochondrial volume allows the endurance athlete to exercise for hours. However, consuming a varied diet that meets energy needs generally provides more protein than required, including any increases that may arise from high-level training.[1,2]

Athletes who severely restrict their energy intakes are at risk of failing to meet their protein needs. These include athletes in weight-restriction sports or aesthetically judged sports as well as athletes with disordered eating patterns. Inadequate protein intake can cause loss of muscle mass and compromise training adaptations and immune function.[2]

Athletes should consume high-quality protein regularly throughout the day to meet their protein requirements.[1] Consuming protein immediately after exercise may help increase net muscle protein balance, promote muscle tissue repair, and enhance adaptations involving synthesis of new proteins.[1-3]

Protein and amino acid supplements offer no advantages over protein-rich foods other than convenience. Although protein powders and amino acid supplements are widely used, they are a potential source for illegal substances such as anabolic steroids, which may not be listed on the ingredient label.[2]

Fat

Fat intake should be sufficient to provide essential fatty acids and fat-soluble vitamins as well as contribute energy for weight maintenance. The Acceptable Macronutrient Distribution range for fat (as established by the Food and Nutrition Board of the Institute of Medicine) of 20 percent to 35 percent of energy intake is appropriate for athletes.[2] Short-term fat adaptation ("fat loading") does not improve prolonged endurance exercise and may impair an athlete's ability to work at high intensities.[2]

Micronutrients

Vitamins and minerals play an important role in energy production, hemoglobin synthesis, maintenance of bone health, adequate immune function, and the protection of body tissues from oxidative damage. Micronutrients are also required to help build and repair muscle tissue following exercise.[2]

Consuming a varied diet that contains adequate micronutrients and energy, getting enough sleep, and reducing life stressors help enhance immunity and reduce the risk of infection.[1]

Athletes at greatest risk of poor micronutrient status usually restrict energy intake (especially over long periods), have severe weight-loss practices, eliminate one or more food groups from their diet, or rely on foods with a low nutrient density.[2]

Athletes should be particularly aware of their needs for calcium, vitamin D, and iron.[1,2] Inadequate dietary calcium and vitamin D increase the risk of low bone mineral density and stress fractures. Low energy availability, insufficient intake of dairy products (and other calcium-rich foods), and menstrual dysfunction greatly increase a female athlete's risk of having low bone mineral density.[1]

Athletes who live at northern latitudes or who train primarily indoors throughout the year, such as gymnasts and figure skaters, are at risk of poor vitamin D status, especially if they do not consume vitamin D-fortified foods. These athletes may benefit from vitamin D supplementation.[1,2]

Iron is required for the formation of hemoglobin, myoglobin, and enzymes involved in energy production. Iron depletion (low iron stores as measured by serum ferritin) is one of the most prevalent nutrient deficiencies observed among athletes, especially females. Iron deficiency, with or without anemia, can impair muscle function and limit work capacity. Athletes should consume a diet with high availability of iron.[2]

Female athletes, long-distance runners, adolescents, and vegetarians should be screened periodically to assess and monitor iron status. The decision to use iron supplements in athletes with depleted iron stores is usually made on an individual basis. Supplements are discontinued when the serum ferritin measurement returns to normal for an individual athlete.[2]

Hydration

Dehydration (loss of more than 2 percent of body mass) can impair performance in most events, particularly in warm and high-altitude environments. Dehydration also increases the risk of heat exhaustion and is a risk factor for heat stroke. Athletes should be well hydrated before exercise and drink sufficiently during exercise to limit dehydration to less than 2 percent of body mass.[1,2]

The amount and rate of fluid replacement depends on an individual's sweating rate, exercise duration, and opportunities to drink. It is not possible to propose a one-size-fits-all fluid and electrolyte replacement schedule due to the multiple factors that influence sweating rate and sweat electrolyte concentrations.[2]

Sports beverages containing carbohydrates and electrolytes may be consumed before, during, and after exercise to help maintain blood glucose concentration, provide fuel for muscles, and decrease the risk of dehydration and hyponatremia.[2] Guidelines for hydration management are as follows:

- **Before exercise:** Athletes should drink about 5 to 7 mL/kg of body weight (2 to 3 mg/lb) four hours before activity.
- **During exercise:** Athletes should monitor changes in body weight during training and competition to establish sweating rates for specific exercise and environmental conditions.[2] Consuming an appropriate amount of fluid during training sessions improves the quality of an athlete's workout and so enhances training adaptations. Athletes should not drink so much that they gain weight during exercise, as this increases the risk of developing hyponatremia.[1,2]
  - Sodium should be included when sweat losses are high, especially when exercise lasts more than about two hours. The average concentration of sodium in sweat is about 35 mmol/L, or about 800 mg/L. Chilled fluids may benefit performance in hot conditions.[1]

- **After exercise:** Athletes should drink 24 oz for each pound lost (1.5 L of fluid for each kilogram lost). To recover from exercise, athletes should replace the water and salt that is lost in sweat. When athletes must compete in several events in a short time period strategies to enhance recovery of fluid are important.[1,2]

Training Diet

Compared with the general population, athletes need additional energy to fuel physical activity and additional fluid to replace sweat losses. As energy requirements increase, athletes should first strive to consume the maximum number of servings appropriate for their energy needs from carbohydrate-rich foods: bread, cereals and grains, legumes, milk/milk alternatives, vegetables, and fruits.[2]

Athletes who are small or have lower energy requirements should focus on making nutrient-dense food choices to obtain adequate carbohydrate, protein, essential fats, and micronutrients.[2]

The food and fluid intake consumed around workouts should be individually determined and based on an athlete's gastrointestinal tolerance as well as the intensity and the duration of a workout.[2]

Preexercise Meal

Eating before exercise improves performance compared with exercising in a fasted state. The size and the timing of the preexercise meal are interrelated; smaller meals should be consumed closer to the event to allow for gastric emptying, whereas larger meals can be consumed when more time is available before exercise or competition. A carbohydrate feeding of 1 g/kg is appropriate one hour before exercise, whereas 4.5 g/kg can be consumed four hours before exercise as shown in Table 2.[2,3]

The preexercise meal should be high in carbohydrate (to maintain blood glucose and maximize glycogen stores), relatively low in fat and fiber (to facilitate gastric emptying and minimize gastrointestinal distress), moderate in protein, contain familiar foods, and provide sufficient fluid to contribute to hydration.[2]

If an athlete is unable to eat breakfast prior to early morning exercise, consuming about 30 g of easily digested carbohydrate five minutes before exercise may improve performance.

Table 2 Carbohydrate Recommendations for the Preexercise Meal

- Consume 1 g of carbohydrate/kg one hour before exercise.
- Consume 2 g of carbohydrate/kg two hours before exercise.
- Consume 3 g of carbohydrate/kg three hours before exercise.
- Consume 4 to 4.5 g of carbohydrate/kg four hours before exercise.

Table 3 Carbohydrate Content of Selected Foods

- 1 qt of Gatorade Thirst Quencher = 56 g
- 1 PowerBar Harvest = 43 g
- 2 Vanilla Bean GU gels = 50 g
- 28 Sport Beans = 50 g
- 6 Clif Shot Bloks = 48 g
- 3 large graham crackers = 66 g
- 4 Fig Newtons = 42 g
- 1 banana = 30 g

Fueling During Exercise

Consuming carbohydrate (30 to 60 g/hour) during endurance exercise or stop-and-go sports lasting one hour or more can enhance physical and cognitive performance by maintaining blood glucose levels and carbohydrate oxidation in the latter stages of exercise.[1,2] As the duration of the event increases, so does the amount of carbohydrate needed to optimize performance. Relatively high rates of intake (up to 90 g/hour) are needed to optimize performance in events lasting three hours or more.[2]

The maximum amount of carbohydrate that can be oxidized during exercise from a single carbohydrate source (eg, glucose) is about 1 g/minute or 60 g/hour because the transporter responsible for carbohydrate absorption in the intestine becomes saturated. A series of studies conducted by researchers at the University of Birmingham has shown that consuming between 1.8 to 2.4 g of carbohydrate per minute (108 to 144 g/hour) from a mixture of carbohydrates increases carbohydrate oxidation up to 75 to 104 g of carbohydrate per hour.[4]

Athletes should experiment with different sports drinks and sports foods during training to develop effective fueling strategies for competition. Consuming carbohydrate during training sessions also improves the quality of an athlete's workout and so enhances training adaptations. Choosing sports foods and drinks that contain a mixture of carbohydrates will maximize absorption from the gut and minimize gastrointestinal disturbances.[1] The carbohydrate content of selected foods is listed in Table 3.

Recovery Following Exercise

The restoration of muscle and liver glycogen stores is important for recovery following strenuous training. Athletes commonly engage in prolonged high-intensity workouts once or twice per day with a limited amount of time (six to 24 hours) to recover before the next exercise session. Utilizing successful refueling strategies following daily training sessions helps to optimize recovery and promote the desired adaptations to training.[1,2]

During the early period of recovery (up to four hours) after glycogen-depleting exercise, an athlete should consume about 1 g of carbohydrate/kg/hour.[3] When there are less than eight hours between exercise sessions, start consuming carbohydrate immediately after exercise to maximize recovery time. Recovery meals and snacks contribute to an athlete's daily carbohydrate requirements of 5 to 12 g of carbohydrate/kg/day.[3]

Table 4 Recovery Nutrition Strategies

- During the early period of recovery after glycogen-depleting exercise, consume 1 g of carbohydrate/kg/hour.
- When there are less than eight hours between exercise sessions, start consuming carbohydrate immediately after exercise to maximize recovery time.
- Consume 15 to 25 g of high-quality protein after each training session to stimulate muscle protein synthesis/repair.

Consuming foods or drinks providing 15 to 25 g of high-quality protein after each training session enhances muscle protein synthesis, promotes maintenance of lean tissue, and aids muscle repair.[1] Recovery meals and snacks contribute to an athlete's daily protein requirements of 1.2 to 1.7 g of protein/kg/day.[2] Table 4 provides recovery nutrition strategies.

Supplements and Ergogenic Aids

Vitamin and mineral supplements are not needed if adequate energy to maintain body weight is consumed from a variety of foods.[2] The use of supplements does not compensate for poor food choices and an inadequate diet.[1] Supplements that provide essential nutrients may be a short-term option when food intake or food choices are restricted due to travel or other factors.[1] The consumption of large amounts of some micronutrients via supplements may be harmful. Vitamin D may be needed in supplemental form when sun exposure is inadequate, particularly for those living in extreme northern latitudes.

Athletes seek that "secret ingredient" that will enhance their workout and give them the edge over their competitors. They want to believe in something magical that can improve performance more than hard training or a prudent diet. In many events, the difference between winning and losing is in divisions of seconds, so it is not surprising that athletes are susceptible to miraculous claims for sports supplements.

An enormous array of nutritional ergogenic aids are available to athletes. The desire for that elusive "magic bullet' may cause athletes to abandon sound nutrition practices and become victims of nutrition quackery. A few nutritional ergogenic aids (eg, creatine, caffeine, sodium bicarbonate) perform as claimed and may enhance athletic performance when used properly. Most, however, do not perform as claimed or give athletes the results they want. Some sports supplements may contain banned substances or be detrimental when taken in high doses for prolonged periods.[1,2]

Dietary supplements do not undergo evaluation for safety and effectiveness by the FDA prior to being marketed. Thus, nutritional ergogenic aids should be used with caution and only after careful product evaluation for safety, efficacy, potency, and legality (doping). Some supplements contain ingredients (anabolic steroids and stimulants) not declared on the label that are prohibited by national and international sports governing bodies. Innocent ingestion of prohibited substances is not an acceptable excuse; athletes are ultimately responsible for the product they ingest and any consequences.[1,2]

The use of supplements by young athletes should be discouraged. The focus should be on consuming a nutrient-dense diet to promote growth as well as a healthy body composition.[1]

Vegetarian Athletes

Vegetarian athletes may be at risk of low intakes of energy, protein, fat, and key micronutrients such as iron, calcium, vitamin D, riboflavin, zinc, and vitamin B12. Women in particular are vulnerable for nonanemic iron deficiency, which may limit endurance performance. Consultation with a sports dietitian is recommended to avoid these nutrition problems.[2]

Sports Dietitians

All athletes can benefit from the guidance of qualified sports nutrition professionals regarding their individual energy, nutrient, and fluid needs and developing sport-specific nutritional strategies for training, competition, and recovery.[1,2] In 2005, the Commission on Dietetic Registration created a specialty credential for food and nutrition professionals who specialize in sports dietetic practice. The board certified specialist in sports dietetics (CSSD) credential is designed as the premier professional sports nutrition credential in the United States. Specialists in sports dietetics provide evidence-based nutrition assessment, guidance, and counseling for health and performance for athletes, sport organizations, and physically active individuals and groups. The credential requires current RD status, maintenance of RD status for a minimum of two years, and documentation of 1,500 sports specialty practice hours as an RD within the past five years.[2]

Final Thoughts

Athletes should adopt nutrition strategies that optimize physical and mental performance and support good health. The proper amount of food, the composition of the meal, and the timing of food intake can help athletes train and perform more effectively and reduce the risk of illness and injury.

Athletes should consume adequate energy and macronutrients (especially carbohydrate and protein) during times of heavy physical activity to maintain body weight, replenish glycogen stores, and provide adequate protein to build and repair tissue. Athletes should also ingest adequate food and fluid before, during, and after exercise to maintain blood glucose concentration during exercise, maximize exercise performance, and optimize recovery. Athletes should be well hydrated before exercise and drink enough fluid during exercise (based on individual sweat rates) and after exercise to replace their fluid losses.

Vitamin and mineral supplements are not needed if an athlete consumes adequate energy to maintain body weight from a variety of foods. Nutritional ergogenic aids should be used cautiously and only after meticulous product evaluation for safety, effectiveness, potency, and legality.

A qualified sports dietitian (in the United States, a CSSD) should provide individualized nutrition guidance and counseling following a comprehensive nutrition assessment.[2]

References

1. International Olympic Committee Consensus Statement on Sports Nutrition. October 27, 2010. Available at: www.olympic.org/Documents/Reports/EN/CONSENSUS-FINAL-v8-en.pdf.
2. Rodriguez NR, Di Marco NM, Langley S, et al. Position of the American Dietetic Association, Dietitians of Canada, and the American College of Sports Medicine: Nutrition and athletic performance. *J Am Diet Assoc.* 2009;109(3):509–527.
3. Nutrition Working Group of the Medical Commission of the International Olympic Committee. Nutrition for athletes. June 2003. Available at: www.olympic.org/Documents/Reports/EN/en-report-1251.pdf.
4. Currell K, Jeukendrup AE. Superior endurance performance with ingestion of multiple transportable carbohydrates. *Med Sci Sports Exerc.* 2008;40:275–281.

Critical Thinking

1. Contrast carbohydrate and protein needs in athletes compared to a person with low physical activity.
2. Describe the benefit of consuming carbohydrates and protein after exercise.
3. Identify the micronutrients that should be of utmost importance among athletes.
4. Summarize the recommendations for hydration before, during, and after exercise.

From *Today's Dietitian*, vol. 13, no. 3, March 2011, pp. 46. Copyright © 2011 by Today's Dietitian. Reprinted by permission.

Snack Attack

Evaluating and Rating Snacks for Athletes

Snacking has been described as the fourth meal, but for many athletes, snacking is also the fifth and sixth meals. Athletes often need extra calories and nutrients to support training and fuel competition and replace losses after a hard workout. Athletes should be encouraged to choose snacks that provide more than energy by selecting snacks that meet their nutritional needs and provide nutrients that may be lacking in their diets. This article reviews snacking and snacking occasions and suggests some snacks that might benefit athletes. Evaluation of snacks from fast-food and quick-service restaurants, energy bars, and weight-loss and weight-gain snacks is presented as well as the top 10 best snacks for athletes. Nutr Today. 2011;46(3):106–115

CHRISTINE ROSENBLOOM, PhD, RD, CSSD

Athletes often ask "what is good snack food?" Good is a relative term; for a dietitian "good" means a healthful, nutritious snack that is nutrient dense, but for an athlete, it means a food that is tasty, convenient, and satisfying. The 2 definitions should not be mutually exclusive, but how do we get athletes to meet their nutritional needs while providing fuel and fluids for good performance through the snacks they choose?

This article reviews snacking in the United States among adults and provides an evaluation of a variety of snacks that athletes can consume to gain, lose, or maintain weight. It also reviews the many options available from fast-food and quick-service restaurants to energy bars and beverages.

The Fourth Meal

Harry Balzer, vice president of the market research company NPD Group, labels snacking as the "fourth meal," but whereas evening snacking at home is still the time when most snacks are consumed, there is a shift to morning snacking, and food manufacturers are responding by providing more snack foods to appeal to the breakfast skippers.[1] Research from NPD found that 1 in 5 meals is snacks and that Americans are becoming a nation of grazers. For athletes, specialty products—bars, gels, drinks, shakes—are a growing business and target the busy athlete with snacks designed to boost stamina, build muscle, lose fat, sustain energy, and replenish losses before, during, and after training and competition. The global sports nutrition market is estimated to be $4.7 billion, with North America contributing $3.2 billion of the revenue.[2]

There is a paucity of research on snacking, in part because it is hard to define a "snack." Couple that with the difficulty in collecting accurate food recall information, and it is easy to understand why we know so little about snacking. However, Piernas and Popkin[3] recently published an article on snacking and have shown an increase in snacking from 1977 to 2006. Using data from nationally representative surveys—Nationwide Food Consumption Survey, Continuing Survey of Food Intake by Individuals, and the National Health and Nutrition Examination Survey 2003–2006—the researchers analyzed 2-day intakes from 44 754 adults. They defined a snack as (1) if the participant identified the meal occasion as a snack, (2) if the participant labeled the eating occasion as a food or coffee break, and (3) all foods consumed outside what the respondents listed as breakfast, lunch, and dinner. If the participant met any of those 3 criteria in the 2 days of recorded food intake, he or she was labeled as a "snacker."

Overcoming snack attacks with healthy snacks is easy.

The prevalence of snacking increased for all adults from 71 percent in 1977 to 97 percent in 2003 to 2006. The energy intake from snacks also increased over the same time, so that by 2006 almost a quarter of energy intake was coming from snacking, or about 500 calories. The top snacks were desserts (cakes, cookies, pies, and ice cream), salty snacks (pretzels, chips, crackers, and popcorn), sweetened beverages (soft drinks, fruit drinks, and sports drinks), and other snacks such as nuts, candy, and ready-to-eat cereals. There was a small downward shift in consuming dairy food snacks (besides ice cream) and fruit.[3]

In determining what makes a good snack for athletes, I got guidance from the Position Paper on Sports Nutrition and Athletic Performance from the American Dietetic Association, Dietitians of Canada, and the American College of Sports Medicine.[4] The bottom line is that athletes should

- consume adequate energy to maintain weight and maximize training effects;
- consume carbohydrate in the range of 6 to 10 g/kg (2.7–4.5 g/lb);
- consume protein in the range of 1.2 to 1.7 g/kg (0.5–0.8 g/lb);
- consume fat in the range of 20 percent to 35 percent of total calories;
- drink adequate fluids to prevent dehydration and replenish losses;
- obtain vitamins and minerals from foods; and
- be cautious about the use of performance-enhancing supplements.

Based on those guidelines, snacks for athletes should provide a nutrient-dense, but moderate energy snack that provides carbohydrate, protein, and some fat and contains vitamins and minerals needed for activity. For women, calcium and iron are of special concern, and snacks rich in these nutrients would be advantageous. Vegetarian athletes are at risk for low intakes of calcium, iron, vitamin D, riboflavin, zinc, and vitamin B_{12}.[4]

Energy Bars

With so many choices available and with so many snacking opportunities, how can athletes make healthy choices for snacks? Table 1 lists some popular energy bars that are frequently consumed by athletes. The choices listed in this table represent some of the best selling bars but is by no means complete. I chose 8 of the most popular bars and only 1 or 2 from each manufacturer. I also chose to display nutrients per bar instead of per 100 g because athletes, like most consumers, will eat what is in the package. When analyzed per 100 g, calories range from 350 to 450, with the "lite" bars containing calories at the lower end of the range. Manufacturers' Web sites for energy bars make claims that are often unsubstantiated, such as "all natural" or containing special proprietary blends of ingredients that promote slow release of nutrients that sustain energy. There is nothing magical about any energy bar, and if they were marketed as "calorie bars," sales would probably not be very good. What these bars do have is convenience and portability, and that is appealing to athletes. It is easy to toss a bar in a gym bag or backpack for easy consumption. One question an elite, professional, college, and/or athlete who is competing in sport where drug testing occurs (even some of the master's-level athlete competitions are drug testing older athletes) should be: "Is this bar free of banned substances?" Over-the-counter sports supplements have been found to contain illegal substances, although most of the contamination occurs in pills and powders claiming to boost testosterone or provide anabolic substances.[5] One of the makers of energy bars, EAS, an Abbott Nutrition company, has products tested and certified by NSF.

Energy bars differ—some are good, and some not from the nutritional standpoint.

NSF International developed a certification program to test products for banned substances and receive the NSF Certified for Sport logo. However, even with certification, a supplement could be contaminated with trace amounts of a banned substance and might be problematic if an athlete takes more than the manufacturer's recommended serving. Although this certification is useful to help athletes make an informed choice, products that are not certified can also be safe. Athletes must weigh the risks with the potential benefits anytime they take a supplement. The NSF maintains an online database of products that have received the certification, and it is available at www.nsf.org/consumer/athletic_banned_substances/index .asp?program=AthleticBanSub.

The Food and Drug Administration has recognized the concerns about dietary and food supplements and has issued a broad warning about potential dangerous supplements. Common types of illegal supplements fall into 3 categories: weight-loss products, body-building products, and sexual enhancers. The Food and Drug Administration issued more than 300 alerts in the past few years because of finding anabolic steroids in body-building products, among other contaminants. Muscle-building supplements have also been found to contain aromatase inhibitors (a drug that is used as a post-breast cancer drug) because it prevents conversion of anabolic hormones into estrogen.[6]

A specific concern for collegiate athletes, a source of confusion for athletes and college athletic association administrators, is the National Collegiate Athletic Association permissible and nonpermissible supplements, including energy bars, weight-gain shakes, and recovery products. Any product with more than 30 percent of calories from protein is impermissible.[7] However, what that really means is that a product greater than the "30 percent rule" cannot be purchased by the athletic association and distributed to athletes. Athletes can purchase products with more than 30 percent protein on their own and use them, but this "rule" is often misinterpreted by coaches, athletic trainers, and strength and conditioning coaches. (Several makers of popular supplements have reformulated products to develop a "collegiate" series that contains <30 percent protein.) Athletes should still be cautious about any supplement that purports to boost testosterone, increase anabolic stimulus to muscle growth, or melt body fat as they could contain banned substances.

When recommending an energy bar for athletes, keep the athlete's goals in mind. For example, SOYJOY energy bar (Pharmavite, LLC, Mission Hills, CA) is lower in calories and appeals to athletes who want to lose weight or maintain a lower weight for sports such as cross-country, diving, or gymnastics. Higher-calorie bars, such as EAS Myoplex (EAS Sports Nutrition, Abbott Park, IL) or Clif Builder's (Clif Bar & Company, Emeryville, CA), are favored by male athletes who are trying to gain weight, such as football or baseball players. Another consideration is taste—for example, female athletes tend to like the taste and consistency of the Luna Bar (Clif Bar & Company,

Table 1 Energy Bars for Athletes[a]

Product	Calories	Carbohydrate, g	Sugar, g	Protein, g	Fat, g	SFA, g	Pros	Cons
Balance Bar Original (50-g bar)	210	22	17	15	7	4	Fortified with vitamins and minerals with 25 percent vitamin D; 8 flavors available; Ratio of 40 percent carbohydrates, 30 percent protein, and 30 percent fat	No evidence to support 40-30-30 as the "perfect" ratio of nutrients for athletes
Clif Bar (68-g bar)	260	42	21	11	6	1.5	Fortified with 25 percent DV calcium and 25 percent DV iron; 18 flavors available	Claims to be "100 percent all natural" but with only 70 percent organic ingredients
Clif Builder's Bar (60-g bar)	270	30	20	20	8	5	Contains 4 g of fiber; High-protein content at 29.6 percent of calories but still NCAA permissible	One of the higher SFA contents for a bar, equal to the SFA found in a serving of cream cheese
EAS Myoplex Strength Formula Nutrition Bar (75-g bar)	280	35	15	25	8	6	Fortified with 30 percent DV calcium and 40 percent DV iron; EAS products are NSF Certified for Sport	With 35 percent of calories from protein, this bar is not permissible by NCAA rules; High in SFA equal to 3 tablespoons of stick margarine
EAS Lite Nutrition Bar (54-g bar)	190	28	15	15	4.5	3	Lower-calorie bar with less fat may appeal to some athletes who are trying to maintain or lose weight	The smaller-size bar at 54 g contributes to its being "lite"; Same amount of sugar as EAS Strength Formula
G Series Pro Nutrition Bar by Gatorade (60-g bar)	230	38	16	10	4	1	One of the lowest-fat and SFA bars for athletes; Available in 3 flavors	Contains 31.5 percent calories from protein; This bar has been hard to find in retail stores but is currently more widely available in sports goods stores and natural food stores
Luna Bar (48-g bar)	180	28	13	8	5	2.5	Bar was designed for women and has 35 percent DV for calcium and 30 percent DV; 16 flavors	Labeled as "all natural" but has only 70 percent organic ingredients
Power Bar Harvest (65-g bar)	250	43	22	10	5	2	One of the original energy bars for athletes; 5 g of fiber; Whole oats is first ingredient; 11 different types of Power Bars available	One of the highest-sugar-containing bars
Power Bar Protein Plus (78-g bar)	360	33	30	30	11	4.5	Contains a blend of whey, soy, and casein proteins with added leucine, thought to be an anabolic stimulus	High in sugar; 33 percent of calories from protein makes it not permissible by NCAA
SOYJOY (30-g bar)	130	16	11	4	6	3.5	2 g of fiber per bar; Made with ground whole soybean with 8 g of soy per bar; Gluten-free	Lower in protein than most bars
Zone Perfect Classic (50-g bar)	210	23	17	15	7	3.5	4 lines of Zone Bars with 21 flavors	Contains only 10 percent DV for calcium

Abbreviation: DV = daily value.

[a]All nutrient information gathered from nutrition facts panel provided on company Web site or product package.

20

Emeryville, CA) or SOYJOY bar, whereas athletes such as endurance athletes tend to like the original Power Bar during long-distance events. (One long distance cyclist I worked with liked to wrap the gooey, sticky Power Bar (Nestle, Glendale, CA) around her bike's handlebars so she could pinch off a piece and eat it on long-distance rides.) Conducting taste tests with athletes can narrow down the favorite flavors, textures, and types of energy bars. Some bars (not included in Table 1) are no more than glorified candy bars and are not worth the extra cost.

Healthy Fast-Food Snacks

Healthy fast food is not an oxymoron, and although many would prefer athletes steer clear of the Golden Arches and fast-food drive through windows, the reality is that athletes are going to eat fast food. McDonald's, Wendy's, Burger King, Pizza Hut, and Taco Bell were described to me by an athlete as the basic 5 food groups. I ask athletes if they are what they eat: Are they fast, cheap, and easy? The good news is that healthy choices can be made at every restaurant—fast-food fare or otherwise. Not only are fast-food restaurants on every corner, but also they are in many college cafeterias. Table 2 shows some healthy snacks at some popular fast-food restaurants. In 2009, *Health Magazine* rated the top 10 healthiest fast-food establishments, and McDonald's made the list.[8] The top 10 were Panera Bread, Jason's Deli, Au Bon Pain, Noodles & Company, Corner Bakery Café, Chipotle, Atlanta Bread, McDonald's, Einstein Bros. Bagels, and Taco del Mar. To be sure, unhealthy choices can be made at all of these restaurants, and the challenge is to steer athletes to the healthier fare and discourage the supersizing and add-ons that can derail a healthy choice (that means "no" to the French fries and large, sugary soft drinks).

One challenge at the fast-food window is the pricing of the "value" meals—a healthy option can turn ugly. Adding fries and a large soft drink with unlimited refills can sabotage a healthy snack. Ask athletes to consider what value really means—it is no value if the choices they make derail their performance or body composition goals. Value is more than just monetary value.

Value meals may not be worth the price if they are chocked full of calories or other ingredients the athlete doesn't need.

Almost all fast-food snacks are high in sodium, but some athletes who lose sodium in sweat may need extra salt. Even so, it is hard to justify sodium levels of more than 1 g in many single items. Another issue is the extras—Subway and Taco Bell both offer healthy snacks, but when the oil, olives, and cheese are added to a low-fat sub, or a healthy chicken taco is stuffed with sour cream and guacamole, and a side of cheese-covered nachos is eaten, the calories and fat can skyrocket.

As more restaurants provide calorie information, we can use that to educate athletes about good choices. Calorie disclosure

in restaurants may be controversial but eating establishments with 20 or more outlets will have to display calories, fat, sodium, and sugar. Some establishments, such as Starbuck's, have already begun to display the calorie information, but soon others will, as required by a provision in the health care reform bill.[9] Currently, most national chains have very informative Web sites that allow a user to assemble a virtual meal and view nutrient information in an interactive way. Substitutions can be made to the meal to show how to reduce calories, fat, sugar, and so on. When conducting team nutrition seminars, I find out the favorite fast-food restaurants of the team and use the restaurant Web site to show athletes how to make a better meal choice than their usual favorites.

Weight-Gainer Shakes

I included weight-gainer shakes as "snacks" because these should be consumed between meals as a way to boost calories. Weight-gain plans should include 3 meals and 3 snacks. Drinking high-calorie and high-protein weight-gainer shakes with meals can lead to less food consumed as these drinks can be very filling. Athletes who want to gain weight might consider using liquid or powder weight-gain supplements between meals as a convenient way to boost calories. There are hundreds of weight-gain supplements, but Table 3 shows some of the most popular shakes and drinks for athletes. The table also includes one whey protein powder as this is another popular option with athletes. The ready-to-drink supplements range in calories from 17 to 45 per ounce, and they can be expensive. Athletes can choose to get extra calories and protein from food, but many like the convenience of a ready-to-drink supplement. Most of the drinks are heavily fortified with vitamins and minerals, and that can impart a "chemical" smell to the product that some athletes dislike. All of the products taste better when chilled, and all need to be thoroughly shaken before consumed or a "sludge" forms on the bottom of some of the containers.

Weight-gainer shakes deserve a careful look before they are bought.

Most contain blends of milk protein, casein and whey, and these 2 proteins have been shown to help athletes accrue lean muscle mass when combined with sufficient energy (calorie) intake and progressive, resistance exercise.[10] Whey is considered a "fast" protein, meaning that it rapidly appears in the bloodstream and helps to stimulate muscle anabolism, and casein is a "slow" protein, leading to a slower rate of appearance in the blood. Because milk protein contains both fast and slow protein, it may provide a more potent stimulus to muscle building than other types of protein. (For a detailed review of protein for athletes, see *Nutrition Today*® 2009;44:204–210.)

Most of the products are not inexpensive, although many can be found in discount warehouse stores and ordered online through Amazon.com.

Table 2 Best Fast-food/Quick Service Restaurant Snacks

Product	Calories	Carbohydrate, g	Sugar, g	Protein, g	Fat, g	SFA, g	Pros	Cons
McDonald's Strawberry Banana Smoothie (medium)	260	60	54	2	1	0	A fruit-yogurt based drink with 90 mg of calcium and 40 mg of sodium	High in sugar from fruit blends Low in protein
McDonald's Egg McMuffin	300	30	3	18	12	5	Fairly healthy on-the-go breakfast with egg, cheese, ham, and English muffin Low in sugar	High in cholesterol at 260 mg and high in sodium at 820 mg
McDonald's Honey Mustard Snack Wrap (grilled)	260	27	4	18	9	3.5	Provides 110 mg calcium and good-quality protein Low in sugar	High in sodium at 800 mg
Wendy's Chicken Grill Wrap	260	25	3	20	20	3.5	High protein snack	High in sodium at 750 mg
Wendy's Broccoli and Cheese Potato	330	25	3	11	2	1	Provides a day's worth of vitamin C at 105 mg Moderate sodium at 470 mg	Not a handheld snack
Wendy's Chili (small)	220	22	6	18	7	3.5	Nutrient-dense snack with 8 mg iron and 350 mg calcium; also a good source of vitamins A and C	Not a handheld snack
Chik-Fil-A Yogurt Parfait With Granola	290	53	39	7	6	2	Provides 200 mg calcium and 45 mg vitamin C	High in sugar but some from natural sugar in yogurt
Chik-Fil-A Chargrilled Chicken Sandwich	300	38	10	29	3.5	1	A low-fat snack option with high-quality protein	Very high in sodium at 1120 mg and even higher with added sauce
Chik-Fil-A Chick-n-Minis (3)	280	31	6	16	10	2.5	Lower in sodium than other options at 640 mg	Fried chicken provides more fat than other fast-food choices
Taco Bell Fresco Grilled Steak Taco	160	21	3	9	4.5	1.5	Fresco menu offers healthy alternatives to regular menu items	The add-ons such as sour cream and cheese make this a high-calorie, high-fat snack
Taco Bell Ranchero Chicken Soft Taco	170	22	3	12	4	1.5	Low in fat and saturated fat snack	High in sodium at 680 mg
Starbuck's Perfect Oatmeal With Dried Fruit Medley	240	49	20	1	2	0.5	A good breakfast snack that is low in fat, high in carbohydrates with 9 mg iron	Low in protein
Starbuck's Strawberry & Blueberry Parfait With Granola	300	60	39	7	3.5	0	High-calcium snack with 300 mg, made with fat-free vanilla yogurt	Sugar content high but mostly from fruit
Starbuck's Chicken Flatbread With Hummus Artisan Snack	250	27	3	17	9	0	Great airport snack with healthy fat and quality protein	Not available at all retail locations
Einstein Bros. Bagels, Power Bagel With Fruit & Nuts	310	61	16	11	5	0.5	Higher in protein than regular bagels, low in saturated fat with 4 mg iron	Best to eat this plain without added fat of cream cheese
Subway 6" Veggie Delite	230	45	5	8	2	0.5	A good way to sneak in veggies without much fat	The add-ons (oil, cheese, or olives) can push the calories up
Subway 6" Turkey Breast	280	47	6	18	3.5	1	A low-fat, high-protein, and high-carbohydrate snack	High in sodium at 910 mg

Abbreviation: SFA = saturated fatty acid.

22

Table 3 Weight-Gain Shakes[*]

Product	Calories	Carbohydrate, g	Sugar, g	Protein, g	Fat, g	SFA, g	Pros	Cons
Boost Plus (Nestle Nutrition) 1 bottle (237 mL)	360	45	22	14	14	1.5	Contains milk and soy protein Fortified with vitamins and minerals Contains 350 mg calcium per serving	High in sugar Lower in protein than other shakes at 15 percent of calories Cost about $2.40 per bottle
Designer Whey Protein Powder (Designer Whey) 1 scoop (26 g)	100	3	2	18	0	0	Contains whey protein concentrate and isolate Contains 90 percent DV for thiamine and vitamin B$_6$	Has to be mixed with 5 oz of water, making it less convenient than ready-to-drink Costs about $1.35 per serving
G Series Pro Nutrition Shake (Gatorade) 1 container (11 oz)	370	54	34	20	8	1.5	Contains milk proteins Fortified with about 25 percent DV for most vitamins and minerals 300 mg of calcium per serving 22 percent of calories from protein	Available through 2 retail outlets so not as readily available as other shakes High in sugar Costs about $3.10 per container
Go Shakes (Go Healthy, Inc) 1 container (330 mL)	310	45	30	20	5	2	Contains milk proteins Lactose-free High in calcium at 630 mg per serving	High in sugar Costs about $1.25 if a college or pro team or about $2.20 retail price
Myoplex Original Ready-to-Drink (EAS, Abbott Nutrition) 17-oz container	300	19	2	42	7	1	High in fiber (6 g) Low in sugar High in protein Fortified with vitamins and minerals at about 50 percent of DV	56 percent calories from protein so not permissible by NCAA Costs $2.40 per serving
Muscle Milk Ready-to-Drink (Cytoport) 14-oz container	240	14	3	25	9	1.5	Contains milk protein Fortified with vitamins and minerals at about 25 percent of DV High in potassium with 1090 mg per serving	42 percent of calories from protein so not permissible by NCAA; however, there is a "collegiate" series of same product with 18 g protein or 29 percent protein

[*]All nutrient information gathered from nutrition facts panel provided on company Web site or product package.

Table 4 Snacks for Weight Loss

Snack	Why This Snack?
Hard-boiled egg and mini–whole-wheat bagel	Eggs may be high in cholesterol, but they are very low in saturated fat and contain high-quality protein. Pair with a mini bagel (100 calories) for carbohydrates and fiber.
Laughing Cow Light Cheese Wedges (2) with 6 Triscuit crackers	Individual portions of cheese (35 calories per wedge) in flavors such as Queso Fresco Chipolte, French Onion, Garlic and Herb, and Creamy Swiss, paired with whole-grain crackers, provide protein, carbohydrates, and fiber in a portable snack.
Quaker Hearty Medleys Fruit and Nuts Instant Oatmeal	A quick snack with 130 calories, no fat, and 3 g of fiber. Flavors such as apple cranberry almond will appeal to athletes.
Smoothie King's Slim-N-Trim 20-oz smoothies	Order a "skinny" smoothie, and a 20-oz snack has 153 calories, 7 g of protein, and 3 g of fiber.
String Cheese (low-fat) and 15 Kashi Original 7 Grain Crackers	Low-fat string cheese has about 50 calories per piece with 6 g protein; pair with a whole-grain cracker.
Yoplait Original Yogurt (6 oz)	Yoplait Original has 170 calories in 6 oz and comes in 25 flavors. It is the only yogurt with 50 percent of the DV for calcium and vitamin D.

Weight-Loss Snacks

When trying to lose weight, it seems counterproductive to recommend snacks, but Americans are a nation of snackers; Table 4 lists some nutrient-dense snacks that athletes can use to boost nutrients and keep hunger away. The key to a healthy snack for athletes trying to lose body fat is portion control, some protein and fiber for satiety, and of course, it has to taste good. The introduction of 100-calorie pack snack foods might help some keep portions in check, but they are expensive. The snacks in Table 4 do not use 100-calorie packs, but do include some individually portioned foods, such as cheese wedges or string cheese. All of these snacks are nutrient-dense and include some of the nutrients, such as

Table 5 Top Ten Best Snacks for Athletes

Snack	Why This Snack?
Almonds	1 oz (23 almonds) provides 6 g protein, 3.5 g fiber, 75 mg calcium, and 7.4 mg vitamin E (highest of all nuts) and heart-healthy fats. Almonds are high in antioxidants. Snacking on almonds provides satiety between meals and provides nutrients needed by athletes.
Cereal and milk and fruit	A whole-grain cereal paired with low-fat milk and fresh fruit provides carbohydrate and protein, along with vitamins and minerals. Choose a cereal that has the "whole-grain" seal, lists a whole grain as the first ingredient, and has at least 3 g of fiber per serving. Top with fruit—banana or berries to boost healthy phytonutrients.
Greek yogurt with low-fat granola	Low-fat Greek yogurt is thicker than other yogurt and contains more protein per serving (up to 20 g of protein per cup) but slightly less calcium than regular yogurt. Add a handful of low-fat granola for crunch and carbohydrates.
Fig bars or oatmeal raisin cookies	Athletes like cookies, and these 2 contain some nutritional value; complex carbohydrates and the benefits of dried fruits such as figs and raisins to boost fiber. These are good postworkout snacks to replenish muscle glycogen.
Fresh fruit paired with low-fat cheese	Apple or pear slices with a couple of ounces of reduced-fat cheese, like Cabot Vermont 50 percent reduced fat jalapeno cheese or Laughing Cow Mini Babybel Light, provide protein, calcium, and the natural sugars and fiber of fresh fruit.
Low-fat chocolate milk	Low-fat chocolate milk is a hot sports recovery drink, and many teams are using it after a workout to provide high-quality protein and carbohydrates to stimulate muscle growth. Milk provides 9 essential nutrients, 160 calories and 8 g of protein in 8 oz (1 cup).
Peanut butter sandwich	Peanut butter on whole-grain bread is a high-energy, tasty, portable snack. Peanut butter has heart-healthy fat and is high in protein.
Pistachios	1 oz of pistachios is 49 nuts—the most nuts per serving and low in calories with 160. Also high in fiber, vitamin B_6, and phytonutrients leutein and zeazanthin.
Popcorn sprinkled with parmesan cheese	Low-fat microwave popcorn is whole-grain snack; when sprinkled with 2 tablespoons of grated parmesan cheese, this snack adds protein and 120 mg of calcium.
Trail mix	The key to this healthy snack is keeping the portions in check and finding or making a trail mix with dried fruit, nuts, seeds, and whole-grain cereal. Avoid the trail mix with candy pieces to reduce fat.

calcium and vitamin D, which may be lacking in a female athlete's diet. There are many yogurt-like products (yogurt shakes, yogurt drinks, and yogurt-in-a-tube) that might also appeal to athletes, but most yogurts do not have vitamin D, so I recommended 6-oz Yoplait original for added vitamins and minerals.

Top Ten Snacks

Table 5 lists my favorite top 10 snacks for athletes based on my experience working with this active group. I chose foods that are easy to find in any grocery store or convenience store; college athletes who live in dorms and are not on meal plans may find that a gas station convenience store is the closest store in walking distance. There are many more snack options available, but I also tried to consider price as well as taste.

Convincing athletes to plan and pack snacks is a challenge. Athletes often tell me they know they should take food with them when they leave the house or dorm room in the morning but often do not know what to take. The snacks listed in Table 5 are all portable, and many do not require refrigeration. One busy athlete came up with a novel approach to eating cereal and milk as a snack; he took a sandwich bag full of Cheerios with him and bought a chug of low-fat milk in the college cafeteria. Sitting in the classroom, he would eat a handful of cereal and take a swig of milk for a portable milk-and-cereal snack. Once athletes see the benefit of snacking (more alert, more energy for practice and conditioning sessions, and less hungry during the day), they often will plan to conquer the snack attack with healthy choices.

Expect to see more healthy snacks on the market this year. The New Nutrition Business Ten Key Trends for 2011 predict that energy and "feel the benefit" foods will be hot, and ultra-convenient will be important in the market place.[11]

References

1. Hills S. Snacks are the fourth meal of the day. Food Navigator. October 10, 2008. www.foodnavigator-usa.com/content/view/print/222356. Accessed December 3, 2010.
2. Virtual Sports Nutrition Conference 2011. www.sportsnutritionconference.com/index.php. Accessed December 15, 2010.
3. Piernas C, Popkin BM. Snacking increased among U.S. adults between 1977 and 2006. *J Nutr.* 2010;140:325–332.
4. American Dietetic Association. Position of the American Dietetic Association, Dietitians of Canada, and the American College of Sports Medicine: Nutrition and Athletic Performance. *J Am Diet Assoc.* 2009;109:509–527.
5. Maughan R. Contamination of dietary supplements and positive drug tests in sport. *J Sports Sci.* 2005;23:883–889.
6. Wilson D. F.D.A. issues new warning on illegal supplements. *The New York Times.* December 15, 2010. Health Section, http://prescriptions.blogs.nytimes.com/2010/12/15/f-d-a-issue-new-warning-on-illegal-supplements/. Accessed December 12, 2010.
7. NCAA issues notice about nutritional-supplement provision. NCAA News. May 23, 2005. http://fs.ncaa.org/Docs/NCAANewsArchive/2005/Association-wide/ncaa+issues+notice+about+nutritional-supplement+provision+-+5-23-05+ncaa+news.html. Accessed December 10, 2010.
8. Minkin T, Renaud B. America's top 10 healthiest fast food restaurants. Health Magazine. February 19, 2009. www.health.com/health/article/0,,20411588,00.html. Accessed December 3, 2010.
9. Grotto D, Zied E. The standard American diet and its relationship to the health status of Americans. *Nutr Clin Pract.* 2010;25:603–612.
10. Tang JE, Phillips SM. Maximizing muscle protein anabolism: the role of protein quality. *Curr Opin Clin Nutr Metab Care.* 2009;12:66–71.
11. Starling S. "Feeling the benefit" guides 2011 trends. Food Navigator.com. December 16, 2010. www.foodnavigator.com/content/view/print/347936. Accessed December 17, 2010.

Critical Thinking

1. Explain why it is difficult to track or conduct research on snacking habits.
2. Identify the six micronutrients that vegetarian athletes are at risk for inadequate intake.
3. Describe the purpose of the certification program developed by the NSF.
4. Identify the three types of supplements that commonly contain illegal ingredients.

CHRISTINE ROSENBLOOM, PhD, RD, CSSD, is professor emerita of nutrition at Georgia State University. She currently serves as the sports dietitian for Georgia State athletes and runs a consulting business, Chris Rosenbloom Food and Nutrition Services, LLC (www.chrisrosenbloom.com).

UNIT 2
Childhood Nutrition

Unit Selections

Learning Outcomes

After reading this Unit, you will be able to:

- Identify the nutrients that are commonly consumed in inadequate amounts in the diet of U.S. children.

- Explain the state of nutrition, dietary intake, eating behavior, and physical activity among U.S. children.

- Summarize how the federal school lunch program has changed over the years since it was formed in 1946.

- Assess whether the Healthy, Hunger Free Kids Act will impact the state of childhood nutrition.

- Describe how families and teachers can improve food behavior of kids during lunch or snack time.

- Identify the six signs that a child or adolescent may exhibit if he or she is developing disordered eating.

- Summarize the "food environment" in the United States. Explain why many health professionals refer to our food environment as toxic.

- Develop recommendations of how families can effectively impact the nutrition and health of their children.

- Judge if marketing non-nutritious foods as fun and entertaining to kids will have long-term consequences on health.

Student Website

www.mhhe.com/cls

Internet References

Centers for Disease Control and Prevention—Obesity Trends
www.cdc.gov/obesity/data/trends.html
Centers for Disease Control and Prevention—Healthy Youth
www.cdc.gov/healthyyouth/obesity
Food Science and Human Nutrition Extension
www.fshn.uiuc.edu
U.S. Dept of Health and Human Services
http://aspe.hhs.gov/health/reports/child_obesity
U.S. Dietary Guidelines
www.cnpp.usda.gov/DGAs2010-DGACReport.htm

According to the Centers for Disease Control, childhood obesity has more than tripled in the past 30 years. In the United States 20 percent of 6- to 11-year-olds and 18 percent of 12–19 year olds are considered obese and 30 percent of U.S. children are considered overweight. Because of this, childhood obesity has gained much needed attention in the media and in health and political arenas.

A great deal of funding and resources are going to curtail the childhood obesity epidemic in the United States. Efforts are being focused on the environmental factors, improving the quality of foods available to kids, and increasing physical activity. This unit concentrates on environmental factors such as the impact of parents and teachers as role models for proper nutrition, the state of foods served in schools, and how foods are marketed to kids.

Think of the foods that are commonly eaten by children in the United States: chicken nuggets, fries, pizza, hamburgers, sweetened cereals, sweetened snacks, and the occasional carrot stick with ranch dressing will come to mind. The problem of childhood obesity and unhealthy "kid friendly" foods marketed to kids in the United States is in the forefront of many nutrition professionals and policymakers. "Healthy Food Looks Serious: How Children Interpret Packaged Food Products" by Charlene Elliott will show a different perspective on the marketing techniques of "fun foods" to kids. Our food environment for childhood nutrition is in the process of change, albeit slow change.

Considering the prevalence of U.S. children and adolescents who are overweight or at risk, the most cost-efficient and effective method of action is prevention. Prevention efforts are geared toward curtailing obese children from maturing into obese adults who burden our current healthcare system and government supported healthcare reimbursement programs with exorbitant costs of obesity-related chronic diseases. The major health consequences of obesity are heart disease, diabetes, gallbladder disease, osteoarthritis, and some cancers.

Although obesity occupies much of the media and political spotlight, the crisis of eating disorders and food restriction in adolescents continues to affect many young people. Two articles in this unit address how eating disorders are still prevalent in this obesocentric environment.

The articles in Unit 2 were compiled to demonstrate different views of the childhood obesity problem. Many of the articles provide solutions to the problem; however, solving the obesity epidemic in the United States is a challenging task. The problem

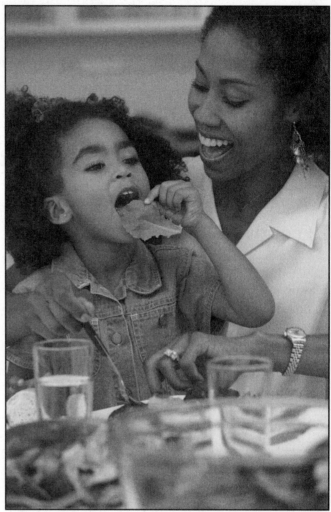

© Rolf Bruderer/Blend Images LLC

is multifactorial and took decades to occur. The solutions, which will essentially be a change in our entire societal culture, will also have to be multifactorial and will take years to see marked results. The articles in this unit can be used as supplemental information for topics on childhood nutrition and the obesity epidemic.

The State of Family Nutrition and Physical Activity

Are We Making Progress?

AMERICAN DIETETIC ASSOCIATION AND AMERICAN DIETETIC ASSOCIATION FOUNDATION

Executive Summary

Ten years ago, the U.S. Surgeon General released a landmark report: "The Call to Action to Decrease and Prevent Overweight and Obesity." The Surgeon General warned that, if overweight and obesity were not controlled, the number of obesity-related deaths would soon surpass the number of tobacco-related deaths.[1] This news caught the nation's attention and led to many public and private efforts targeting two of the root causes of overweight and obesity: poor nutrition and lack of physical activity.

The Surgeon General's report, and many subsequent government and science-based institutions' reports, called for changes in five key areas: communities and families, schools, healthcare, worksites and media. As these reports have concluded, poor nutrition and inactivity stem from many factors deeply rooted in our culture, factors that have become part of the societal norm. Changes will not necessarily come quickly and will require ongoing, vigilant attention from public and private sectors.[2]

In a major step to drive changes further, First Lady Michelle Obama launched the Let's Move! initiative, and the White House convened a Task Force on Childhood Obesity Prevention. In May 2010, the task force released 70 recommendations for childhood obesity prevention and announced the goal of reducing the childhood obesity rate from the current 17 percent to 5 percent by 2030.[3] The recommendations for government, healthcare, communities, schools and families help to focus resources, and the Let's Move! campaign brings the vital momentum required to keep prevention efforts moving forward.

Over the past decade, the American Dietetic Association (ADA) and its Foundation (ADAF) committed resources toward efforts to treat, reduce and prevent childhood over weight and obesity. This commitment is further strengthened now with the launch of *Kids Eat Right,* a platform designed to ensure that sound nutrition recommendations are part of childhood obesity prevention. A member-driven public education campaign, *Kids Eat Right* mobilizes ADA's 71,000 members to support families, schools and communities in their pursuit of quality nutrition for all children—especially for our most at-risk populations.

With all of this exciting momentum, we must also give care and consideration to actions taken and messages sent regarding food and nutrition. It is critical that nutrition policies and practices take a total diet approach that supports all the foods required for optimal growth and development. An inadequate amount of food or lack of nutrient-dense foods may negatively affect children's health today and disease prevention for the future.[4] Without daily consumption of foods providing the necessary nutrients, children are at risk for iron-deficiency anemia, poor academic performance, development of psychosocial difficulties and an increased likelihood of developing chronic diseases such as heart disease, diabetes and osteoporosis during adulthood.[5]

Nutrition policies and practices need a total diet approach supporting eating patterns that provide nutrients required for normal growth and development.

Kids Eat Right **is designed to ensure that sound nutrition recommendations are part of childhood obesity prevention. This initiative mobilizes the American Dietetic Association's 71,000 members to support families, schools and communities in their pursuit of quality nutrition for all children— especially for our most at-risk populations.**

Review of recent food consumption data from the National Health and Nutrition Examination Survey (NHANES) indicates that there are gaps between children's recommended and actual intake of key nutrients, gaps that sadly are the same as ten years ago, despite increasing efforts to close them.[6,7,8] Along with low intake of vitamins and minerals, these data show higher-than-recommended consumption of sugar and saturated fat. The consumption of sweetened beverages, desserts and snack foods adds calories without necessary nutrients and may also displace the eating of nutrient-dense foods, resulting in a negative effect on the quality of kids' diets and their nutritional status.[9,10] Failure to address these nutritional gaps puts the nation at risk of raising a generation of children who suffer negative consequences to their social and physical well-being regardless of their weight.

We must assess, re-calibrate and redouble our efforts to address children's total nutrient needs while promoting healthy weights. *Kids Eat Right* recognizes the powerful role that registered dietitians can play in this effort. With a unique blend of skills and knowledge, dietitians can balance the concurrent needs of normal growth and development along with prevention of chronic illnesses.

This report outlines the premise behind *Kids Eat Right* and highlights the eating and activity habits of families and subsequent nutritional gaps or deficiencies in kids' eating patterns. A newly released survey conducted by the ADAF—the *Family Nutrition and Physical Activity Survey* of children and their parents—reveals that families have made changes since the initial survey in 2003 and are ready to make more changes. The child-parent pairs were asked the same questions to determine if parents were aware of behaviors and if they connected with children's views. Obviously, being aware of eating and activity habits is the starting point; without that, change cannot occur. The survey provides insight into eating and activity behaviors and can help to explain why kids' diets are inadequate in key nutrients. Kids are not always eating three meals a day and eat many times throughout the day. This is reflected in the NHANES data that documents kids' snack foods are often high in calories without

necessary nutrients; this may lead to unhealthy weights in kids.[11,12] Importantly, the survey indicates that there are many opportunities for positive change. By building on children's and parents' desire to eat healthy and be active—and by identifying drivers of positive habits— solutions to the chronic problems associated with under-nourishment, inactive lifestyles and unhealthy weights can be more successful.

The time is now. With communities across America focused on the issue, with the Let's Move! initiative in place and with children and their parents showing a new stage of readiness for change, this is the time to help *Kids Eat Right*.

Are We Making Progress?

The December 2001 Surgeon General's report made headlines: it found that 13 percent of 6- to 11-year-old children and 14 percent of 12- to 19-year-olds were obese (at that time, the terminology was overweight).[1] Since then, information about obesity and two of the primary causes—poor nutrition and inactivity—has been regularly in the news. Although researchers say the rapid rise in obesity is leveling off, nearly a decade later 17 percent of 2- to 19-year-olds are obese, with the highest prevalence among Mexican American boys (27 percent) and African American girls (29 percent).[13,14]

Since 1980 when the first Dietary Guidelines for Americans were released, there have not been the types of improvements in the diets of Americans as hoped for by health professionals working as advisors on the Guidelines.[15] The aim of the Guidelines is to provide advice about how good dietary habits can promote health and decrease risk for major chronic disease.[16] The messages have been generally consistent: Americans have been called upon to maintain a healthy weight, to limit sugar, sodium and saturated fat and to eat plenty of fruits, vegetables, whole grains and low-fat and fat-free dairy foods. Unfortunately, the majority of children do not meet the recommended servings from the five food groups, and adults consume below recommended intake on four or more nutrients.[17]

In light of these trends, this *Kids Eat Right* report examines the state of family nutrition and physical activity using data from the National Health and Nutrition Examination Survey (NHANES 2005–2006, 2007–2008),[17,18] statistics from the Centers for Disease Control and Prevention 2009 Youth Risk Behavior Surveillance Survey[19] and new findings from the American Dietetic Association Foundation's (ADAF) *Family Nutrition and Physical Activity Survey*. Conducted initially in 2003 and again in 2010, the ADAF survey assesses children's attitudes and behaviors related to nutrition and physical activity and parents' understanding

Family Nutrition and Physical Activity Survey Methodology

The American Dietetic Association Foundation Family Nutrition and Physical Activity Survey was developed to gain a better understanding of factors related to healthy weights. The survey explored children's attitudes and behaviors regarding nutrition, eating habits and physical activity, as well as parents' awareness of their children's attitudes and behaviors.

The survey was first fielded in January 2003 to 615 pairs of children and parents representative of the U.S. population. In 2010, the survey instrument was amended to include new content domains based on results from an environmental scan, literature review on factors related to childhood obesity and prevention as well as information and insights gained from focus groups conducted in spring 2009 with parents (low-income white, Hispanic, African American, men and women) and their children of middle-school age (boys and girls).[20] Changes to the survey instrument included adding questions about potential drivers of healthful behaviors and the role of registered dietitians. Nearly two-thirds of the original questions were repeated in the 2010 survey.

Knowledge Networks, a custom survey research company, administered the 2003 and 2010 surveys. Beginning in 1999, Knowledge Networks recruited and established the first online research panel through probability-based sampling. Panel members were randomly recruited through random-digit dialing and address-based sampling methods and were representative of the entire U.S. population. To cover both online and offline populations, households were provided with access to the Internet and hardware if needed.

The most recent survey was administered online in February 2010 to three population samples of youth aged 8 to 17 and their parents. The population samples included 754 pairs of children and parents who are representative of the U.S. population, 230 Hispanic pairs and 209 African American pairs. The participants were randomly selected from Knowledge Networks' panel, and the survey was offered in English or Spanish.

A sample of 420 white child-adult pairs taken from the 754 pairs in the U.S. population sample was used to assess differences between white, Hispanic and African American child-adult pairs. For analysis by race and income, income brackets were matched to the USDA's nutrient data. "Low" income includes household incomes below $25,000, "medium" income includes household incomes between $25,000 and $74,999, and "high" income includes household incomes of $75,000 or more.

of and connectedness to their children's behaviors. (See sidebar for more information on the ADAF survey.)

What Kids Are Not Eating

At the same time that many children are overweight or obese, many children have diets that are deficient in one or more nutrients, leaving them in a state of under-nutrition, or malnourishment.[21] Data from the National Health and Nutrition Examination Survey (NHANES) from 2007–2008 indicate that 90 percent of children over 8 years of age do not consume recommended servings of vegetables and that 75 percent consume less than recommended amounts for fruits. For milk and milk products, more than 50 percent of boys aged 9 to 18 years and over 90 percent of girls do not consume recommended amounts.[21] The grain group now distinguishes between refined and whole grain foods, and while all kids exceed recommended servings for refined grains, 95 percent do not consume the recommended amount of whole grains. Lastly, consumption of meat, poultry, fish, eggs, soy products, nuts and seeds is low for 75 percent of girls aged 9 to 18 years, while other kids meet or exceed recommended servings.[21]

At the same time that many children are overweight or obese, many children have diets that are deficient in one or more nutrients, leaving them in a state of under-nutrition, or malnourishment.

The 2010 Advisory Committee to the Dietary Guidelines for Americans is concerned about the food kids do *not* eat. Because kids do not consume recommended amounts of core food groups, their diets are low in Vitamin D, calcium, potassium and dietary fiber.[21] Eighty percent of girls and 75 percent of boys ages 4 to 18 have inadequate intake of calcium, and nearly half of all kids' diets are deficient in Vitamin D. The low intake of vegetables, whole grains and fruits is evident in the inadequate consumption of dietary fiber and potassium by 95 percent of all kids.[21] This is not a new problem. Over the past decade, children's eating patterns have been markedly low in vitamins A, C, D and E.[22,23,24]

Poor eating habits not only contribute to unhealthy weights, but negative effects from poor nutrition may also include learning and behavior problems, lowered immunity or resistance to colds and flu and dental caries.[4,5] These nutrition-related problems can affect children's academic achievement due to missed days of school, poor classroom behavior and diminished ability to concentrate and problem solve.[25,26,27] Chronic under-nutrition and/or not eating breakfast before going to school (or work) can have a negative effect on problem solving and other cognitive tasks.[28,29] A review of studies linking nutrition and learning found that even a well-nourished child who misses breakfast could have diminished problem-solving capacity to a degree that lowers test scores.[30]

The State of Childhood Overweight and Obesity

According to the National Health and Nutrition Examination Survey (NHANES), prevalence of overweight and obesity has doubled among 2- to 11-year-olds and tripled among 12- to 19-year-old adolescents.

Among children surveyed in NHANES 2003–2006, 16 percent of 2- to 19-year-old children and teens were obese, with body mass index (BMI) levels at or above the age and gender-specific 95th percentile, and almost one-third were over-weight or obese, with BMI levels at or above the 85th percentile.

Based on 2007–2008 NHANES data, obesity is more prevalent among Hispanic males aged 6 to 19 years (27 percent) than among non-Hispanic white (18 percent) and non-Hispanic African American (19 percent) males in that same age group. For females, obesity is more prevalent among non-Hispanic African American females (26 percent) than among non-Hispanic white females (16 percent). No significant differences in prevalence of overweight by race and ethnicity were observed among either males or females aged 6 to 19 years.[31]

Weight Status	Percentile Range
Underweight	Less than the 5th percentile
Healthy weight	5th percentile to less than the 85th percentile

Weight Status	Percentile Range
Overweight	85th percentile to less than the 95th percentile
Obese	*Equal to or greater than the 95th percentile*

Definition of Overweight and Obesity

For children and adolescents (aged 2 to 19 years), the BMI value is plotted on the CDC's growth charts to determine the corresponding BMI-for-age percentile.

- Overweight is defined as a BMI at or above the 85th percentile and lower than the 95th percentile.
- Obesity is defined as a BMI at or above the 95th percentile for children of the same age and sex.

These definitions are based on the 2000 CDC Growth Charts for the United States and expert committee. A child's weight status is determined based on an age- and sex-specific percentile for BMI rather than by the BMI categories used for adults. Classification of overweight and obesity for children and adolescents are age- and sex-specific because children's body composition varies between boys and girls and by age.

For more information, see Prevalence of Obesity Among Children and Adolescents: United States, Trends 1963–1965 Through 2007–2008 *by Cynthia Ogden, Ph.D., and Margaret Carroll, M.S.P.H., Division of Health and Nutrition Examination Surveys (www.cdc.gov/mmwr/preview/mmwrhtml/mm5940a7.htm).*

What Kids Are Eating

Most children and teens eat enough calories, and some eat more calories than needed for their activity level, which could lead to unhealthy weight gain. The majority of kids, whether at a healthy weight or not, are not eating the right foods—those foods that provide "quality calories." The NHANES survey of 1977–1978 and 2001–2002 identified, major changes in food and drink choices during this period of time; these changes coincided with increases in weight in all age-sex categories. Children shifted from drinking milk to high-sugar drinks and ate more foods that were higher in calories yet lower in nutrients.[9] More kids now eat food from outside the home, and daily snacking has increased, with calories in the snacks increasing as well. As noted above, consumption of the food groups kids need more of did not increase over this period. [21,23,24]

Foods that provide the most calories in children's diets are also high in solid fats and/or added sugar. In fact, about one-third of total calories consumed by 2- to 18-year-old U.S. children and adolescents come from the intake of solid fats and added sugars that are commonly viewed as nutrient-poor calories. Grain-based desserts, such as cakes, cookies, donuts, pies, cobblers and granola bars, are the largest source of calories for adults and kids, without contributing any important nutrients.[9,10,21]

The shift toward consumption of sweetened beverages, desserts and snack foods is a major contributor to daily calorie intake without contributing valuable nutrients.[10,21,32] Substituting nutrient-dense foods, such as vegetables, fruits, low-fat and nonfat dairy and non-dessert whole grain foods, would benefit calorie balance and diet quality.

The chart on page 32 lists foods that represent the largest source of calories from sugar in kids' diets. The results vary slightly by race/ethnicity and income levels but are generally consistent among all groups of kids.[32] Dominating the list are soda/energy/sports drinks, which contribute nearly one-third of the calories in children's diets.[21,32]

Foods that provide the most calories from saturated fat include the grain-based desserts (11 percent calories from solid fat), regular cheese (8 percent), sausage, franks, ribs and bacon (together 7 percent), pizza (6 percent), French fries (6 percent) and dairy-based desserts (5 percent). Kids ages 14 to 18 get more solid fat calories from French fries and beef.[9,10,21] The Advisory Committee recommends that no more than 5 percent to 15 percent of total

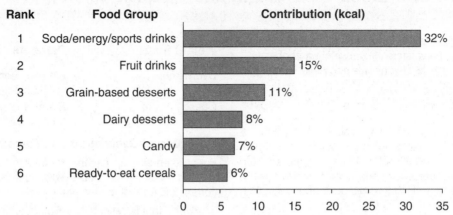

Percent Contribution of Foods to Calories from Added Sugar in Kids' Diets

Rank	Food Group	Contribution (kcal)
1	Soda/energy/sports drinks	32%
2	Fruit drinks	15%
3	Grain-based desserts	11%
4	Dairy desserts	8%
5	Candy	7%
6	Ready-to-eat cereals	6%

Source: Mean Intake of Added Sugar & Percentage Contribution (kcal) of Various Foods Among US Children & Adolescents, by Race/Ethnicity & Family Income, NHANES 2005-06. National Cancer Institute. See http://riskfactor.cancer.gov/diet/foodsources/added_sugars/table4a.html. Accessed Oct. 11, 2010.

calories come from solid fats and added sugar to allow for more nutrient-dense foods and maintain caloric balance.

To both meet recommended nutrients and limit added sugar and solid fat, major changes to eating patterns will be required. Changing the foods kids eat requires attention to taste-appeal. Because taste drives eating habits, modifying favorite foods to improve kids' total diet is a key prevention strategy, especially when those preferred foods are also a good source of nutrition. For example, popular "kids foods" like pizza and whole milk provide Vitamin D, calcium and potassium, although because kids eat these at higher frequency, they are also a source of saturated fat. Reduced-fat and fat-free alternatives to whole milk are available, and many school lunch programs now serve pizzas made with whole grain crusts and lower fat cheese. On the other hand, some of the sources of saturated fat, like grain-based desserts, do not provide beneficial nutrients. Focusing on increasing the foods and drinks that supply missing nutrients could displace foods that provide a high amount of "nutrient-poor calories".[33]

The chronic nature of low nutrient consumption combined with higher intake of sugar and solid fats is cause for alarm. Poor nutrition from the over-consumption of foods high in calories and low in required nutrients can result in weight gain along with low nutrient intake. However, it is important to note that, whatever a child's weight, it is likely that the child is not consuming the recommended servings from all required food groups.[21,31]

Physical Activity Stagnates

Nutrition and physical activity are addressed simultaneously for healthy weights and overall health. As with nutrition, time kids spend being physically active and their fitness levels are important determinants of health;

higher fitness levels are also correlated with better moods, behaviors, concentration and learning.

The 2009 Youth Risk Behavior Surveillance Study (YRBSS) found that the percentage of high school students who had been physically active for a total of at least 60 minutes per day on seven days has not significantly changed in the past half decade.[19] In the 2005 YRBSS, only 18 percent of high school students were active at least 60 minutes on all seven days, and in 2009, 18 percent of students reported seven days of activity.[19] Additionally, the percentage of students who do not participate in 60 minutes of physical activity on any day decreased from 25 percent in 2005 to 23 percent in 2009, although this too was not statistically significant.[19]

Inactivity is just as important to monitor as activity. YRBSS data show a significant increase in the percentage of students using computers three or more hours a day for non-school work such as video games: 22 percent fit this description in 2003 while the figure increased to 25 percent in 2009.[19] Concurrent with this increase in computer time has been a significant decrease in the percentage of students who watch three or more hours per day of television, from 43 percent in the 1999 YRBSS to 33 percent in the 2009 YRBSS.[19] It may be that sedentary activities are traded one for another and that it is harder for youth to switch to being physically active on most, if not all, days of the week.

Similarly, the ADAF *Family Nutrition and Physical Activity Survey* finds mixed results to questions about physical activity. For example, between 2003 and 2010, there was a significant increase in the percentage of kids being physically active with their parents three or more days a week (from 16 percent in 2003 up to 31 percent in 2010). However, during the same time period, there also was a significant increase (from 57 percent in 2003 to 64

Children's and Parents' Beliefs about Nutrition and Weight

"In general, people think they eat better than they do." So says Gayle Coleman, MS, RD, nutrition educator, University of Wisconsin-Extension, Cooperative Extension.

The *Family Nutrition and Physical Activity Survey* confirms Coleman's claim. Both children and their parents report that children are eating nutritious foods. In fact, the majority of children (59 percent) perceive themselves as eating healthy foods (up from 46 percent in 2003). In 2010, kids rank their food intake as being significantly more nutritious (p <.001) than they did in 2003, and in 2010, parents are more aligned with ranking the healthfulness of their children's diets than they were in 2003. However, while children report that they are eating nutritious foods, studies demonstrate that children's diets have serious nutrient shortfalls.

Children also have misperceptions of their body size. Significantly more children in 2010 report being at the "right weight" than in 2003, with 22 percent of the surveyed children reporting that they are overweight, down from 32 percent in 2003. Registered Dietitians interviewed explained that many over-weight adults underreport their weight; this is happening with some kids too. The national data do not agree that kids are slimming down quite like kids tell us: over the 2003-2010 period, weight was still increasing, though in some categories it was starting to stabilize.[13, 14, 31]

These disconnects may reflect a shift in what is perceived as "normal" food intake and body weight. Because high-calorie, low-nutrient foods are more available than high-nutrient options, poor food choices have become the standard. At the same time, society in general has become desensitized to over-weight. Lucille Beseler, MS, RD, LD/N, CDE, president and founder of the Family Nutrition Center of South Florida, points out that television commercials now more often feature overweight children. Seeing overweight kids, she says, has become "the norm."

"A big piece of prevention is educating parents and communities and having the trickle-down effect."

Yet despite these gaps, registered dietitians find that parents want to help their children eat healthier foods and maintain appropriate body weight. "It's not that parents don't understand their child is overweight," Beseler says. "They're busy and overwhelmed without a lot of time or a lot of resources." Coleman agrees. People have a "general sense of what's healthy and what they should do," she says, but they may need help putting that information into action.

"Many, if not the majority of, parents want to know what they can do to improve their families' diets," says Beseler. This desire for greater nutrition literacy gives registered dietitians a real opportunity to help parents understand the most healthful food choices and recognize healthy weights.

"A big piece of prevention is educating parents and communities and having the trickle-down effect," Beseler remarked about her experiences working with families for over 20 years.

Parents are the behavior leaders at home, and as the Let's Move! initiative also calls for, we must empower parents to be the best role models possible. Registered dietitians can help to improve parents' self-efficacy by teaching skills and information essential for putting a balanced meal on the table. We need to help parents see the immediate benefits of eating and serving healthier options consistently.

percent in 2010) in the number of kids and parents spending time watching TV, viewing a movie or playing a video game together three or more days a week.

In 2010, the percentage of kids who played on a sports team or participated in group physical activity decreased a few percentage points, although not significantly (from 63 percent in 2003 to 60 percent in 2010). Also in 2010, there was an increase in the number of kids preferring outdoor activities to sedentary indoor activities (21 percent preferring out door activities in 2010 compared to 15 percent in 2003), although it was also not statistically significant. The *Family Nutrition and Physical Activity Survey* also finds that the percentage of children having 60 minutes of physical activity seven days a week was similar to the national YRBSS findings. The survey further finds that parents' knowledge of their kids' activity level is consistent with their children's self-report, with no differences by race: 17 percent white, 17 percent Hispanic and 16 percent African American kids report getting 60 minutes of activity daily.

Between 2003 and 2010, there was a significant increase in the percentage of kids being physically active with their parents, according to the *Family Nutrition and Physical Activity Survey* results.

Ready for Change

The *Family Nutrition and Physical Activity Survey* results provide a new level of confidence that changes are occurring and will continue to occur. Perhaps the most compelling survey finding is that children and their parents are at a different place in awareness and that they are even trying new behaviors, more so than they were in 2003.

When the *Family Nutrition and Physical Activity Survey* was first conducted in 2003, a primary aim was to understand the child-parent connection as it related to activity and eating attitudes and behaviors. The big news in 2003 was the disconnect that existed between parents and their children.

This year's survey results show a marked improvement in the parents' connection to eating and activity patterns for their kids. Child-parent pairs are much more aligned, showing an awareness that was not there in 2003. Changes in kids' behaviors cannot take place without parents being aware and making nutrition and activity important priorities for the family. There was statistically significant agreement in the child-parent pairs in 2010 on nearly every question. This alignment signals a shift in children's and parents' connectedness on these topics. This higher awareness relates to a new stage of "readiness" to make healthy changes.[36]

The "Stages of Change Model" is a framework that can help visualize the process or sequence of behavior states or stages that occur between not knowing there is a problem to a changed behavior that has now become a habit. This framework can help explain changes in population samples too. Until there is an awareness of a behavior—precontemplation—there is not a move forward.[36,37] Precontemplation moves to contemplation once there is an awareness of the problem.

The Family Factor

For youth to experience lasting changes in nutrition and physical activity, the entire family system needs to change.[38] Generational habits and behaviors can prevent change from happening, so it's important to have buy-in from the family system.[40] As such, slow and gradual changes usually are more effective. It is also important to identify which family behaviors can help meet the goals of healthy weights and quality nutrition.[38,39,40] Research over the past decade has identified child-parent interactions that can promote healthy or unhealthy weights.[38,39,40,41] Eating family meals at home has positive benefits, while eating away from home can have a negative effect on the quality of kids' diets.[42,43,44,45] Other positive effects on healthy eating habits are seen with regular daily routines and with children and parents spending time together.[46,47]

"Both parents and children are aware that there is a problem and that they need to be eating healthier and they're willing to think about eating healthier. I think this is a major step. In my experience over the decades in treating overweight children and their families, a lot of times the hardest thing is to move a person from a stage of inaction to a stage of contemplation, to saying 'Gee, maybe I want to do something.' I think that this is the opportunity for dietitians to help patients."

Nancy Copperman, MS, RD, CDN,
Director of Public Health Initiatives, North Shore Long Island Jewish Health System

"It seems like parents are more aware of what the kids are doing. And I think that's good. That's the first little mini-step into trying to do something differently."

Aida Miles, MMSc, RD, CSP, LD, CNSD,
Director of the Coordinated MPH Program,
Division of Epidemiology and Community Health,
University of Minnesota School of Public Health

More family meals

Many benefits are found in sharing meals as a family.[42,43,44,45] Studies of teens who regularly have meals with their families find that these teens are at lower risk of using drugs and that they experience better connectedness at home, enjoy improved mental health and exhibit better eating patterns, including higher consumption of fruits and vegetables.[46,47,48,49] Data indicate that when kids eat meals with their parents/families, without watching television, this meal time is an important opportunity for bonding and teaching good nutrition and eating behaviors.[42,44,49,50,51] The *Family Nutrition and Physical Activity Survey* finds a significant increase in family meals, with 73 percent of families eating at home daily in 2010 up from 52 percent of families in 2003. A closer look at 2010 data reveals significant racial/ethnic differences in the percentage of children eating with their parents at home daily. African American children (61 percent) eat dinner with their parents daily, significantly less often than white (72 percent) and Hispanic children (72 percent).

While the percentage of families eating dinner at home has increased since 2003, the percentage of children reporting that they eat out with their parents has remained constant and much less than the percentage eating at home. Children's and parents' responses to these questions are significantly correlated across all racial groups, indicating a high level of parental awareness and validation of children's responses in 2010.

Increase in regular routines

Another family factor correlated with healthy behaviors is the existence of family routines. Routines—or regular daily activities—are important in organizing daily life and reflect family characteristics.[41,46,47] Family routines, including regular family meals and regular bedtimes, are positively linked to multiple positive child outcomes, including academic achievement, self-esteem and both behavioral and psychosocial adjustment. Families that are organized and have predictable routines produce children with more positive outcomes.[46,47,52]

Changes Between 2003 and 2010: Percent of Children Reporting Behaviors

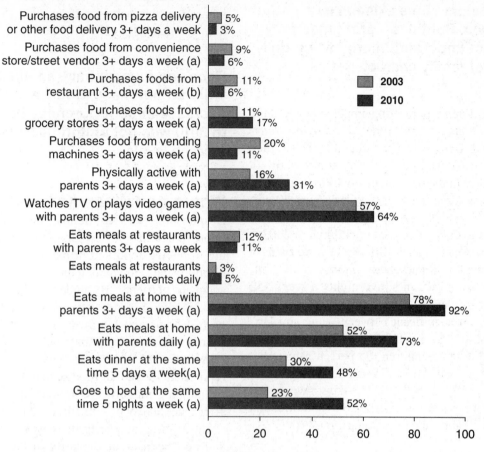

Behavior	2003	2010
Purchases food from pizza delivery or other food delivery 3+ days a week	5%	3%
Purchases food from convenience store/street vendor 3+ days a week (a)	9%	6%
Purchases foods from restaurant 3+ days a week (b)	11%	6%
Purchases foods from grocery stores 3+ days a week (a)	11%	17%
Purchases food from vending machines 3+ days a week (a)	20%	11%
Physically active with parents 3+ days a week (a)	16%	31%
Watches TV or plays video games with parents 3+ days a week (a)	57%	64%
Eats meals at restaurants with parents 3+ days a week	12%	11%
Eats meals at restaurants with parents daily	3%	5%
Eats meals at home with parents 3+ days a week (a)	78%	92%
Eats meals at home with parents daily (a)	52%	73%
Eats dinner at the same time 5 days a week (a)	30%	48%
Goes to bed at the same time 5 nights a week (a)	23%	52%

a: Behaviors are different with statistical significance between 2003 and 2010, p < 0.001.

b: Behaviors are different with statistical significance between 2003 and 2010, p < 0.05.

Source: ADAF Family Nutrition and Physical Activity Survey, *2003 and 2010*

Percent of Kids Reporting Eating with Parents

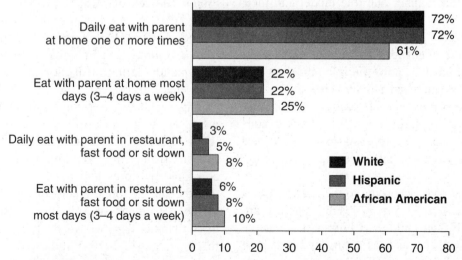

	White	Hispanic	African American
Daily eat with parent at home one or more times	72%	72%	61%
Eat with parent at home most days (3–4 days a week)	22%	22%	25%
Daily eat with parent in restaurant, fast food or sit down	3%	5%	8%
Eat with parent in restaurant, fast food or sit down most days (3–4 days a week)	6%	8%	10%

There are differences among races in the frequency of children and parents eating meals at home, with African Americans having meals together significantly less often than Hispanic and white parent-child pairs, p < 0.05.

Source: ADAF Family Nutrition and Physical Activity Survey, *2010*

Another family factor correlated with healthy behaviors is the existence of family routines. Routines—or regular daily activities—are important in organizing daily life and reflect family characteristics.

Many more children report eating dinner at or about the same time five nights a week in the 2010 *Family Nutrition and Physical Activity Survey* (48 percent) than they did in 2003 (30 percent). The 2010 survey also shows a significant increase in the percentage of children going to bed about the same time five nights a week; over 50 percent of kids in 2010 report regular bedtimes on all school nights compared to only 23 percent of children in 2003.

There are, however, racial differences observed in 2010 survey results. Significantly more white children report regular meal times five nights a week (52 percent) than do African American children (40 percent); the difference is not significant between white and Hispanic children at 48 percent. The 2010 survey also finds significantly more white children (55 percent) than Hispanic (46 percent) and African American (45 percent) children reporting regular bed time five days a week. But overall, daily routines are up—a step in the right direction for healthy eating habits and proper nutrition.[42,46,47]

More time together

Time parents spend with children is an important factor affecting children's health and nutrition for a variety of reasons.[51,52,53] Parents model behaviors, good or bad, and children in both the 2003 and 2010 surveys name their mothers as their number one role model and their fathers as number two. What parents eat, whether they value being physically active and whether they spend time with their children engaged in healthy behaviors—all are examples of positive, powerful role modeling that can shape children's eating and activity behaviors.[43] The quality of the time parents and children spend together is critical. As parents are stretched for time, they can convey all-important lessons by preparing meals with their children, shopping for foods and cleaning up after the meal.[46,47,52,53]

The good news is that, according to the *Family Nutrition and Physical Activity Survey* results, parents are spending time with their children. Children and parents enjoy activities together—such as eating and watching movies or TV—on a daily basis. The increase in parents spending time being physically active three or more days a week is sizable, moving from 16 percent in 2003 to 31 percent in 2010. However, as noted above, more children

and their parents are watching TV and playing video games together three or more days a week, a significant increase in this behavior from 2003 (57 percent of children and parents) to 2010 (64 percent).

Race and income have an effect on where children purchase foods, and the general decrease in poor purchase habits from 2003 to 2010 was not uniform across race and income levels.

Where and When Kids Eat

Despite the positive trends, there is still room for improvement. From skipping meals and frequent snacking to buying food and drinks from a variety of places, troubling patterns stand in the way of children consuming adequate nutrients. By understanding behaviors related to kids' eating and activity, decision makers, health professionals and families are better equipped to make changes that have an impact on the lives of children.

A recent U.S. Department of Agriculture (USDA) report concluded that foods eaten from fast food outlets, restaurants and other commercial sources negatively affect the quality of kids' diets.[45] The study shows that away-from-home eating increases caloric consumption and decreases dietary quality in kids aged 6 to 18.[45] Food consumption data from 2007–2008 show on average that one-third of children's calorie intake is away-from-home food; in 1977, it was less than one-fourth of calorie intake in children.[45,54,56] This is an area where educational efforts are necessary to help improve children's choices of away-from-home foods and beverages.[54]

The 2010 ADAF *Family Nutrition and Physical Activity Survey* indicates that parents and children are infrequently eating meals at restaurants. Survey results show that only 9 percent to 18 percent of children and parents eat away-from-home foods three or more days a week. A significant difference between 2003 and 2010 is the decrease in the percentage of kids buying food or drink from school vending machines and snack bars, convenience stores and restaurants. It is worth noting that the survey found a statistically significant increase in the percentage of kids buying from grocery stores three or more days per week, from 11 percent in 2003 to 17 percent in 2010. Purchase data are not available, making it unclear if an improvement in nutrition follows this trend. However, this is a sign that kids have access to nutrient-dense foods, and this could mean new opportunities for healthier snacking.

Race and income have an effect on where children purchase foods and the general decrease in poor purchase habits from 2003 to 2010 was not uniform across race and income levels. Significantly more African American children from low-income homes (less than $25,000 a year) report buying foods from vending and snack bars at school, convenience stores and restaurants. Low-income African American children buy food three or more days a week from pizza or other food delivery (22 percent), significantly more often than Hispanic children at all income levels (5–7 percent) and white children in medium- (1 percent) and high-income (2 percent) households.

Kids eat day and night

Meals aside, most kids report eating several times throughout the day. The majority of kids eat snacks after school at least some of the time (81 percent white, 88 percent Hispanic and 87 percent African American). Kids eat while watching TV, doing homework, playing computer games and talking on the phone; however, some kids do so more than others. African American children report snacking more often—while watching TV (significantly more than white children), while doing homework, while playing computer games, while talking on the phone (significantly more than white and Hispanic) and before bedtime (significantly more than Hispanic children).

Recently published data on kids' snacking patterns find that the overall quality of the diet, or nutrient density, lowers as snacking increases.[11,12,32] Foods eaten as snacks provide more sugar and saturated fat and fewer vitamins and minerals.[9,10,11,12] Since the late 1970s, the percentage of 12- to 19-year-olds who snack increased from 61 percent to 83 percent, the number of snacks increased from 1.0 to 1.7 snacks per day, and daily calories from snacks increased from 300 to 526.[12,57]

Three Square Meals a Day— Not Always

The meal kids skip most frequently is breakfast, probably the worst meal to miss given the connection between breakfast and learning and given that after a night's sleep immediate

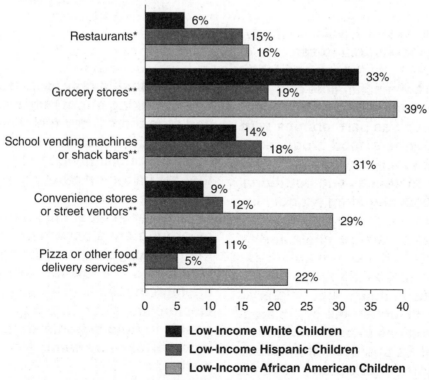

Percent of Low-Income Kids Purchasing Snacks and Meals
Kids purchase foods three or more days a week from the following places ...

Restaurants*
- 6%
- 15%
- 16%

Grocery stores**
- 33%
- 19%
- 39%

School vending machines or shack bars**
- 14%
- 18%
- 31%

Convenience stores or street vendors**
- 9%
- 12%
- 29%

Pizza or other food delivery services**
- 11%
- 5%
- 22%

■ **Low-Income White Children**
■ **Low-Income Hispanic Children**
■ **Low-Income African American Children**

*Statistically significant differences by race, p < 0.05
* * Statistically significant differences by race, p < 0.001
Source: ADAF Family Nutrition and Physical Activity Survey, 2010

Percent of Kids Eating All, Most or Some of the Time ...

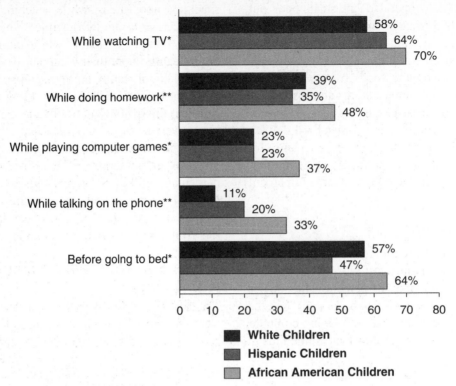

* Statistically significant differences by race, p < 0.05
** Statistically significant differences by race, p < 0.001
Source: ADAF Family Nutrition and Physical Activity Survey, 2010

"The *[Family Nutrition and Physical Activity]* study tells us that for children to eat healthier foods, they have to look and taste good. Schools have financial, time and other resource-related limitations. We need new approaches, such as partnerships with local restaurants, farmers, food producers and local dietetic associations, especially to address cultural preferences and nutritional issues of the children attending schools in those communities."

"For example, restaurateurs, chefs and registered dietitians in the community could help schools make culturally relevant tasty meals that also meet dietary guidelines for the children. Help in the area of food and nutrition has to be continuous if it is going to make a positive difference in the children's nutritional status and their acceptance of school foods."

Judith Rodriguez, PhD, RD, FADA, LDN, President, American Dietetic Association

"A lot of people only look at macronutrients when thinking about nutrient standards and stop there. They feel that if we meet our macronutrient goals, then the food is okay. I think the public needs to look at guidelines that are based on meeting micronutrient standards as well."

"In order to meet micronutrient and macronutrient standards, schools would then be supported in offering more fruits, vegetables and low-fat dairy products that are high in folic acid, Vitamin C, Vitamin A, calcium and fiber. One way of meeting this goal is to fund schools so that they can incorporate more whole foods into their menus."

Nancy Copperman, MS, RD, CDN, Director of Public Health Initiatives, North Shore Long Island Jewish Health System energy stores in the body are running low. The *Family Nutrition and Physical Activity Survey* asked kids if they eat breakfast all of the time and results indicate that many children do not do so. Significantly more African American children do not eat breakfast all of the time (59 percent) compared to white and Hispanic children (42 percent). Even higher numbers of low-income whites and medium-income African Americans (both at 67 percent) do not eat breakfast all of the time. It is of particular concern when lower income children miss breakfast, as many would be eligible for the free or reduced price School Breakfast Program if their school offered it.

The USDA School Breakfast Program provides one-fourth of the Recommended Dietary Allowance for protein, calcium, iron, Vitamin A, Vitamin C and calories.[58,59] Studies have shown that children who eat breakfast on a regular basis are less likely to be overweight.[58] Schools that provide breakfast in the classroom to all students have shown decreases in tardiness and suspensions as well as improved student behavior and attentiveness.[28] Which foods are eaten for breakfast also has an impact on learning.[60] One study showed that eating foods high in fiber and low in sugar helped students sustain the cognitive effects of breakfast.[61]

Children also have an opportunity to participate in the National School Lunch Program, which is available at most schools. While school lunch often gets a "bad rap," it offers the most nutritious foods available at school. The *Family Nutrition and Physical Activity Survey* results reveal that 44 percent of white children, 35 percent of Hispanic children and 25 percent of African American children do not eat from the school lunch line on most days. Kids report not eating school lunch because they "do not like what is served or how it tastes" (50 percent white, 59 percent Hispanic and 63 percent African American) or because "their parents want them to bring lunch from home" (56 percent white, 45 percent Hispanic and 37 percent African American). Of those not eating the school lunch, most bring their lunch from home (88 percent white, 70 percent Hispanic and 60 percent African American).

One of the few areas in which parents are disconnected from what their kids are doing is that of alternative lunch sources. For kids who do not eat from the school lunch line each day, African American children more than white or Hispanic children buy food from vending machines (27 percent) or from stores or restaurants close to school (29 percent). And of those African American children who do not eat lunch from the school lunch line, more than a third—34 percent—do not eat lunch at all.

Dinner is a meal many parents and kids say is their healthiest because it is eaten at home. Despite the high numbers reporting regular meal times and eating at home with parents, a good percentage of kids report they do not eat dinner all of the time: 22 percent of white children, 38 percent of Hispanic children and 34 percent of African American children report not eating dinner every night.

Taste Matters

"Food has to look good and taste good," says Lucille Beseler, MS, RD, LD/N, CDE, president and founder of the Family Nutrition Center of South Florida. "If it doesn't look good and taste good, kids are not going to eat it."

In other words, kids eat for taste. But while taste can be a potential barrier to eating nutrient-rich foods, it can also be a draw if we help kids develop a taste for these healthier foods. To meet kids' taste expectations while also providing healthy foods, registered dietitians say we need to think about cultural preferences, work gradually to help kids change their taste buds and prepare healthier versions of the foods kids like.

Again and again, the *Family Nutrition and Physical Activity Survey* found that kids eat—or don't eat—based on taste. When asked why they ate, the majority of children selected hunger and taste over other reasons. Eating "all of the time" because "food tastes good" significantly increased, from 23 percent in 2003 to 31 percent in 2010. Likewise, a majority of kids who don't eat from the school lunch line said they do not do so because they don't like how the school meal tastes. And an overwhelming majority of kids (89 percent white, 90 percent Hispanic and 94 percent African American) reported that they'd eat healthier foods if those foods tasted better.

However, trying to decipher what kids mean by "taste" can be challenging.

One key factor in taste is cultural preference, says Nancy Copperman, MS, RD, CDN, director of Public Health Initiatives at North Shore Long Island Jewish Health System. Kids are used to certain flavors that are associated with particular cultural foods. As we prepare school meals, she asks, "are we really bringing in the cultural foods that these particular ethnicities enjoy as taste?"

Just as they are accustomed to certain cultural flavors, kids also become accustomed to certain tastes from processed foods. "As we help kids shift to healthier foods with lower sugar and salt content," says Gayle Coleman, MS, RD, nutrition educator, University of Wisconsin-Extension, Cooperative Extension, "we need to realize that taste for many foods is acquired. Healthier foods, like vegetables, may not meet kids' taste needs initially, but they can learn to like them." Thus, change needs to be gradual.

When asked why they ate, the majority of children selected hunger and taste over other reasons.

Judith Rodriguez, PhD, RD, FADA, LDN, President, American Dietetic Association, notes that taste has always been an important factor. "It may be because of an increased availability of sweet and saltier foods that choice for those foods is impacted," she says. "If a child has a greater access to foods that are high in sugar, fat and sodium and also has preference for it, he or she is likely to select it. Over time, if other foods do not have that sweet and salty taste, they will not taste as good as what is now preferred. It is an interesting research question: does the taste take on greater significance because there is more choice? Also, how does the exposure to a variety of flavors and tastes impact choices and preferences? The data seem to indicate that it does, so early education and modeling are important."

Finally, it's important to give kids great-tasting, healthier versions of their favorite foods, argues Elizabeth M. Ward, MS, RD, nutrition consultant, mother of three and author of several books about feeding children. For example, Ward says, "Pizza is the number one food on kids' plates, and that's a good thing because pizza supplies several nutrients, such as protein, calcium and magnesium. However, there are ways to reduce the calories, total fat and saturated fat in pizza that preserve the important nutrients while better promoting good health."

As we work with cultural food preferences and help kids get used to new tastes and create healthier versions of kids' favorite foods, we need to remember that change won't come overnight, Copperman says. "It's kind of retraining the taste buds."

Perspectives from the Field

Registered dietitians from around the country were interviewed about their reactions to the *Family Nutrition and Physical Activity Survey*. These leading professionals reflected on the survey and shared their observations of the current nutrition environment.

> People have general knowledge, but they need skills, techniques, tips they can use within their lifestyle. They need to know how to make changes that work with the way they live. The survey data on why children eat were striking relative to hunger and taste. Taste is always a primary factor, and it may seem more important because of greater access to tasty foods. The increase in hunger needs to be looked at because hunger is a physiological response, where taste or appetite is a sociological phenomenon because something looks, appealing.

> *Judith Rodriguez, PhD, RD, FADA, LDN, President, American Dietetic Association*

> We need strategies that are flexible enough to accommodate different types of families and culture.

> *Gaye Coleman, MS, RD, University of Wisconsin-Extension, Cooperative Extension*

There seems to be a need and a readiness. Both parents and children have a new level of awareness that there is a problem and a willingness or desire to make changes. This is the opportune time for registered dietitians to help families.

> *Nancy Copperman, MS, RD, CDN, Director of Public Health Initiatives, North Shore Long Island Jewish Health System*

A big piece of prevention is educating families and communities. All health professionals have to be saying the same thing when addressing healthy eating and healthy weights for children. It is imperative to find a way for registered dietitians to share their expertise while educating other professionals. This could be a vital role for dietitians—training other health professionals. Getting more dietitians into the community does require us to be innovative, creative educators. As part of my business, I have had great response to registered dietitians being part of sports events, health fairs and festivals. There are tremendous opportunities to reach parents where they are, even in health fairs in retail outlets.

> *Lucille Beseler, MS, RD, LD/N, CDE, President and Founder of the Family Nutrition Center of South Florida*

Staying positive about healthy eating means focusing on what kids should include in their diets on a daily basis, rather than what to avoid. Taking that approach typically displaces high-calorie foods that offer little in the way of nutrients that kids need to grow and develop to their fullest potential. The data say that soda is the number one contributor of sugar in children's diets, yet flavored milks, which are often the nutritional scapegoat, don't even make the list of the top five sources. Any type of milk provides vital nutrients, including calcium, potassium and vitamin D, three nutrients that experts say kids do not get enough of. We want kids to drink milk, and their preference for flavored milk should be taken into consideration at home and at school.

> *Elizabeth M. Ward, MS, RD, Nutrition Consultant and Author*

"The data say that soda is the number one contributor of sugar in children's diets, yet flavored milks, which are often the nutritional scapegoat, don't even make the list of the top five sources."

Elizabeth M. Ward, MS, RD, Nutrition Consultant and Author

> "Staying positive about healthy eating means focusing on what kids should include in their diets on a daily basis, rather than what to avoid."
>
> *Elizabeth M. Ward, MS, RD,*
> *Nutrition Consultant and Author*

We're looking at prevention and we're looking at what's going to make a difference 20 years from now, but we still have the now. Policy and environmental change efforts may be a bit longer term. We need short-term strategies that help parents or schools immediately too. Students are working with local grocery chains and chefs to collaborate in developing nutritious meals that match the weekly food sales; cooking demonstrations are given by the chef, and the student dietetic professionals walk people through the menu for that week.

Aida Miles, MMSc, RD, CSP, LD, CNSD, Director
of the Coordinated MPH Program, Division of
Epidemiology and Community Health, University
of Minnesota School of Public Health

Moving Forward: Opportunity Areas

The *Family Nutrition and Physical Activity Survey* finds several key "opportunity areas"—family habits and children's behaviors. Parents' increased connectedness with their children on wellness as well as parents' improved understanding and awareness of their children's behaviors signal a shift in "readiness" to change eating and physical activity habits. Additionally, the majority of children responded positively to approaches that would help them eat healthier.

Parents also responded positively toward seeing a registered dietitian to get help with making better food choices and preparing healthier meals for their children. These drivers to positive change should be at the forefront of efforts to educate, support and work with children and their parents to improve kids' healthy eating and activity habits.

Opportunity #1: Parent Power

The majority of children identified their parents as their number one role model, with mothers as the first choice and fathers as the second choice. If parents display healthful eating and activity habits themselves, children are likely to emulate those behaviors. Indeed, children say that it would help them eat healthier foods if their parents ate these foods at home, with significantly more Hispanic and African American children reporting that this would help them.

Parents have many opportunities to set a good example when it comes to healthy habits. According to the *Family Nutrition and Physical Activity Survey* results from 2010, parents spend time with their children in numerous ways and thus have many opportunities to have an impact on children's health behaviors, especially when they eat together. Despite the prevalent belief that children and parents do not eat at home any more, the 2010 survey shows that more than 80 percent of white, Hispanic and African American children and parents say they eat meals at home together at least three days a week. Families that eat at home daily comprise the largest segment of this group, with 72 percent of white and Hispanic children and 61 percent of African American children reporting eating at home with family at least once a day. Not only does eating together as a family lead to lower rates of overweight and obesity as well as higher quality, more nutrient-dense diets;[42] mealtimes are also an excellent time to demonstrate healthy eating choices. Even the away-from-home eating could be improved with education, especially the times, although infrequent, that parents and kids are eating out together.[40,43,45]

Kids name their parents as the number one role model. More than 70 percent of kids said that, if parents ate healthy at home, this would help them do the same.

Kids Who Say Their Number One Role Model Is ...	White	Hispanic	African American
Their Mother	18 percent	23 percent	30 percent
Their Father	17 percent	18 percent	16 percent

Nearly all parents base purchases on nutrition, fat and calorie content. Parents report that health attributes are important determinants to foods brought home.

The *Family Nutrition and Physical Activity Survey* finds that, in the majority of households, mothers have primary responsibility for meals. Moreover, in their role as primary food preparer, mothers buy food for the family's meals and snacks. As the number one role model and primary meal provider, mothers have a great responsibility to model

Percent of Parents Finding Health Attributes as "Very Important" When Buying Food

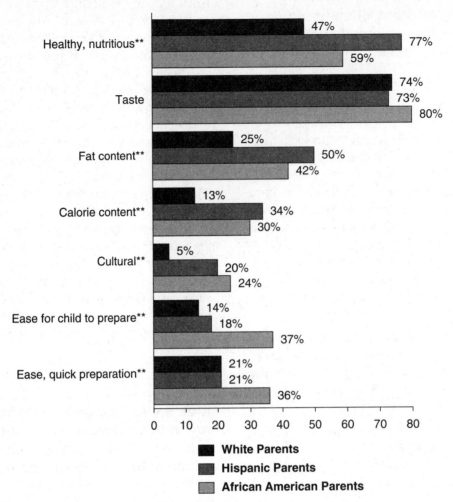

** Statistically significant differences by race, p < 0.001

Source: ADAF Family Nutrition and Physical Activity Survey, *2010*

healthy behaviors. Thus, working with mothers through nutrition and health education efforts should pay dividends in teaching healthy dietary habits to young people.

Parents play an especially important role as they make decisions about which foods to purchase—both for the nutrient quality of food that is available in the home and for the example they set as they select foods. Although not statistically different than others, more African American parents selected taste as a very important reason for buying foods. Parents have other "very important" reasons for purchasing foods, reasons that differ significantly by race (see chart on this page). For example, a significantly higher percentage of African American parents reported ease of preparation for their child and ease in general more than for white or Hispanic. Even more important to parents, however, are the health attributes of the foods they purchase, with significantly more Hispanic parents ranking the nutritious aspects of a food as a "very important" determinant. Similarly, fat and calorie

content is significantly less important to white parents than to Hispanic or African American parents—yet when combining responses for "somewhat important" and "very important," nearly all parents use nutrition, fat and calorie content to determine which foods are purchased.

Overall, parents have a powerful opportunity to model healthy behaviors for their children. Whether they're shopping for nutritious groceries or playing with their kids outside, parents set the tone for their families. Thus, parent education can be a key factor in improving children's healthy eating and activity habits.

Opportunity #2: The Rhythm of Family Routines

As noted throughout this report, children exhibit a range of healthy behaviors when their families observe regular routines.[46,47] When kids eat meals at home, when they eat with their parents regularly, when they spend time with their parents and when they go to bed at about

Hispanic Families: Positive Signs

Maria C. Alamo, MPH, RD, is president and founder of Salud Consulting Inc. She works with clients to develop culturally relevant communications, translate nutrition and health information into Spanish and develop recipes for nutritious meals for Hispanic families. Alamo explains that the primary characteristics of Hispanic meals are flavor, color and presentation of the foods. Hispanic cooks, she says, "are used to lengthier recipes with many ingredients including a variety of spices and longer cooking times. They are not afraid of a long recipe. The freshness of the ingredient is very important, so going to the grocery store several times a week is not unusual."

The Hispanic parents' responses to survey questions about talking to a registered dietitian are good to see, says Alamo, although not that much of a surprise. "The Hispanic culture has a lot of respect for medical professionals," she says, "so it is easy to see why they want to meet with a registered dietitian."

Alamo comments that the overall responses by Hispanic children and parents are encouraging. She points to several very positive behaviors revealed in the survey: the higher frequency of meals eaten at home, the pattern of eating at regular meal times and the practice of eating as a family. Hispanics "are health conscious and want to learn how to make the most nutritious meals for their family," Alamo observes. "The gaps in nutrition and foods that are missing from kids' diets can be addressed with the Hispanic community because there is an openness and readiness."

Alamo concludes that the survey findings indicate unmet needs that can specifically be addressed by registered dietitians due to their background in food and nutrition.

---

the same time each night, they are more likely to have healthier behaviors, including eating behaviors.[38,42,47]

Sharing meals as a family improves mental health and leads to better eating patterns; this important bonding time can be a great opportunity to teach good nutrition and eating behaviors.[40,42,43,44] Quality time spent together as a family—whether cooking a meal or playing outside—can enhance children's well-being; new research shows it may be protective against higher than normal weight gain.[45,53,55] And family routines—such as regular bedtimes—can lead to stronger academic achievement and higher self-esteem.[46,47,52]

The *Family Nutrition and Physical Activity Survey* results indicate there are differences in the percentage of families that practice these behaviors by race and income. Regular schedules may be more difficult for lower- and middle-income parents; some may have several jobs, varying work schedules and longer transportation times to and from work.[51,52] Families could benefit from learning cooking techniques and skills for parents and older children.[51,55] Overall, the trend for all races is quite promising, though significantly fewer Hispanic and African American families have the same regularity of routines as white families. These regular rhythms can provide a strong foundation as we seek to improve children's healthy eating and activity habits.

Opportunity #3: Kids' Desire to Move More

We know that the majority of children don't get the recommended 60 minutes of physical activity each day—but kids tell us they would move more if they had more opportunities to do so.[19]

In the *Family Nutrition and Physical Activity Survey* children report that they would be more physically active if there were fun activities after school. Other motivations they mention for being more physically active are: if their friends wanted to do something physically active, if there were activity breaks during class, if there were a safe place to play in their neighborhood, if there were a way to get home after staying late after school and if there were fun activities before school.

Significantly more minority children than white children express an interest in opportunities to be physically active before, during and after school. Other motivators include transportation home from afterschool activities and safe places to play; these motivators are significantly less important to whites than to Hispanic and African American children. These findings show that children want to be more physically active, and they need encouragement and support to do so.

Opportunity #4: Quality Nutrition, Wherever Kids Eat

The *Family Nutrition and Physical Activity Survey* results from 2010 indicate a decrease in kids purchasing foods at restaurants, vending and other commercial locations from 2003 survey results. However, a large majority of kids are purchasing foods away from home at least some of the time each week. Children say that they would eat healthier foods at school and other locations if the foods tasted better. Additionally, results show it would help kids eat healthier if healthy food and drinks cost less money, if their parents ate healthy foods at home and if there were less "junk food" in stores on the way to and from school.

Percent of Children Who Would Be More Active If ...

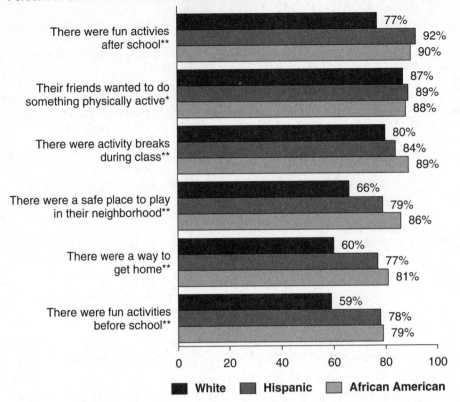

*Statistically significant differences by race, p < 0.05

**Statistically significant differences by race, p < 0.001

Source: ADAF Family Nutrition and Physical Activity Survey, *2010*

Percent of Children Who Would Eat Healthier If ...

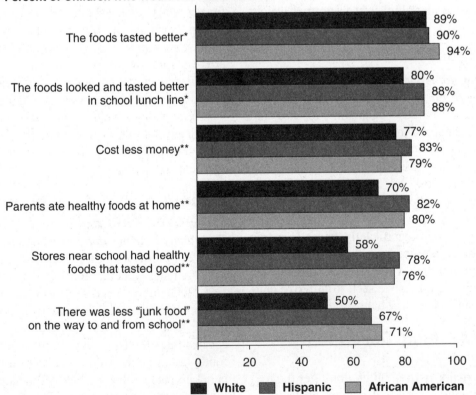

*Statistically significant differences by race, p < 0.05

** Statistically significant differences by race, p < 0.001

Source: ADAF Family Nutrition and Physical Activity Survey, *2010*

Percent of Parents Wanting to Meet with a Registered Dietitian to Discuss . . .

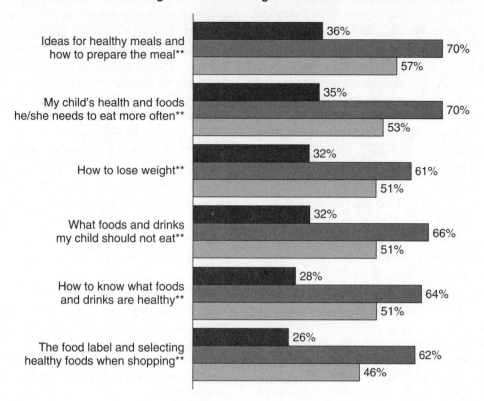

Percent of Children Wanting to Meet with a Registered Dietitian to Discuss . . .

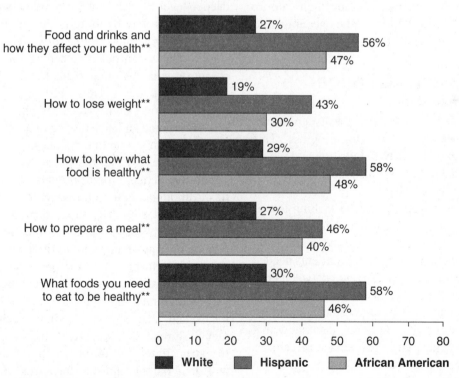

** Statistically significant differences by race, p < 0.001

Source: ADAF Family Nutrition and Physical Activity Survey, *2010*

Because kids do eat at school and do purchase foods away from home, we need to ensure that these foods are both healthy and kid-appealing.[45,57] Kids want foods that taste good—and public/private partnerships can take steps to enhance the flavor of the foods kids need to consume more of. Working together, community restaurants, registered dietitians and chefs can help schools improve the flavor and presentation of the foods they offer through their meal programs. Local funding could be made available so that schools could purchase fresh ingredients, use more scratch cooking and reduce dependence on processed foods. Local stores and restaurants—especially those near schools—can be encouraged to carry healthier foods that kids will eat.

Along with where the food is prepared, when kids eat is also an important consideration. Survey findings indicate that kids snack throughout the day. Current snacking patterns are problematic because of the food choices; however, snacking can be an opportunity to increase kids' consumption of the foods they need to eat more of—the nutrient-dense options.

If we focus on providing access to the nutrient-dense foods kids need to eat, making them look and taste great, these foods may displace high-sugar, high-calorie, low-nutrient foods.[33] This "displacement theory" may work in reverse too, unfortunately, as high-calorie, low-nutrient foods may displace nutrient-dense foods. In short, eating snacks does not have to mean eating high-calorie, low-nutrient foods.[33] Instead, kids can be encouraged to snack on foods that are good for them.

Poised for Healthy Change

It has been nearly a decade since the release of the Surgeon General's pivotal report on the obesity epidemic. Now is the time to ask: Are we making progress? This question must look beyond weight to nutrition and physical activity patterns in children. We also must ask: Are we addressing this comprehensively?

On one level, it would seem that we're making few, if any, strides. Looking at the current landscape, epidemic numbers of kids are overweight or obese, and the majority of kids' diets are deficient in one or more nutrients needed for growth and development.[4,6,21] The gap between children's recommended and actual intake of key nutrients remains alarmingly wide, regardless of weight status. Along with low intake of vital nutrients, data show that kids continue to consume a large percentage of calories from foods with sugar and saturated fat.[9,10]

The gap between children's recommended and actual intake of key nutrients remains alarmingly wide, regardless of weight status.

Additionally, the *Family Nutrition and Physical Activity Survey* shows kids' eating behaviors are inconsistent. Kids are grazing on foods throughout the day; frequent snacking throughout the day and evening is the norm, and there are less consistent patterns for meals for some kids, especially when race and income are factors. Recent food consumption data from NHANES found that increased snacking leads to lower quality of children's diet based on snack food choices high in calories and low in nutrients.[11,12] Snacking still occurs during school, with food purchased from school snack bars and vending machines. There are more kids who could benefit from school meal programs, so there are opportunities to increase participation. To do this, more attention on the taste and kid-appealing qualities of the foods is necessary, especially considering cultural differences in flavor and presentation of foods.

At the same time that kids' eating behaviors are less than optimal, activity levels are not adequate either.[19] In fact, the vast majority of youth are not achieving the national recommendation of 60 minutes of physical activity daily. This was the finding from the *Family Nutrition and Physical Activity Survey* and from the YRBSS 2009 results.[19]

Despite these real trouble spots, the *Family Nutrition and Physical Activity Survey* also reveals that on a deeper level the news about children's eating and activity behaviors may be more promising than first appears. Representing a crucial move forward, the survey findings suggest that a significant percentage of children and their parents are making or are ready to make changes in eating and activity patterns. How did we get to this new readiness for change, and how can we make the most out of this occurrence and not miss an opportunity?

The nation's attention to obesity and its causes has steadily increased over the last ten years, resulting in new policies, practices, food products and healthcare priorities. Although slight with respect to the magnitude of the problem, it seems that the national attention and subsequent changes have translated into more children and parents making changes in nutrition and physical activity on multiple levels. For example, compared to the 2003 report, children are engaging in healthier behaviors, such as maintaining more regular schedules and purchasing meals and snacks from vending machines and convenience stores less frequently. Children also say they want to eat healthier and be physically active. Both children and their parents indicate their trust in registered dietitians as credible sources as well as their desire to see them for guidance on what to eat and drink for health and wellness. All of this suggests that parents and children are ready to be supported as they work toward healthier behaviors.

Kids Eat Right

Kids Eat Right is the American Dietetic Association and Foundation platform of childhood obesity prevention initiatives. As part of **Kids Eat Right,** registered dietitians are mobilizing to support First Lady Michelle Obama's Let's Move! campaign and are working to ensure that childhood obesity prevention efforts are taking a quality nutrition approach.

Kids Eat Right recognizes that registered dietitians can provide evidence-based nutrition guidance supporting quality nutrition and healthy weights. Registered dietitians are uniquely qualified—through years of education and training—to advocate, educate and demonstrate the importance of meeting the total nutrient needs of all youth.

The public outreach effort brings more registered dietitians into community and school settings with tools and resources for shaping positive, lifelong habits of good nutrition and physical activity in youth. As part of this effort, registered dietitians are providing families with the tips they need to "Shop Cook Eat" to support quality nutrition and healthy weights in children.

The public education component shines a light on the deficiencies in nutrients that have become a common occurrence in children's diets along with unhealthy weights. Research shows that, while childhood obesity is at epidemic proportions, even higher numbers of youth are not eating the recommended number of servings from all food groups and therefore are missing nutrients vital to normal growth and development. ADA members are fighting these trends by working with families, parents, children, schools, community settings and media.

Bottom line, the 2010 survey indicates new areas for intervention and support from registered dietitians. It also points to a shift in children's and parents' readiness for change that must be taken advantage of by efforts currently underway.

We must focus renewed attention on the total diet, ensuring that nutrient requirements are met as part of obesity prevention and health promotion efforts. The chronic poor eating habits have become intertwined with the problems of undernourishment and overweight. Kids' diets need to be shaped around eating the nutrient-dense food first. This approach can help to ensure kids consume the more than 50 nutrients necessary for proper growth, development and good health while simultaneously addressing obesity and undernourishment.[17,62] We need to encourage them not only to avoid unhealthy foods but also to eat plenty of nutrient-rich foods: fruits, vegetables, whole grains and low-fat and fat-free dairy foods, meat and beans.

As we work together to educate parents, support schools, reach out to children and take a "total diet" approach, we must call upon the expertise of registered dietitians, who are uniquely qualified to apply the science of food and nutrition to increase health and to prevent and treat disease.

The *Family Nutrition and Physical Activity Survey* makes clear that children and their parents are poised for healthy change. It's time to build on this readiness for change, to seize this positive momentum. Together, we can tackle the twin problems of obesity and undernourishment—and help *Kids Eat Right.*

Special thanks to the following:

VANGUARD NETWORK
Kathryn A. Brown, EdD, RD, LD
Constance Brown-Riggs, MSEd, RD, CDE, CDN
Ruth Ann Carpenter, MS, RD
Gayle Coleman, MS, RD, CD
Jessica Donze-Black, RD, MPH
Robin Hamre, RD, MPH, LD
Kim Stitzel, MS, RD
Dorcas Ukpe, MS, RD, LD
Elizabeth M. Ward, MS, RD

RD COMMUNICATOR NETWORK
Maria C. Alamo, MPH, RD, LD
Stacey A. Antine, MS, RD
Susan T. Borra, RD
David Grotto, RD, LDN
Janet Helm, MS, RD
Cathy Kapica, PhD, RD, LD, CFCS, FACN
Shelley Maniscalco, MPH, RD
Susan D. Moores, MS, RD
Mary Mullen, MS, RD, LDN
Carolyn O'Neil, MS, RD
Jodie Shield, M.Ed, RD, LD
Liz Weiss, MS, RD

CONTRIBUTORS
Lucille Beseler, MS, RD, LD/N, CDE
Leslie Bonci, MPH, RD, CSSD, LDN
Nancy Copperman, MS, RD, CDN
Sheri Doucette, RD, LDN
Tab Forgac, MS, RD
Debra French, RD, CD
Niki Gernhofer, MS, RD
Lorry Luscri, MPH, RD, LDN
Aida Miles, MMSc, RD, CSP LD, CNSD
Theresa Nicklas, DrPH
Jean Ragalie, RD
Judith Rodriguez, PhD, RD, FADA, LDN
Bonnie Spear, PhD, RD

DIETETIC PRACTICE GROUPS
Food and Culinary Professionals
Sanna Delmonico, MS, RD
Amy Myrdal Miller, MS, RD

Hunger and Environmental Nutrition
Christopher Wharton, PhD, RD

References

1. US Department of Health and Human Services, Public Health Service, Office of the Surgeon General. The Surgeon General's call to action to prevent and decrease overweight and obesity. www.surgeongeneral.gov/topics/obesity/. Published 2001. Accessed August 31, 2010.

2. Koplan JP, Liverman CT, Kraak VI, eds. *Preventing Childhood Obesity:* Health in the Balance. Washington, DC: The National Academies Press; 2005.

3. White House Task Force on Childhood Obesity Report to President. Solving the problem of childhood obesity within a generation, www.letsmove.gov/obesitytaskforce.php. Published May 2010. Accessed September 15, 2010.

4. American Dietetic Association. Position of the American Dietetic Association: Nutrition guidance for healthy children ages 2–11. J Am Diet Assoc. 2008;108:1038–1047.

5. American Dietetic Association. Position of the American Dietetic Association: Child and adolescent nutrition assistance programs. J Am Diet Assoc. 2010;110:791–799.

6. US Department of Agriculture. What we eat in America, NHANES 2007–2008: Nutrient intakes from food: Mean amounts consumed per individual, by gender and age. Agricultural Research Service Web site, www.ars.usda.gov/ba/bhnrc/fsrg. Published 2010. Accessed October 15, 2010.

7. US Department of Agriculture. Dietary Guidelines for Americans, 1980 to 2000. Center for Nutrition Policy and Promotion Web site. www.cnpp.usda.gov/DGAsPreviousGuidelines.htm. Published May 30, 2000. Accessed October 1, 2010.

8. Report of the Dietary Guidelines Advisory Committee on the Dietary Guidelines for Americans, 1990, Letter to the Secretary of Agriculture and the Secretary of Health and Human Services. Center for Nutrition Policy and Promotion Web site. www.cnpp.usda.gov/DGAs1990Guidelines.htm. Published May 14, 1990. Accessed August 25, 2010.

9. Williams C. Report of the Dietary Guidelines A dvisory Committee on the Dietary Guidelines for Americans, 2010: Resource 1: Children's dietary intakes. US Department of Agriculture, Center for Nutrition Policy and Promotion Web site. www.dietaryguidelines.gov. Accessed October 20, 2010.

10. Reedy J, Krebs-Smith SM. Dietary sources of energy, solid fats, and added sugars among children and adolescents in the United States. J Am Diet Assoc. 2010;110(10):1477–1484.

11. US Department of Agriculture. What we eat in America, NHANES 2007–2008: Snacks: Distribution of snack occasions, by gender and age. Agricultural Research Service Web site. www.ars.usda.gov/ba/bhnrc/fsrg. Published 2010. Accessed October 15, 2010.

12. US Department of Agriculture. Beltsville Human Nutrition Research Center. Food Surveys Research

Group Dietary Data Brief. Snacking patterns of US adolescents: What we eat in America, NHANES 2005–2006. agricultural Research Service Web site. http://ars .usda.gov/Services/docs.htm?docid-19476. Published 2010. Accessed October 18,2010.

13. Ogden CL, Carroll MD, Curtin LR, Lamb MM, Flegal KM. Prevalence of high body mass index in US children and adolescents, 2007–2008. *JAMA*. 2010;303:242–249.

14. Ogden CL, Carroll MD, Flegal KM. High body mass index for age among US children and adolescents, 2003–2006. *JAMA*. 2008;299(20):2401–2405.

15. US Departments of Agriculture and Health and Human Services. Nutrition and your health: *Dietary Guidelines for Americans, 1980.* Center for Nutrition Policy and Promotion Web site. www.cnpp.usda.gov/ DGAs1980Guidelines.htm. Accessed September 1, 2010.

16. Report of the Dietary Guidelines Advisory Committee on the *Dietary Guidelines for Americans, 1990,* to the Secretary of Agriculture and the Secretary of Health and Human Services. Center for Nutrition Policy and Promotion Web site. www.cnpp.usda.gov/ DGAs1990Guidelines.htm. Published May 14, 1990. Accessed August 25, 2010.

17. Report of the Dietary Guidelines Advisory Committee on the *Dietary Guidelines for Americans, 2010.* Part D. Section 2: Nutrient Adequacy. Center for Nutrition Policy and Promotion Web site. www.cnpp.usda.gov/ DGAs2010-DGACReport.htm. Published June 15, 2010. Accessed September 2, 2010.

18. US Department of Agriculture. What we eat in America, NHANES 2007–2008: Nutrient intakes from food: Mean amounts consumed per individual, by family income (in dollars) and age. Agricultural Research Service Web site. http://www.ars.usda.gov/ba/bhnrc/fsrg. Published 2010. Accessed October 10, 2010.

19. Eaton D, Kann L, Kinchen S, Shanklin S, Ross J, Hawkins J, Harris W, Lowry R, McMahnus T, Chyen D, Lim C, Whittle L, Brener N, Wechsler H. Youth risk behavior surveillance - United States, 2009. *MMWR* 2010;59(SS-5):1–142.

20. MEE Productions, Juzang I, Moag-Stahlberg A, Ellis K. Multi-cultural audience research. Copyright National Dairy Council, 2009. Published MEE Productions, May 2009. Philadelphia, PA.

21. Report of the Dietary Guidelines Advisory Committee on the Dietary Guidelines for Americans, 2010. Part D. Section 2: Nutrient adequacy. Center for Nutrition Policy and Promotion Web site. www.cnpp.usda.gov/DGAs2010-DGACReport.htm. Accessed August 22, 2010.

22. US Department of Agriculture. What we eat in America, NHANES 2007–2008: Nutrient intakes from food: Mean amounts consumed per individual, by family income (in dollars) and age. Agricultural Research Service Web site. www.ars.usda.gov/ba/bhnrc/fsrg. Published 2010. Accessed October 10, 2010.

23. Report of the Dietary Guidelines Advisory Committee on the *Dietary Guidelines for Americans, 2005,* Part

D: Science base. US Department of Health and Human Services Web site. www.health.gov/dietaryguidelines/ dga2005/report/default.htm. Accessed August 25, 2010.

24. Report of the Dietary Guidelines Advisory Committee on the *Dietary Guidelines for Americans, 2000.* Center for Nutrition Policy and Promotion Web site. www.cnpp. usda.gov/DGAs2000Guidelines.htm. Accessed August 25, 2010.

25. Taras H. Nutrition and student performance at school. *J School Health.* 2005;75(6):199–213.

26. Taras H, Potts-Datema W. Obesity and student performance at school. *J School Health.* 2005;75(8):291–295.

27. Bryan J, Osendarp S, Hughes D, Calvaresi E, Baghurst K, van Klinken JW. Nutrients for cognitive development in schoolaged children. *Nutrition Reviews.* 2004;62(8):295–306.

28. Basch CE. Healthier students are better learners: A missing link in school reform to close achievement gap. *Equity Matters: Research Review* 2010 Mar;6A. www.equitycampaign.org/i/a/document/12557 _ EquityMattersVol6_Web03082010.pdf. Accessed September 30, 2010.

29. Black M. The evidence linking zinc deficiency with children's cognitive and motor functioning. *Journal of Nutrition.* 2003;133(5)(Supp.1):1473S-6S.

30. Action for Healthy Kids. The learning connection: The value of improving nutrition and physical activity in our schools. Action for Healthy Kids Web site. www. actionforhealthykids.org/resources/learningconnection. Published 2004. Accessed June 2, 2010.

31. Fryar C, Ogden C. Prevalence of underweight among children and adolescents: United States, 2007–2008. *NCHS Health EStat* 2010 Oct. National Center for Health Statistics Web site. www.cdc.gov/nchs/data/hestat/ underweight_child_07_08/underweight_child_07_08. htm. Accessed October 25, 2010.

32. Sources of calories from added sugars among the US population, 2005-06: Mean intakes and percentage contribution of foods among children and adolescents. Applied Research Program. National Cancer Institute. Risk Factor Monitoring and Methods Branch Applied Research Program Web site. http://riskfactor.cancer.gov/ diet/foodsources/added_sugars/. Accessed August 22, 2010.

33. Epstein LH, Paluch RA, Beecher MD, Roemmich JN. Increasing healthy eating vs. reducing high energy-dense foods to treat pediatric obesity. *Obesity.* 2008;16:318–326.

34. Centers for Disease Control and Prevention. Student health and academic achievement: The association between school-based physical activity, including physical education, and academic performance. National Center for Chronic Disease Prevention and Health Promotion Web site. www.cdc.gov/HealthyYouth/health_ and_academics/index.htm. Published 2010. Accessed August 22, 2010.

35. McCormack Brown K, Alfonso ML, Bryant CA. *Obesity Prevention Coordinators' Social Marketing Guidebook.* Tampa, FL: Florida Prevention Research Center at the University of South Florida; 2004.

36. Huang TT, Drewnowski A, Kumanyika SK, Glass TA. A systems-oriented multilevel framework for addressing obesity in the 21st century. *Prev Chronic Dis.* 2009;6(3). www.cdc.gov/pcd/issues/2009/jul/09_0013.htm. Accessed May 10, 2010.

37. Glanz K, Rimer BK. *Theory at a Glance: A Guide for Health Promotion Practice.* 2nd ed. National Institutes of Health, U.S. Department of Health and Human Services. National Cancer Institute Web site. www.cancer.gov/PDF/481f5d53-63df-41bc-bfaf-5aa48ee1da4d/TAAG3.pdf. Published 2005. Accessed August 12, 2010.

38. Chen AY, Escarce JJ. Family structure and childhood obesity, Early Childhood Longitudinal Study–Kindergarten Cohort. Prev Chronic Dis. 2010;7(3). www.cdc.gov/pcd/issues/2010/may/09_0156.htm. Accessed July 15, 2010.

39. Rhee K. Childhood overweight and the relationship between parent behaviors, parenting style, and family functioning. *The ANNALS of the American Academy of Political and Social Science.* 2008;615:11.

40. Patrick H, Nicklas TA. A review of family and social determinants of children's eating patterns and diet quality. *Journal of the American College of Nutrition.* 2005;24(2):83–92.

41. Parenting and Family Life: A National Profile. Child and Adolescent Health Measurement Initiative, 2007. National Survey of Children's Health, Data Resource Center for Child and Adolescent Health. Published October 2009.

42. Rollins BY, Belue RZ, Francis LA. The beneficial effect of family meals on obesity differs by race, sex, and household education: The National Survey of Children's Health, 2003–2004. *J Am Diet Assoc.* 2010;110:1335–1339.

43. Boutelle KN, Birkeland RW, Hannan PJ, Story M, Neumark-Sztainer D. Associations between maternal concern for healthful eating and maternal eating behaviors, home food availability, and adolescent eating behaviors. *J Nutr Educ Behav.* 2007;39:248–256.

44. Cason KL. Family mealtimes: More than just eating together. *J Am Diet Assoc.* 2006;106(4):532–533.

45. Mancino, L, Todd JE, Guthrie J, Lin B-H. How food away from home affects children's diet quality. US Department of Agriculture, Economic Research Service Web site. www.ers.usda.gov/publications/err104/. Published October 2010. Accessed October 25, 2010.

46. Dickstein S. Family routines and rituals–the importance of family functioning. *Journal of Family Psychology.* 2002;16(4): 441–444.

47. Denham SA. Relationships between family rituals, family routines, and health. *Journal of Family Nursing.* 2003;9(3):305–330.

48. Befort C, Kaur H, Nollen N, Sullivan DK, Nazir N, Choi WS, Hornberger L, Ahluwalia JS. Fruit, vegetable, and fat intake among non-Hispanic black and non-Hispanic white adolescents: Associations with home availability and food consumption settings. *J Am Diet Assoc.* 2006;106:367–373.

49. Boutelle KN, Lytle LA, Murray DM, Birnbaum AS, Story M. Perceptions of the family mealtime environment and adolescent mealtime behavior: Do adults and adolescents agree? *Journal of Nutrition Education.* 2001;33:128–133.

50. Feldman S, Eisenberg ME, Neumark-Sztainer D, Story M. Associations between watching TV during family meals and dietary intake among adolescents. *J Nutr Educ Behav.* 2007;39:257–263.

51. Guthrie J, McClelland K. Working parents outsource children's meals. *Amber Waves.* 2009;7(1):5. www.ers.usda.gov/AmberWaves. Accessed August 15, 2010.

52. Heymann SJ, Earle A. The impact of parental working conditions on school-age children: The case of evening work. *Community, Work & Family.* 2001;4(3):305325.

53. US Department of Agriculture. Economic Research Service. Food and Nutrition Assistance Research Program. Parental time, role strain, and children's fat intake and obesity-related outcomes. Contractor and Cooperator Report No. 19. June 2006.

54. Sebastian RS, Enns CW, Goldman JD. US adolescents and MyPyramid: Association between fast-food consumption and lower likelihood of meeting recommendations. *J Am Diet Assoc.* 2009;109(2):226–235.

55. Manchino L, Newman C. Who has time to cook? How family resources influence food preparation. US Department of Agriculture, Economic Research Service Web site. www.ers.usda.gov/Publications/ERR40/. Published May 2007. Accessed October 1, 2010.

56. US Department of Agriculture. What we eat in America, NHANES 2007–2008: Away from home: Percentages of selected nutrients contributed by foods eaten away from home, by family income (in dollars) and age. Agricultural Research Service Web site, www.ars.usda.gov/ba/bhnrc/fsrg. Accessed October 15, 2010.

57. Hair E, Ling T, Wandner L. School food unwrapped: What's available and what our kids actually are eating. *Child Trends Research Brief.* 2008(Nov). www.childtrends.org/Files//Child_Trends-2008_11_17_RB_SchoolFoodPolicy.pdf. Accessed August 29, 2010.

58. Rampersaud GC, Pereira MA, Girard BL, Adams J, Metzl JD. Breakfast habits, nutritional status, body weight, and academic performance in children and adolescents. *J Am Diet Assoc.* 2005;105(5):743–760.

59. Murphy JM, Pagano M, Nachmani J, Sperling P, Kane S, Kleinman R. The relationship of school breakfast to psychosocial and academic functioning: Cross-sectional

and longitudinal observations in an inner-city sample. *Archives of Pediatric and Adolescent Medicine.* 1998;152:89–907.

60. Wesnes KA, Pincock C, Richardson D, Helm G, Hails S. Breakfast reduces declines in attention and memory over the morning in schoolchildren. *Appetite.* 2003;41(3):329–331.

61. Affenito SG, Thompson DR, Barton BA, Franko DL, Daniels SR, Obarzanek E, Schreiber GB, Striegel-Moore RH. Breakfast consumption by African-American and white adolescent girls correlates positively with calcium and fiber intake and negatively with body mass index. *J Am Diet Assoc.* 2005;105:938–945.

62. American Dietetic Association. Position of the American Dietetic Association: Total diet approach to communicating food and nutrition information. *J Am Diet Assoc.* 2007;107:1224–1232.

Critical Thinking

1. What is meant by "quality calories"?

2. Based on data from NHANES 1977–1978 and 200–2002, describe the major changes in dietary intake of children between these two time periods.

3. Identify the foods that provide the most calories from saturated fat in children's diet. What is the percentage of calories from solid fat for each of these foods?

4. Identify the nutrients that are inadequate in the typical child's diet.

Acknowledgments—This report outlines the premise behind *Kids Eat Right,* the first joint effort of the American Dietetic Association and American Dietetic Association Foundation. The *Kids Eat Right* initiative is the result of a year-long process that included discussions with ADA volunteer leadership, diverse groups of members and ADA-ADAF staff, survey of members' interests, data collection from published research and gleaning of members' food and nutrition expertise. *Kids Eat Right*—whose public education campaign elements include the 2003 and 2010 ADAF *Family Nutrition and Physical Activity Survey* and subsequent report on "The State of Family Nutrition and Physical Activity: Are We Making Progress?"—would not have been possible without the many leading registered dietitians who have generously contributed their knowledge and time to the effort.

It is with much gratitude that I thank all who have contributed to the development of Kids Eat Right. *Many ADA members were especially helpful in creating the foundational elements of* Kids Eat Right *and this touchstone report.*

With regard and esteem, Alicia Moag-Stahlberg, MS, RD, LD, Consultant, Campaign Director, Kids Eat Right

---

Underage, Overweight

The federal government needs to halt the marketing of unhealthy foods to kids.

SCIENTIFIC AMERICAN

The statistic is hard to swallow: in the U.S., nearly one in three children under the age of 18 is overweight or obese, making being over-weight the most common childhood medical condition. These youngsters are likely to become heavy adults, putting them at increased risk of developing cardiovascular disease, type 2 diabetes and other chronic ailments. In February First Lady Michelle Obama announced a campaign to fight childhood obesity. Helping parents and schools to instill healthier habits in kids is an important strategy in this battle. But the government must take further steps to solve the problem.

In an ideal world, adults would teach children how to eat healthily and would lead by example. But in reality, two thirds of U.S. adults are themselves overweight or obese. Moreover, the food and beverage industry markets sugar- and fat-laden goods to kids directly—through commercials on television, product placement in movies and video games, and other media. Its considerable efforts—nearly $1.7 billion worth in 2007—have met with sickening success: a recent study conducted by researchers at the University of California, Los Angeles, found that children who see more television ads tend to become fatter. You might expect that watching TV, being a sedentary activity is responsible for obesity but the study found that obesity is correlated not with television per se but with advertising. The more commercial programming children watched, the fatter they got compared with those who watched a comparable amount of public television or DVDs. The majority of products marketed during children's programming are foods.

As nutritionist Marion Nestle of New York University has written, society needs to "create a food environment that makes it easier for parents and everyone else to make better food choices." Protecting children from junk-food marketing would help create conditions conducive to achieving a healthy weight.

Unfortunately like the tobacco industry before it, the food industry cannot be trusted to self-regulate in this regard. In a study published in the March *Pediatrics,* investigators looked at the prevalence of food and beverage brands in movies released between 1996 and 2005. They noted, for instance, that although

Coca-Cola and PepsiCo have pledged to not advertise during children's television programming, their products routinely appear in movies aimed at kids.

Likewise, in the March *Public Health Nutrition,* researchers reported a 78 percent increase from 2006 to 2008 in the use of cartoon characters, toys and other child-oriented cross promotions on food packaging—much of it for nutritionally bereft foods. A whopping 55 percent of these cross promotions came from food manufacturers that have opted into the Children's Food and Beverage Advertising Initiative, sponsored by the Council of Better Business Bureaus, which promises to limit advertising to kids but allows participants to decide for themselves whether to restrict in-store marketing. Such examples of ineffectual commitments on the part of the food industry abound.

In December a group of U.S. agencies—the Federal Trade Commission, the Centers for Disease Control and Prevention the Food and Drug Administration, and the Department of Agriculture—proposed standards for foods and beverages that are marketed to children between the ages of two and 17. The agencies sensibly recommended that such foods must provide a meaningful contribution to a healthy diet by meeting specified requirements; that the amounts of saturated fat, trans fat, sugar and salt in these foods must not exceed limits set by the group; and that certain clearly healthy foods-such as those that are 100 percent fruits, vegetables or whole grains—may be marketed to kids without meeting the other two standards.

The interagency working group is due to submit a report containing its final recommendations to Congress by July 15. The standards are worthy but have one problem: as they stand, they would be voluntary. They should be mandatory, not optional, and the FDA should implement and enforce them.

The estimated cost of treating obesity-related ailments in adults was $147 billion for 2009. With the health care system already faltering, allowing companies to decide for themselves whether to peddle junk food to kids is a fox-and-henhouse policy this country simply cannot afford any longer.

Critical Thinking

1. Which nutrients are being targeted by the Federal Trade Commission, the Centers for Disease Control, and Food and Drug Administration as being unhealthy for children and, thus, should not be marketed to kids between the ages of 2 to 17?

2. From 2006 to 2008, what percentage increase was observed in the use of cartoon characters, toys, and kid-oriented promotion on food packaging?

3. How have Coca-Cola and PepsiCo addressed the popular opinion to decrease marketing of unhealthy products to kids?

The Impact of Teachers and Families on Young Children's Eating Behaviors

Erin K. Eliassen

Young children depend on their families and teachers to support their well-being and promote positive development, including eating behaviors. Children's food preferences and willingness to try new foods are influenced by the people around them (Bellows & Anderson 2006).

The eating behaviors children practice early in life affect their health and nutrition—significant factors in childhood overweight and obesity (Clark et al., 2007)—and may continue to shape food attitudes and eating patterns through adulthood (Birch 1999; Campbell & Crawford 2001; Westenhoefer 2002). Eating environments—mealtime and snack—that make food fun, offer new foods and a variety, and encourage children to taste and choose the foods they want let children develop food attitudes and dietary practices that ultimately support good health (Campbell & Crawford 2001).

Developing Eating Behaviors

The development of eating behaviors is a dynamic process that begins in infancy and continues throughout life. In this article, *eating behaviors* refers to food preferences, patterns of food acceptance and rejection, and the types and amounts of food a person eats. Genetics and the contexts in which foods are presented are two key factors that underpin the development of eating behaviors. Although parents provide a child's biological predisposition, which may affect factors like taste perception, they are not the only adults influencing the development of a child's eating behaviors. Every family member and caregiver interacting with a child at meals or snacks has the potential to do so.

In center- and home-based child care settings, teachers and family child care providers influence children's eating behaviors by the foods they offer, the behaviors they model, and their social interactions with children at snack and mealtimes (Savage, Fisher, & Birch 2007). Here are a few examples of how these factors influence eating behaviors.

Repeated exposure to a new food reduces a child's fear of the food and helps increase acceptance. Observing families and teachers eating and enjoying a variety of foods makes these foods more appealing to children. In contrast, children who are pressured to eat specific foods learn to dislike them. Restricted access to some foods, such as cookies or potato chips, often results in overconsumption of those foods when children are free to choose them (Savage, Fisher, & Birch 2007).

Educators and Families are Role Models

Based on research, the following six subsections discuss food fears, care environments, food behavior models, food restriction, pressures to eat, and food as a reward or celebration. Each area offers suggestions for educators and families to help children develop positive, early eating behaviors.

Food Fears

Most children naturally demonstrate fears of new foods. Neophobia, or fear of the new, is a protective behavior observed in omnivores, including humans, that helps prevent consumption of harmful substances (Birch 1999). Teachers help decrease children's fears by creating supportive environments with enjoyable, nutritious, and fun early food experiences.

For example, teachers could involve families by encouraging each family to bring every child a tasting sample of a unique food their child enjoys (or the teacher may offer suggestions of foods to taste). The teacher can arrange a tasting schedule, with a different family sharing a food tasting each week. Once every family has had an opportunity to share, host a classroom tasting party with all of the foods and invite parents to enjoy the event with their children. Although experiments vary, researchers tell us that offering a food 10 to 15 times appears necessary to increase a child's food acceptance (Savage, Fisher, & Birch 2007). Activities like tasting parties expose children to foods from different cultures and provide opportunities to learn more about their friends.

Researchers tell us that offering a food 10 to 15 times appears necessary to increase a child's food acceptance.

The acceptance of new foods is a slow process. Particularly through the ages 2 to 5, persistence is essential (Birch 1999; Satter 2008). A teacher/caregiver may think it is best to hold off on introducing food variety until children's fearful responses decrease. Instead, it is important to continue introducing a variety of foods throughout early childhood. Although children are skeptical of many foods during these early years, the variety of foods they accept is greater in this developmental phase than it is in later childhood (Skinner et al., 2002).

Enjoyable or satisfying experiences with a food highly influence a child's subsequent selection of the food on given occasions or its adoption into his or her regular diet. These experiences are as simple as frequent family meals during which the television is off and parents or caregivers are tuned in to the mealtime experience by talking and enjoying the foods themselves. Positive exposure to multiple foods helps children develop a taste for more foods, choose them as regular mealtime selections, and have needed dietary variety—whole grains, fruits, and vegetables. Many children lack opportunities to taste a variety of healthful foods, compared to the numerous chances our culture makes available for tasting high-fat, calorie-dense foods (Savage, Fisher, & Birch 2007).

Care Environments

Child care settings foster positive development of eating behaviors for 2- to 5-year-olds. Caregivers introduce variety in the foods served at meals and snacks and encourage families to do the same when they send lunches from home. Programs can guide parents by sharing comprehensive lists of foods that present a variety of grains, fruits, vegetables, nuts and seeds, and meats and beans, and an illustration of their nutritional value. For instance, using MyPyramid (www.mypyramid.gov) food groups helps families categorize foods and prepare lunches with variety and nutritional balance. Teachers can share examples of simple, creative lunches with variety in color, texture, and taste to appeal to young children.

Being persistent and providing repeated exposures to foods is important for both teachers and families. Avoid temptations to remove healthy foods from the program's meal or snack menus just because children reject them. Support families in continuing to offer lunch items even if their child does not consume the food on a given day. When serving a new item such as snap peas at snack time, include it two or three times a month and encourage children to look, smell, touch, and taste the new food. It is perfectly acceptable for a child to avoid a new vegetable the first several times it is offered. Inviting children to touch and smell the food helps them take small steps toward tasting. Encouraging rather than requiring children to eat a food is the key objective.

Food Behavior Models

Families are typically children's first significant models of eating behavior (Golan & Weizman 2001). Child care providers also are early role models. Positive role modeling correlates with an increased interest in food and less food fussiness among children (Gregory, Paxton, & Borzovic 2010). Poor role

---

Ten Steps to Positive Eating Behaviors

1. Provide a variety of foods at meals and snacks, especially whole grains, vegetables, and fruits.
2. Offer repeated opportunities to taste new foods.
3. Share with families nutrition resources, such as lists of foods (by category) to guide their food selections and offer new ideas for meals sent from home.
4. Apply the same guidelines to food selections in teachers' lunches brought from home.
5. Sit with children at meals, and enjoy conversation. Talk about the taste, texture, appearance, and healthful aspects of foods.
6. Plan adequate time for all children to finish eating.
7. Respect a child's expression of satiety or sense of being full.
8. Develop a routine for serving snacks, applying the same rules whether offering carrots, crackers, or cookies.
9. Wash hands before snack and mealtime; encourage touching and smelling a food as a step toward tasting.
10. Find alternatives to using food as a reward or serving foods high in fat, sugar, or salt as part of a celebration.

---

models influence children's perceptions of foods and mealtimes (Matheson, Spranger, & Saxe 2002). For example, negative comments about the taste or texture of a food will make a child less willing to try it. On the other hand, a child is more likely to try a food if he or she observes an adult enjoying it.

Teachers and caregivers become role models by engaging with children at mealtime and sitting down and eating with them. This practice is often called family-style dining. When early childhood programs provide meals, teachers and staff can model healthy eating behaviors by eating the same foods the children eat.

Staff who bring their lunches can model the same kinds of healthy eating as described in the guidelines the program suggests for families who send lunches with their children. For example, if parents send a fruit and a vegetable item, then teachers can include both of these items in their lunches. If children have milk, water, or 100 percent fruit juice as a beverage, teachers should drink these same beverages.

Interesting and engaging mealtime conversations create greater food enjoyment (Hughes et al., 2007). Adults can talk positively about the foods they are eating and also invite the children to describe colors, tastes (sweet, sour, salty), and textures (crunchy, smooth, stringy). However, the conversation should not be about the food alone. Also engage children in conversation about other appropriate topics, such as animals or family activities. Too much emphasis on the foods may decrease the children's interest.

Teachers and care-givers become role models by engaging with children at meal-time and sitting down and eating with them.

Food Restriction

Many well-meaning adults try to control the way children eat. They may believe that restricting or forbidding unhealthy foods will decrease children's preference for them, but the opposite is true (Satter 2008). Pressuring a child to eat one type of food (such as fruit or vegetables) leads to resistance. When an adult restricts access to certain foods (such as sweets or french fries), a child may become preoccupied with the restricted food.

A study on the effect of restricted access to foods among a population of 3- to 6-year-olds (Fisher & Birch 1999) found that the children focused great attention on the visible but inaccessible food through spontaneous clapping and chanting. In a similar study (Fisher & Birch 1999), restricting a desired, palatable snack food substantially increased children's selection of that food compared to times when both it and similar foods were freely available.

Avoid making comments about children's frequency or quantity consumption of a given food. For example, when serving cookies for snack, offer them as all other snacks are served. Their quantity should not be restricted unless the quantity of all snack foods is restricted. Early childhood educators can develop routines for offering all snacks, both unfamiliar and favorite foods, in the same unbiased way.

Pressure to Eat

When families or teachers pressure children to eat at mealtimes, the practice negatively influences a child's food intake as well as attitude toward food (Galloway et al., 2006). Gregory, Paxton, and Brozovic (2010) report that children pressured to eat were less interested in food over time; whereas, when parents modeled healthy eating, the children expressed greater interest in food and less food fussiness. Coercion to eat specific quantities or types of foods may mean that children eat more at the given meal, but over time they will likely avoid the targeted food (Satter 2008).

In a study involving adults, Batsell and colleagues (2002) traced common food dislikes to the adults' childhood experiences in being pressured to consume certain foods. Galloway and colleagues (2006) learned that refraining from the use of pressure and simply eating with and talking to the children had a more positive impact on children's attitude toward the food offered.

While pressure to eat contributes to a dislike of certain foods, emphasis on having a "clean plate" may hinder children's recognition of the internal cues of hunger and satiety and contribute to overeating (Satter 2008). It is important for adults to respect the child's expression of food preference and fullness (particularly if the child tastes a food) and to follow a schedule that gives children enough time to eat.

Food as a Reward or Celebration

Food as reward or celebration is common in some early childhood settings. Such practices may be well intentioned but can have negative consequences and impact long-term eating behaviors (Birch 1999; Brown & Ogden 2004). Food rewards or party treats are often sweets or other "desired" snack items. Giving a desired food as a reward enhances a child's preference for the food (Puhl & Schwartz 2003).

By establishing guidelines for the use of food in the classroom, early childhood programs encourage families to provide alternatives to fast-food lunch parties or cupcake celebrations and to bring instead, for example, fruits or muffins. Class celebrations or everyday activities also give young children opportunities to prepare their own foods in the classroom. Children enjoy making edible art fruit or vegetable skewers, or snacks resembling animals.

Alternative practices for recognition and celebration are growing in variety in early childhood settings. Instead of food, teachers recognize children by giving them special opportunities, such as selecting a song for the group to listen or dance to, choosing a game to play with friends, or having first choice of equipment for gross motor play. Non-food-related activities, like bringing a favorite book or game to class to read or share with friends, are other ways to acknowledge individuals.

Conclusion

Early childhood educators who understand the importance of their role in the development of children's healthful eating behaviors can help improve the lifelong health of the children they serve. They can offer meaningful, positive experiences with food, including growing, preparing, and eating foods with children. Regardless of the foods offered at home, the early childhood educator has the opportunity to model selection and enjoyment of a variety of foods. Food in the program should be associated with opportunities and fun experiences rather than rules and restrictions. Tasting activities help children learn about foods, manners, and even other cultures.

Everyone caring for children needs to be aware that some food strategies have negative effects on the development of eating behaviors. Food practices involving pressure and restriction may not only affect childhood health but also have long-lasting implications, such as problematic behaviors of binge eating and dietary restraint among adults (Puhl & Schwartz 2003).

Regardless of the foods offered at home, the early childhood educator has the opportunity to model selection and enjoyment of a variety of foods.

A supportive, caring early childhood environment offers guidance through adult modeling, serving a variety of nutritious foods at meals and snacks, and exposing children to new foods in the classroom. These practices encourage children's development of healthy eating attitudes and behaviors and promote positive long-term health outcomes.

References

Batsell, R., A. Brown, M. Ansfield, & G. Paschall. 2002. "You Will Eat All of That! A Retrospective Analysis of Forced Consumption Episodes." *Appetite* 38 (3): 211–19.

Bellows, L., & J. Anderson. 2006. "The Food Friends: Encouraging Preschoolers to Try New Foods." *Young Children* 61 (3): 37–39. www.naeyc.org/yc/pastissues/2006/may.

Birch, L. 1999. "Development of Food Preferences." *Annual Reviews of Nutrition* 19 (1): 41–62.

Brown, R., & J. Ogden. 2004. "Children's Eating Attitudes and Behaviour: A Study of the Modeling and Control Theories of Parental Influence." *Health Education Research* 19 (3): 261–71.

Campbell, K., & D. Crawford 2001. "Family Food Environments as Determinants of Preschool-Aged Children's Eating Behaviors: Implications for Obesity Prevention Policy. A Review." *Australian Journal of Nutrition and Dietetics* 58 (1): 19–25.

Clark, H., E. Goyder, P. Bissel, L. Blank, & J. Peters. 2007. "How Do Parents' Child-Feeding Behaviours Influence Child Weight? Implications for Childhood Obesity Policy." *Journal of Public Health* 29 (2): 132–41.

Fisher, J., & L. Birch. 1999. "Restricting Access to Palatable Foods Affects Children's Behavioral Response, Food Selection, and Intake." *American Journal of Clinical Nutrition* 69 (6): 1264–72.

Galloway, A., L. Fiorito, L. Francis, & L. Birch. 2006. "'Finish Your Soup': Counterproductive Effects of Pressuring Children to Eat on Intake and Affect." *Appetite* 46 (3): 318–23.

Golan, M., & A. Weizman. 2001. "Familial Approach to the Treatment of Childhood Obesity." *Journal of Nutrition Education* 33 (2): 102–07.

Gregory, J., S. Paxton, & A. Brozovic. 2010. "Maternal Feeding Practices, Child Eating Behavior and Body Mass Index in Preschool-Aged Children: A Prospective Analysis." *The International Journal of Behavioral Nutrition and Physical Activity* 7: 55–65.

Hughes, S., H. Patrick, T. Power, J. Fisher, C. Anderson, & T. Nicklas. 2007. "The Impact of Child Care Providers' Feeding on Children's Food Consumption." *Journal of Development & Behavioral Pediatrics* 28 (2): 100–07.

Matheson, D., K. Spranger, & A. Saxe. 2002. "Preschool Children's Perceptions of Food and Their Food Experiences." *Journal of Nutrition Education and Behavior* 34 (2): 85–92.

Puhl, R., & M. Schwartz. 2003. "If You Are Good You Can Have a Cookie: How Memories of Childhood Food Rules Link to Adult Eating Behaviors." *Eating Behaviors* 4 (3): 283–93. www.faeriefilms.com/images/Schwartz_-_If_You_Are_Good.pdf.

Satter, E. 2008. *Secrets of Feeding a Healthy Family.* Madison, WI: Kelcy Press.

Savage, J., J.O. Fisher, & L. Birch. 2007. "Parental Influence on Eating Behavior: Conception to Adolescence." *Journal of Law, Medicine & Ethics* 35 (1): 22–34.

Skinner, J., B. Carruth, W. Bounds, & P. Ziegler. 2002. "Children's Food Preferences: A Longitudinal Analysis." *Journal of the American Dietetic Association* 102 (11): 1638–47.

Westenhoefer, J. 2002. "Establishing Dietary Habits During Childhood for Long-Term Weight Control." *Annals of Nutrition & Metabolism* 46 (supplement): 18–23.

Critical Thinking

1. Describe how families and teachers can improve food behavior of children during lunch or snack time.

2. Critique common practices in U.S. homes and schools that negate acceptance of consuming a variety of healthy foods.

2. Explain how food restriction affects eating behavior.

ERIN K. ELIASSEN, EdD, RD, LD, is an assistant professor in the Department of Family and Consumer Sciences at Eastern Kentucky University in Richmond. As a registered dietitian, she provides education and training on the topic of child feeding to health care providers, educators, and parents of young children.

Engaging Families in the Fight against the Overweight Epidemic among Children

MICK COLEMAN, CHARLOTTE WALLINGA, AND DIANE BALES

"Epidemic!" "Alarming!" "A threatening storm!" These powerful descriptors have been used by the Centers for Disease Control and Prevention (CDC) (Polhamus et al., 2004), the American Academy of Pediatrics (Committee on Nutrition, 2003; Council on Sports Medicine and Fitness and Council on School Health, 2006), and other medical professionals (Olshansky et al., 2005) to describe the increase in the number of U.S. children who are overweight. Indeed, data compiled from the National Health and Nutrition Examination Survey by the CDC (2007) show that the prevalence of overweight preschool-age children, 2 to 5 years old, increased from 5% in the period 1971–74 to 13.9% in the period 2003–04. During the same time periods, the prevalence of overweight 6- to 11-year-olds increased from 4% to 18.8% and the prevalence of overweight 12- to 19-year-olds increased from 6.1% to 17.4%. Across age groups, the prevalence of overweight children remains higher among low-income and minority groups than among children as a whole (Anderson & Butcher, 2006).

In this article, we provide an update on the overweight epidemic with early childhood educators in mind. We begin with information about the consequences of being overweight for children's health. We then examine the multiple factors that contribute to the overweight epidemic. Next, we look at the case for involving families in the fight against the overweight epidemic among children. Finally, we share three principles and associated strategies that early childhood educators can use to help families guide their children toward a healthy lifestyle.

Consequences Associated with Children Being Overweight

Cardiovascular Disease. It is estimated that a majority (61%) of overweight children from 5 to 10 years old have one or more cardiovascular risk factors (Freedman, Dietz, Srinivasan, & Berenson, 1999), such as high blood pressure, high cholesterol, and hardening of the arteries (Daniels, 2006; Freedman et al., 1999). While these biological processes can take decades to progress to a stroke or heart attack, it is feared that becoming overweight during childhood may accelerate their impact and lead to an early death (Daniels, 2006).

Diabetes

Diabetes in children also is attributed to the increased incidence of children being overweight (Daniels, 2006; Ludwig & Ebbeling, 2001). Diabetes, in turn, can lead to blindness, heart disease, kidney disease, and loss of limbs (The Center for Health and Health Care in Schools, 2005).

Asthma

The risk of asthma is higher among children who are overweight (Gilliland et al., 2003). In addition, overweight children with asthma have been found to use more medicine, make more visits to the emergency room, and spend more days wheezing than non-overweight children with asthma (Belamarich et al., 2000).

Sleep Apnea

Being overweight carries a higher risk of sleep apnea, an abnormal collapse of the airway during sleep, both in adults and children (Daniels, 2006). As a result, overweight children may exhibit daytime sleepiness, which, in turn, can lead to a decrease in physical activity and further heighten the risk for being overweight (Daniels, 2006). In addition, daytime sleepiness can negatively impact children's classroom performance. Over the long term, sleep apnea also can increase blood pressure, further raising the risk of heart disease.

Quality and Length of Life

Overweight children and their parents report significantly lower quality of life scores for physical, emotional, social, and school functioning than do families with children diagnosed as "healthy" (Schwimmer, Burwinkle, & Varni, 2003). Perhaps more alarming, because of the increased incidence of childhood overweight, young children today may live less healthy and shorter lives than their parents (Olshansky et al., 2005). Should this occur, being overweight would indeed prove to be the "threatening storm" that reverses the steady rise in life expectancy observed during previous centuries.

Factors Contributing to the Overweight Epidemic among Children

Children become overweight when they eat too many calories and do not get enough physical activity to burn off those calories (Anderson & Butcher, 2006; U.S. Department of Health and Human Services, 2001). Although genetics and body metabolism both contribute to this imbalance, certain lifestyle factors also must be considered (Anderson & Butcher, 2006; Council on Sports Medicine and Fitness and Council on School Health, 2006).

The Food Environment

Children in the United States have an overwhelming abundance of food choices. Unfortunately, not all foods found in grocery stores are healthy, few fast food meals are healthy, and pre-packaged foods and soft drinks are often high in fat, sugar, and calories. Advertisements also can be confusing and sometimes misleading. For example, although many prepackaged foods are advertised as healthy (e.g., "reduced fat"), they may contain as many or more calories than the foods they are designed to replace (CDC, 2005a). We only need to look at the vending machines at our work sites to realize that milk, juices, and healthy snacks are far less available than their less healthy counterparts. Unfortunately, vending machines and food advertising through television programming remain a fact of life in too many elementary and middle schools, perhaps, in part, because of the added income they bring to schools (Anderson & Butcher, 2006; Cawley, 2006).

Portion Sizes

Yet another factor contributing to the confusing food environment is portion size (Cawley, 2006). Food manufacturers began producing larger portion sizes in the 1970s and continued to do so at an increasing rate through the 1980s and 1990s, leading children and adults to eat more and take in more calories during meals and snacks (CDC, 2005a; Young & Nestle, 2002). It easy to understand why children have difficulty establishing healthy eating patterns.

Schedules

Skipping breakfast and eating fast food are characteristics of a national mindset in which food quantity and convenience override considerations of food quality and health. Even though many ready-to-eat healthy foods are available (e.g., fruits), families often prefer prepackaged foods because they have longer shelf lives, do not require cleaning, and appeal to the tastes of children. Nevertheless, results from research suggest that eating food away from home, especially at fast food establishments, contributes to children becoming overweight (Davis et al., 2007). Likewise, skipping breakfast is a risk factor for becoming overweight (Davis et al., 2007).

Technological Advances and Urban Design

While technology has contributed to the quality of our lives, it also has reduced our level of physical activity. For example, as children spend more time watching television, they spend less time engaged in outdoor physical activities. Likewise, many families live in communities designed more for vehicles than for walking and biking (Fierro, 2002). Urban sprawl, combined with inadequate sidewalks and heavy traffic, prevents children from walking or riding bikes to school and parks (Anderson & Butcher, 2006).

Play and Physical Education

Recess and time for free play have been eliminated or shortened in many school systems (U.S. Department of Health and Human Services, 2004). In addition, rules regarding physical education for elementary school children vary widely (National Conference of State Legislatures, 2005). These changes have come about at least in part due to the increased concern over preparing children to meet mandated test scores (Anderson & Butcher, 2006). In response, such groups as the American Association for the Child's Right to Play (www.ipausa.org) are advocating for the 60 minutes of daily physical activities often recommended by the medical profession (Council on Sports Medicine and Fitness and Council on School Health, 2006; Davis et al., 2007).

The Case for Engaging Families as Health Educators

Increasingly, families are being viewed as essential in the fight against the overweight epidemic among children. Families, more than any other social institution, serve as both mediators and monitors of children's health behaviors.

Families as Mediators

Families mediate their children's eating behaviors through their choice and preparation of snacks and meals, as well as through their decisions of where to eat when outside the home. Families serve as mediators of children's physical activities through the rules they set regarding the amount of time children spend watching television and playing computer games. Likewise, families determine the degree to which children are involved in such physical activities as games, recreational pursuits, home chores, and yardwork.

Families as Monitors

Families also serve as monitors of their children's eating and physical activity patterns. Although some families appear to

Table 1 Families as Health Educators: Guides for Developing Healthy Lifestyle Activities for Families

Family-based Activities. In order to make healthy living truly a family affair, strive to develop activities that involve all family members in a household and not just a child or a parent-child dyad. Otherwise, efforts to fight family overeating and inactivity may not be successful.

Time Efficiency. Because families lead busy lives, develop family involvement activities that can be incorporated into their usual routines (e.g., dinner, bedtime, housework). Families are more likely to try healthy lifestyle activities if they fit into their daily schedules.

Simplicity. The fewer materials and directions needed to complete an activity, the better. Families may not bother to attempt a healthy lifestyle activity if that activity involves numerous materials and directions.

Clarity. Check all printed materials for clarity. If doubt remains about certain words or phrases, ask a few families to read the materials and provide you with feedback. Identify volunteers to translate printed materials into the languages represented in your classroom.

Fun. No one wants to eat bland food or engage in boring or unpleasant physical activities. Use your creativity and consult with community nutritionists and recreation specialists to develop fun and creative activities that reinforce healthy eating and exercise.

Encourage Rather Than Preach. Avoid a "preaching" stance by acknowledging that we all have a right to watch television, play video games, and eat a piece of cake. Disallowing these things altogether will only serve to sabotage families' efforts. Note the importance of moderation, not total elimination, when suggesting activities that help move families toward a more active and healthy lifestyle.

---

have difficulty recognizing the potential health risks associated with being overweight (Young-Hyman, Herman, Scott, & Schlundt, 2000), a number of family-based intervention programs have achieved success in lowering the weight of overweight children (see Epstein, Valoski, Wing, & McCurley, 1994; Golan & Crow, 2004; Golan, Weizman, Apter, & Fainaru, 1998; Harvey-Berino & Rourke, 2003; Lindsay, Sussner, Kim, & Gortmaker, 2006). Indeed, one of the most basic ways that parents can monitor and contribute to their children's development of healthy eating patterns is by establishing a family rule about eating dinner together (Lindsay et al., 2006).

The importance of a family-based approach to addressing the overweight epidemic becomes even clearer when we consider how families must juggle multiple schedules and unique demands, which can interfere with their ability to serve as effective monitors of their children's eating patterns and exercise activities. As a result, consideration must be given to respecting the realities of family life when planning family activities to promote healthy eating and exercise. Table 1 presents guides that we have followed in carrying out training related to healthy living. These guides also were the foundation for our development of the activity ideas found in Table 2 and Figure 1.

Involving Families in the Fight against the Overweight Epidemic

Early childhood educators have the expertise to bridge the gap between factual health information and the application of family involvement practices to promote family-oriented healthy eating and exercise. Three recommendations from the CDC (2005b) for involving families in promoting a healthy approach to eating and physical activity are especially relevant to early childhood teachers' work with families.

Guide 1. Encourage Families to Serve as Role Models

A family-based approach to fighting against the factors contributing to children being overweight is in keeping with current recommendations that recognize the importance of parents as children's most important role models in adapting a healthy lifestyle (Council on Sports Medicine and Fitness and Council on School Health, 2006; Davis et al., 2007; Lindsay et al., 2006). Families that model healthy eating patterns, regularly participate in physical activities, and talk about the benefits associated with a healthy lifestyle set an example for children to follow. Younger children, in particular, are more likely to mimic the behavior of important adults like parents and guardians. Some ideas to share with families to help them model healthy living habits can be found in Table 2.

Guide 2. Encourage Families to Engage in Healthy Activities in Different Settings

Help families discover practical ways to eat healthy meals and exercise throughout the week. Family activity calendars, like the one presented in Figure 1 for families of preschool and kindergarten children, can provide the encouragement families need to work toward a healthy lifestyle within and outside the home.

Guide 3. Advocate for Quality School and Community Physical Activity Programs

Families may not always see themselves as having the knowledge or skills needed to serve as health advocates for their children. Help promote families' knowledge, confidence, and skills in the following ways:

Figure 1   Themes and Ideas for an Activity Calendar

Theme	Mon	Tue	Wed	Thu	Fri
Practice Fundamental Motor Skills	*Trapping.* Sit on the floor and roll a large ball back and forth. Roll it to one side, then the other side. Roll it slowly, then quickly.	*Catching.* Help your child practice catching a large ball by rolling it down a slide or chute. Then, toss the ball back and forth to each other.	*Hopping.* Hop like a rabbit or grasshopper. See how long you can hop on one foot.	*Weaving.* Weave through an obstacle course of chairs or sheets hung over an outdoor line.	*Throwing.* Practice throwing a ball through a hula hoop from different distances and angles.
Encourage Creative Movement	Attach a large scarf to your child's pants or around her waist. Do the same for yourself. Pretend you have been swept up by the wind and are floating in the sky. What do you see below?	Observe how bugs move on the ground. Take turns making up your own creative bug movements.	Use ribbons attached to your wrists as butterfly wings. Fly around and visit your favorite flowers and plants.	Some communities have free introductory dance classes. Take your family to different classes. Which ones do family members enjoy the most?	Put on a fast song. Everyone make up a silly dance, the sillier the better.
Family Relaxation and Recreation	As a family, take a stroll around the neighborhood after dinner. Using hints, play a game of "guess what I see."	As a family, color and decorate heavy paper plates. Use them as frisbees. Aim for a tree or play toss and catch.	Read a book with or to your child. Make up a story together. Be sure to write it down and draw pictures so you can enjoy it again later.	Use the Internet or library to look up dances from different cultures. Try a new dance each week.	As a family, bowl, play a round of miniature golf, ride bikes, dance, etc. Don't make it competitive. Just have fun.
Movement Games	Try walking in a straight line while balancing a balloon or foam ball in your hand. Repeat, this time walking in a circle or along a winding path.	Play "Simon Says" by directing your child to move in different ways. Repeat, with your preschooler giving you directions.	Make up your own family movement game. Remember to keep it simple so everyone can play and have fun.	Divide into pairs and play a game of opposites. If your partner hops forward, you hop backward. If you partner crouches on her knees, you jump up in the air.	As a family, form a line and play a movement game of follow the leader. Take turns being the leader.

61

Table 2 Ideas for Helping Families Become Healthy Role Models

Incorporate the following ideas into classroom newsletters, family workshops, and parent-teacher conferences to help families become healthy role models for their children.

Starting Smart: Teaching Young Children About Healthy Foods While Grocery Shopping

1. Help your child name the different types of vegetables and fruits on display in the produce section. Note that these foods are good for our bodies. When passing by the cookie and candy aisles, note that we should eat only a little of these items, and only occasionally. Help reinforce this message by "skipping" past these aisles with your child as you move on to more healthy foods.

2. Make a shopping list using pictures of healthy foods. Help your child cut out and paste the pictures onto sheets of paper. As your child decorates each page, note that the foods in the pictures are good for our bodies because they give us energy and help our bodies stay strong and healthy. Arrange the pictures in an order that reflects the layout of your grocery store. Hand your child a few pictures of the healthy food you are shopping for before entering each aisle. Your child can use the pictures to help you look for the healthy food. This game will also help distract him from looking for less healthy foods.

3. Point out the different colors, shapes, and textures associated with such foods as bell peppers, apples, onions, grapes, tomatoes, nuts, and lettuces. Help your child pick foods with the colors, shapes, or textures she would like to try in a snack or meal.

Eating In, Eating Out: Managing the Food Environment

1. Make sure that fresh and dried fruit, juice, milk, and water are readily available and easily accessible to everyone in the family. Putting juice and water in colorful pitchers will help catch your child's attention. Ask your child to draw pictures of his favorite fruits. Paste the pictures onto serving bowls to encourage him to go to those bowls for his snacks.

2. Ask your child to name her favorite healthy foods and write these on a large sheet of paper. Work with your child to write her own recipe, using some of the foods from her list. Use the recipe when preparing a family snack or meal.

3. When eating out, help your child find and make healthy choices by limiting your and his choices to only healthy items. Share the healthy choice you have made and repeat the healthy choices available to your child.

Serve as an Exercise Role Model

1. Take your child shopping for your exercise clothing and equipment. Talk about why you wear these clothes and how you use the equipment.

2. When dressing for exercise, talk to your child about why you are stretching, drinking water, and dressing in certain types of clothes. After exercising, talk to your child about how you feel.

3. Allow your child to play with your exercise equipment in a supervised and safe environment. Do not try to teach athletic skills. Instead, let her experiment with different movements.

Exceptions to the Rule

1. Practice moderation, not elimination. Allow your child to eat sweets now and then, explaining the importance of not making them a part of our daily diet. Repeating this message will help your child develop the mindset needed to follow a balanced diet.

2. At the end of holiday celebrations, help your child divide the candy he received into small portions and put them into individual sandwich bags. Give him two bags each week. One can serve as a special snack for the week. Encourage him to share the other bag with a family member. Serve something healthy (milk, water, or an apple) to drink or eat with the candy.

Practices to Avoid

1. Avoid the mindset of "Do as I say, not as I do," as it strikes children as being unfair. When they see adults eating candy or fast food, they have a difficult time understanding why they cannot do the same. Eating healthy is a family affair. Everyone should follow the same rules.

2. Avoid forcing your child to eat foods she does not like. Instead, use a "try me" approach to encourage your child to try new foods. Visit the following United States Department of Agriculture website to learn about the variety of foods you can serve that have similar nutritional qualities: www.mypyramid.gov/pyramid/index.html

3. Avoid using food as a reward. Such rewards often consist of unhealthy sweets, and this can promote unhealthy food choices and eating patterns.

4. Avoid placing your child on a strict diet. This will only interfere with her ability to develop the knowledge, skills, and motivation needed to follow a balanced diet. If you believe your child is overweight, consult with a nutritionist or your family physician to develop a plan of action that addresses both eating and physical activity patterns of behavior.

Television and Electronic Games

1. Follow the recommendation of the Council on Sports Medicine and Fitness and the Council on School Health (2006) of limiting your child's television viewing to no more than 2 hours per day. Help remind your child of this family rule by monitoring his television viewing and using the hands of a clock to show how much time he has left to watch television before it is turned off for the day.

(continued)

Table 2   Ideas for Helping Families Become Healthy Role Models *(continued)*

2. Take inventory of the number of electronic games in your home versus games and materials that promote physical activity, such as bikes, badminton sets, jump ropes, balls, and rackets and bats. Are your purchases more heavily weighted toward sedentary electronic games? If so, make a concentrated effort to balance out your purchases when selecting gifts for your child during the holidays and on her birthday.

3. Take television shows and electronic games outside. Work with your child to plan a version of her favorite television show or an electronic game that can be played outside. Follow two rules. First, the game must be safe and nonviolent. Second, it must involve movement. For example, you may plan a game called the human pinball machine. Friends and family members can take turns serving as stationary "bumpers" located at arm's length from each other (the bumpers cannot move from their spot) and "balls." Each "ball" attempts to run through the pinball machine without being touched by the stationary "bumpers."

- *Note how your center or school promotes healthy eating and physical activity.* Point out classroom menus and outdoor play equipment to families when conducting registration and orientations. Explain how menus and physical activities are developed. Encourage dialogue by asking families about their children's favorite foods and physical activities.

- *Make health part of parent-teacher conferences.* Address children's nutritional habits and physical activities that you have observed in the classroom. Compare your observations to those made by families in the home environment. Provide families with a list of community youth groups that offer free or inexpensive age-appropriate activities, like dance and swimming. Visit with a local school nutritionist or your local cooperative extension agent to gather ideas for quick and healthy snacks for families to try at home. Invite these experts to conduct family night workshops on such topics as childhood nutrition, reading and understanding food labels, using the food pyramid, and identifying misleading food advertisements. Invite professionals from your local department of recreation to demonstrate noncompetitive games that families can play at home, as well as fun activities that promote children's fundamental motor skills, like those presented in Figure 1.

- *Encourage families to share.* Inviting family members to the classroom to share their recreational hobbies is an inexpensive way to introduce children to a variety of physical activities. If children do engage in the activity being demonstrated, pair the visiting parent with an early childhood physical education teacher to ensure that developmentally appropriate practices are followed.

- *Engage families in the learning process.* Recruit families to work with children in growing a garden of herbs and vegetables in pots or raised beds. Families that are unable to come to the classroom can be provided with tip sheets on how to grow herbs and vegetables at home. Invite families to help children prepare healthy salads and other dishes using the herbs and vegetables they harvest.

Conclusion

There are no easy solutions to addressing the epidemic of children who are overweight. The authors hope that the information and ideas presented in this article will help early childhood educators play an active role in working with families to help children develop the eating and activity patterns needed for a healthy lifestyle.

References

Anderson, P. M., & Butcher, K. F. (2006). Childhood obesity: Trends and potential causes. *The Future of Children: Childhood Obesity, 16*(1), 19–45.

Belamarich, P. F., Luder, E., Kattan, M., Mitchell, H., Islam, S., Lynn, H., & Crain, E. F. (2000). Do obese inner-city children with asthma have more symptoms than nonobese children with asthma? *Pediatrics, 106*(6), 1436–1441.

Cawley, J. (2006). Markets and childhood obesity policy. *The Future of Children: Childhood Obesity, 16*(1), 69–88.

Center for Health and Health Care in Schools. (2005). *Childhood overweight: What the research tells us.* School of Public Health and Health Services, The Georgia Washington University Medical Center. Retrieved June 29, 2008, from www .healthinschools.org/~/media/Files/obesityfs.ashx.

Centers for Disease Control and Prevention. (2005a). *Overweight and obesity: Contributing factors.* Retrieved June 29, 2008, from cdc.gov/nccdphp/dnpa/obesity/contributing_factors.htm.

Centers for Disease Control and Prevention. (2005b). *Healthy youth! Promoting better health strategies.* Retrieved June 29, 2008, from www.cdc.gov/HealthyYouth/physicalactivity/promoting _health/strategies/families.htm.

Centers for Disease Control and Prevention. (2007, May 22). *Overweight prevalence.* Retrieved June 29, 2008, from www.cdc.gov/print.do?url=http%3A%2F%2Fwww.cdc .gov%2Fnccdphp%2Fdnpa%.

Committee on Nutrition. (2003). Prevention of pediatric overweight and obesity. *Pediatrics, 112*(2), 424–430.

Council on Sports Medicine and Fitness and Council on School Health. (2006). Active healthy living: Prevention of childhood obesity through increased physical activity. *Pediatrics, 117*(5), 1834–1842.

Daniels, S. R. (2006). The consequences of childhood overweight and obesity. *The Future of Children: Childhood Obesity, 16*(1), 47–67.

Davis, M. M., Gance-Cleveland, B., Hassink, S., Johnson, R., Paradis, G., & Resnicow, K. (2007). Recommendations for prevention of childhood obesity. *Pediatrics, 120* (Supplement 4), S229–S253.

Epstein, L. H., Valoski, A., Wing, R. R., & McCurley, J. (1994). Ten-year outcomes of behavioral family-based treatment for childhood obesity. *Health Psychology, 13*(5), 373–383.

Fierro, M. P. (2002). *The obesity epidemic—How states can trim the fat. Issue Brief.* National Governors Association Center for Best Practices. Online: www.nga.org/portal/site/nga.

Freedman, D. S., Dietz, W. H., Srinivasan, S. R., & Berenson, G. S. (1999). The relation of overweight to cardiovascular risk factors among children and adolescents: The Bogalusa heart study. *Pediatrics, 103*(6), 1175–1182.

Gilliland, F. D., Berhane, K., Islam, T., McConnell, R., Gauderman, W. J., Gilliland, S., Avol, E., & Peters, J. M. (2003). Obesity and the risk of newly diagnosed asthma in school-age children. *American Journal of Epidemiology, 158*(5), 406–415.

Golan, M., & Crow, S. (2004). Targeting parents exclusively in the treatment of childhood obesity: Long-term results. *Obesity Research, 12*(2), 357–361.

Golan, M. A., Weizman, A., Apter, A., & Fainaru, M. (1998). Parents as the exclusive agents of change in the treatment of childhood obesity. *American Journal of Clinical Nutrition, 67*(6), 1130–1135.

Harvey-Berino, J., & Rourke, J. (2003). Obesity prevention in preschool Native-American children: A pilot study using home visiting. *Obesity Research, 11*(5), 606–611.

Lindsay, A. C., Sussner, K. M., Kim, J., & Gortmaker, S. (2006). The role of parents in preventing childhood obesity. *The Future of Children: Childhood Obesity, 16*(1), 169–186.

Ludwig, D. S., & Ebbeling, T. B. (2001). Type 2 diabetes mellitus in children: Primary care and public health considerations. *Journal of the American Medical Association, 286*(12), 1427–1430.

National Conference of State Legislatures. (2005). *Childhood obesity: An overview of policy options in legislation for 2003–2004.* Online: www.ncsl.org/programs/health/childhoodobesity.htm.

Olshansky, S. J., Passaro, D. J., Hershow, J. L., Carnes, B. A., Brody, J., Hayflick, L., Butler, R. N., Allision, D. B., & Ludwig. D. S. (2005). A potential decline in life expectancy in the United States in the 21st century. *New England Journal of Medicine, 253*(11), 1138–1145.

Polhamus, B., Dalenius, K., Thompson, D., Scanlon, K., Borland, E., Smith, B., & Grummer-Strawn, L. (2004). *Pediatric nutrition surveillance 2002 report.* Atlanta, GA: U.S. Department of Health and Human Services, Centers for Disease Control and Prevention.

Schwimmer, J. B., Burwinkle, T. M., & Varni, J. W. (2003). Health-related quality of life of severely obese children and adolescents. *Journal of the American Medical Association, 289*(14), 1813–1819.

U.S. Department of Health and Human Services. (2001). *The surgeon general's call to action to prevent and decrease overweight and obesity.* Rockville, MD: Public Health Service, Office of the Surgeon General.

U.S. Department of Health and Human Services. (2004). *Healthy People 2010 Progress Review: Nutrition and overweight.* Online: www.healthypeople.gov/data/2010prog/focus19/default.htm.

Young, L. R., & Nestle, M. (2002). The contribution of expanding portion sizes to the U.S. obesity epidemic. *American Journal of Public Health, 92*(2), 246–249.

Young-Hyman, D., Herman, L., Scott, D. L., & Schlundt, D. G. (2000). Care giver perception of children's obesity-related health risk: A study of African-American families. *Obesity Research, 8*(3), 241–248.

Critical Thinking

1. What percentage of overweight children, 5–10 years old, have high blood pressure, high cholesterol, and/or hardening of the arteries?

2. What are the six health-related consequences associated with children being overweight?

3. What are three examples of how families can serve as positive role models for overweight kids?

MICK COLEMAN is Professor, CHARLOTTE WALLINGA is Associate Professor, and DIANE BALES is Associate Professor, Department of Child and Family Development, University of Georgia, Athens.

From *Childhood Education*, Spring 2010, pp. 150–156. Copyright © 2010 by the Association for Childhood Education International. Reprinted by permission of the authors and the Association for Childhood Education International, 17904 Georgia Avenue, Suite 215, Olney, MD 20832.

The School Lunch Wars

Sixty-five years ago, the federal school lunch program was created to make American schoolchildren healthier. Today, it's helping to make them fatter. Will a new law change the diets of millions of kids raised on French fries and chicken nuggets?

KRISTEN HINMAN

When Colombia native Beatriz Zuluaga, a professional cook for 20 years, became the admissions director at CentroNía's DC Bilingual Public Charter School in 2007, she thought she was leaving her old career far behind. Then she laid eyes on the trays in the lunchroom. Mashed potatoes from a box, chicken nuggets, chocolate milk—to Zuluaga, the processed fare didn't look fit for growing kids. At her last job, Zuluaga had cooked for 450 people a day. Surely she could take over the school's kitchen, no?

She unpacked her knives and started whipping up from-scratch dishes: lasagna with lentils, peppers stuffed with barley and turkey, roasted beets. The reformation did not go over well. One offense after another set the tongues of parents and teachers wagging. *What is that? How can you serve that to children? Why are you trying to turn my kid into a vegetarian?*

Three years later, Zuluaga has given up on the beets. But American cheese has been scrapped for calcium-rich provolone. White flour has been swapped for whole wheat in pizza crust. Fruit juice, high in sugar, is out. The school nurse is reporting fewer sick kids, and Zuluaga has chuckled at least once when a parent remarked on the new efficacy of her child's bowel movements. More than a third of parents have participated in the school's nutrition workshops.

But when I visited the school last fall, all Zuluaga had to do to temper her optimism was walk into a DC Bilingual lunchroom and discover a chubby, misbehaving fourth grader relegated to a table facing the wall and going to town on his brown-bag lunch: an Oscar Mayer Lunchables "pizza." As the boy perched a piece of pepperoni and some shredded cheese atop a cracker, Zuluaga picked up the packaging to inspect its long ingredient list, then put it back down, crossed her arms, and frowned. I expected her to seize the opportunity for a teachable moment, but she was silent. Later she explained, "He didn't go to the grocery store and buy that."

Zuluaga's education, as it were, mirrors what's occurring in schools across America as proponents of whole—that is, minimally processed—foods try to introduce children to more nutritious diets through the $9.8 billion federal school lunch program, which feeds about 32 million of America's 50 million

schoolchildren every school day. One in three American children and teenagers today is overweight or obese. Last year, in a report titled *Too Fat to Fight,* a group of retired military brass blamed school lunches for the fact that an estimated 27 percent of American youth are too overweight to serve in the armed forces. A study of Michigan sixth graders published in December found that regularly consuming school lunches was a greater risk factor for obesity than spending two or more hours a day watching television or playing video games.

First lady Michelle Obama, a former hospital executive, has made the war on obesity her defining cause, and put the school lunch program in her crosshairs. In December, thanks in part to her lobbying, Congress passed the Healthy, Hunger-Free Kids Act, which awards schools that meet certain nutritional guidelines an extra six cents per student meal. The extra pennies increase federal reimbursements for lunches above the rate of inflation for the first time in three decades. The law, which cuts funds from future federal food-stamp benefits to cover the reimbursement hike, also grants the U.S. Department of Agriculture (USDA) more power to police what's served in school cafeterias. In reality, though, the battle over school lunches is just beginning, as educators confront a culture that prizes its hamburgers and French fries.

How did a program that was designed to improve the nutrition of the nation's children become a culprit in the scourge of childhood obesity?

As early as the 19th century, some American schools operated their own school lunch programs, often with the help of volunteers. In the 1930s, in the midst of the Great Depression, the federal government began providing some funds for school lunches on an ad hoc basis. But many children still didn't get enough to eat. The problem was thrown into stark relief during World War II, when it was discovered that half of all draftees who were deemed unfit for service were rejected because of malnutrition. In 1946, Congress passed the National School Lunch Act "as a measure of national security." The law guaranteed a free or subsidized midday meal for millions of needy children. It was also intended to teach America what to eat. "Not only is the child taught what a good diet consists of," noted a congressional agriculture committee report, "but his parents and family likewise are indirectly instructed."

During the Depression, when farmers were surrounded by mountains of unsold commodities and schools were full of hungry children, New Deal politicos had used the USDA to funnel surpluses to school cafeterias. Thus, when it came time to designate an authority for the new national lunch program, the USDA seemed a natural choice. Schools would receive subsidized commodities and cash reimbursements in exchange for feeding low-income children lunches that met USDA nutrition standards. And so the same law that was supposed to ensure a nutritious midday meal for millions of kids also created an enduring market for American farmers.

It was up to state officials to administer the federal funds. For the first two decades student participation was low, partly because many schools lacked adequate facilities but also because local authorities often established the eligibility threshold with little regard for students' actual need. The poor results prompted Congress in the 1960s to establish a federal eligibility standard linked to the poverty level.

Today, students from families with incomes below 130 percent of the poverty level ($28,665 for a family of four) eat for free. The school receives a federal subsidy of $2.72 per meal. Children from families earning up to 185 percent of the poverty level pay 40 cents per meal, and the subsidy is correspondingly reduced. Other students pay the "full" price, an average of $1.60. The government also provides a small subsidy for these meals, on the principle that child nutrition contributes to national security. (Even so, schools often are not able to cover the production cost of the "full" price meals and essentially make up the difference from the subsidies meant for lower-income kids. A controversial provision of the new law will rectify that by requiring some districts to charge more for full-pay lunches.)

Student participation doubled within the first few years after the federal eligibility standards were set. Educators suddenly found themselves in the food business. Poorer districts, particularly, didn't have functioning kitchens, or the money to improve them. It became standard practice for cafeteria staff to purchase ready-made heat-and-eat meals, whose less-than-palatable qualities made headlines once it was learned that much of the food was being thrown out. These reports, along with the fact that the government was subsidizing lunches for middle-income families that could afford to pay full price, caught the attention of Ronald Reagan's cost-conscious administration. Among the resulting USDA proposals was the reclassification of ketchup as a vegetable—on the theory that replacing broccoli and lima beans with cheap condiments would reduce so-called plate waste. That idea caused a political uproar and was never carried out, but in 1981 Congress slashed school lunch reimbursement rates by a third and eliminated money for equipment.

Already making do with slim resources and now facing more budget pressures, some schools turned to professional vendors to replace the cafeteria ladies of old. At the same time, many schools added "à la carte" items that could be sold to anyone who could pay. Since the government didn't reimburse for à la carte fare, and thus didn't regulate its nutritional content, school officials were free to offer French fries, nachos, and pizza. Some items were branded by fast-food companies such as Domino's Pizza and Taco Bell. Many schools also allowed companies to install vending machines that dispensed snack foods, candy, and soda, from which the schools kept a portion of the sales.

Consumption of government-subsidized school lunches began to fall off because of the "needy" stigma associated with the reimbursable meals. Kids who had once purchased meals at full price switched to the more tempting à la carte line. Some lower-income students simply went without. In response, cafeteria managers goosed the offerings to make them more enticing. Out went baked chicken, in came chicken nuggets; roasted potatoes gave way to Tater Tots. Cheap commodities were available from the government, in all the processed forms kids were believed to covet. USDA nutrition standards were lax enough that it was possible to satisfy the grain and protein requirements with, say, breaded and fried fish sticks, or the fruit requirement with sugar-laced canned peaches.

In 1990, only one percent of schools were serving meals that met the USDA's dietary guidelines for percentage of calories from fat.

In 1990, the USDA commissioned a comprehensive analysis of the school lunch program to see how it stacked up against the agency's Dietary Guidelines for Americans. In yet another bureaucratic oddity of the program, schools had to meet a different, and looser, set of nutrition standards. "The results were disturbing," recounts sociologist Janet Poppendieck in *Free for All* (2010), a survey of the politics surrounding school lunch programs. "On average, school lunches were deriving not [the recommended] 30 but 38 percent of calories from fats, not [the recommended] 10 but 15 percent from saturated fats. The meals were also found to be high in sodium. . . . Only one percent of schools were serving, on average, meals that complied with the dietary guidelines for percentage of calories from fat—one percent!"

Without allocating more money, Congress in 1994 required that school menus meet the USDA's Dietary Guidelines for Americans. But what was on the plate changed very little. Today, less than 20 percent of schools cook lunch from scratch. Eighty percent of schools exceed the fat allowance per meal. The average high school lunch has 1,600 milligrams of sodium—100 milligrams more than the daily amount deemed within healthy limits for children.

In the late 1990s, some school districts around the country quietly began removing vending machines or putting the kibosh on minimally nutritious à la carte programs. But the reformers who eventually drew national attention were two chefs who had far more ambitious goals. Alice Waters, whose Berkeley restaurant Chez Panisse was in the vanguard in serving seasonal and local cuisine, won over the California state superintendent of education with Edible Schoolyard, a garden project at a Berkeley middle school. By 2002, produce gardens had been established in more than 2,000 of California's 9,000 schools. The same year, Waters convinced the Berkeley Unified School District to hire Ann Cooper, who became known as "the Renegade Lunch Lady," to revamp its food service program with whole foods. (Cooper has since gone to work for the Boulder Valley School District in Colorado.)

To the California duo, the biggest culprit in the child nutrition crisis is the transformation of agriculture since World War II and the rise of agribusiness. Livestock is raised in mechanized indoor facilities rather than pastures, cash-crop monoculture has replaced the diversified family farm, and the food industry has undergone far-reaching consolidation. Today, only two percent of Americans—supported by government subsidies—produce food, and they do so at prices so low that the other 98 percent don't have much incentive to question the system. Pervasive marketing by fast-food companies pitching cheap children's "Happy Meals" and other convenience foods to working parents has helped establish a drive-through culture. The eat-your-vegetables ethos has given way to an emphasis on food that can be put on the table quickly (if it's consumed at a table at all) and that children will eat without a battle royale every evening.

The view that poor-quality school lunches are the result of a broken food system has led food activists to see the USDA as part of the problem. How, they ask, can an authority responsible for helping agribusiness produce and market its output also be an effective nutrition watchdog in school cafeterias?

In 2009, two months after moving into 1600 Pennsylvania Avenue, Michelle Obama planted an organic kitchen garden on the White House lawn, a step of both symbolic and practical significance. With her backing, the USDA dusted off projects that promote local and regional food systems, rolling out a local-foods marketing campaign called "Know Your Farmer, Know Your Food." Another initiative aims to help small and medium-size farms sell their products to schools.

What elevated Obama's whole foods advocacy above the charges of impracticality and foodie snobbery leveled at Waters and Cooper was the rollout last February of a campaign dubbed "Let's Move" that puts the focus squarely on health—and on those responsible for the well-being of children. "Our kids didn't do this to themselves," Obama said when she announced the wellness plan. "Our kids don't decide what's served to them at school or whether there's time for gym class or recess. Our kids don't choose to make food products with tons of sugar and sodium in supersized portions, and then to have those products marketed to them everywhere they turn. And no matter how much they beg for pizza, fries, and candy, ultimately they are not, and should not be, the ones calling the shots at dinnertime. We're in charge. We make these decisions."

In placing the blame for the obesity epidemic on corporate food processors, educators, and parents, Obama picked the right targets. Conventional agriculture isn't the main problem. If there were greater demand for less-processed ingredients, agribusiness companies could produce them. Nor is the USDA's jurisdiction of the program a real obstacle to reform. In the 1970s and again in 2001, the department pressed Congress for more regulatory authority over à la carte and vending machine offerings—only to come up short against the soft drink and snack food lobbies. The real problem—and the solution—is a lot closer to the school lunch lines than Washington, or America's feedlots and farm fields.

About five years ago Linda Henke, superintendent of the Maplewood–Richmond Heights School District in suburban St. Louis, decided to start mingling with her high schoolers in the lunchroom. When she saw the array of Pop-Tarts, candy, and "cheese fries" that had been mainstays on the à la carte menu for years, she was disgusted. "It was the fish not seeing the water," she says of her years-long inattention to what her students were eating. She started to lay the groundwork for some drastic changes.

Three years ago, with the help of her congressman, Russ Carnahan, a local university, and a group of family farmers desperate for new markets, Henke began making over the district's food program. She prohibited candy and chips in the cafeterias and had all vending machines but one removed. She required that all the starches come from whole grain sources and banned the purchase of chicken patties and nuggets—processed chicken, period. Whenever possible, ingredients were to be Missouri grass-fed beef and pesticide-free produce. Local sourcing would allow the staff to order whole foods, which is not always an option when purchases are made through the USDA or a distributor. This way, the district could prepare the foods as desired—apples for applesauce, tomatoes for marinara and salsa, for example—while controlling for calorie, fat, and sodium content. An à la carte line was preserved at the high school, but it no longer serves cheese fries and other junk food.

When I visited last fall, I was struck by the positive vibe around the revamped program. A teacher said he'd lost seven pounds by eating in the high school cafeteria every school day for the previous three months. A senior girl who had embraced the changes from the beginning observed that even she was surprised when football players started eating salads. The elementary school's cook of 14 years told me her job is now harder, but it's rewarding. She recounted a recent visit to the school her sister's kids attend in Indiana. "They had all this processed food that we don't serve anymore, and I was thinking, 'This is farm country! If we're city people and we can cook, why can't they?'"

These reforms have not come cheaply. The meals cost from $3.75 to $4.25 apiece to prepare. Henke's board of education has allowed her to run the program at a deficit equal to roughly one teacher's salary. But if she wants to keep using local food sources, she has to convince a consortium of schools to buy in. The farms that have been supplying Maplewood–Richmond Heights on an experimental basis need to sell their food at great volumes to turn a profit. One of Henke's selling points to other school officials? Her cafeterias are selling 10 percent more lunches.

Administrators such as Henke, Beatriz Zuluaga, and others in Kentucky, Wisconsin, and Texas have revealed some important principles. It takes a tough-minded school leader to assert that nutrient-rich food is the right choice for kids—and that it's an appropriate use of government dollars. Kids will complain initially but will come around. And a number of collateral benefits follow when students eat well. Anecdotal reports from schools with healthful and flavorful food indicate that teachers have started eating with students, attendance rates are higher, and fewer students fall asleep in class or commit vandalism and violence at school.

So far, these cafeteria visionaries are the exception. Since 2004, the USDA has administered the HealthierUS School Challenge, awarding distinction, but no money, to schools that voluntarily improve the healthfulness of their meals. By last fall, only a paltry 841 of the 101,000 schools in the National School Lunch Program (less than one percent) had received awards. That leaves a lot of schools that are still promoting Tater Tot Day and reheating frozen pizzas.

Food activists hope that the passage of the Healthy, Hunger-Free Kids Act will make a big difference. More money will buy better ingredients and pay for more staff to prepare foods from scratch. At least as important is the USDA's increased authority over the nutrition standards of all food served in schools, and the department's proposal to establish more rigorous standards, including two vegetables per meal, strict sodium limits, and, for the first time, maximum calorie counts.

It could take another generation to see meaningful change in the waistlines of American children. Yes, reform will require more government money. But at least as important is a stomachs-and-minds campaign aimed at the nation's adults: food service directors who cling to the argument that a child won't drink low-fat milk, so cookies 'n' cream–flavored milk is better than no calcium at all; parents who ask, *Why do you want to turn my kid into a vegetarian?;* and teachers who snort, *How can you serve beets to students?*

Critical Thinking

1. How much does the federal school lunch program cost the U.S. government? How many children are fed every day by this program?

2. Describe the Healthy, Hunger-Free Kids Act. How is the increased reimbursement going to be funded?

3. Explain why school lunches have changed from scratch-made food to processed, easy-to-prepare foods.

4. Compare the amount of reimbursement schools receive from the federal government with the costs of buying lunch in a restaurant.

KRISTEN HINMAN is a journalist based in Washington, D.C., who writes frequently about food. Her work has been published in *The Atlantic, The Washington Post,* and *Slate.*

Kids Who Won't Eat

KELLEY KING HEYWORTH

The cheerful drawings depicted carrots, broccoli, and other vegetables, and the childish scrawl over them read, "Good Foods!" When 9-year-old Lily showed them to her mother, Maria Adams, one spring afternoon, Adams did what any health-conscious mom might: She grinned with pride. "Lily and her friend had started 'The Healthy Eating Club,' and this was their information packet," says Adams, of Columbia, South Carolina. "I was big on natural foods, smart fats, that sort of thing. I thought, 'How cute that she's taking after me.'"

Even more impressive was Lily's follow-through. Later that day, Adams served the girls a snack of ice cream. As her playmate gobbled it up, Lily primly pushed the bowl away. "It's a bad food, Mom," she said. Over the next few weeks, Lily started refusing all treats, and at mealtime, she moved more food around her plate than she put in her mouth. "I'm not hungry" or "I just want to eat healthy," she'd say, when her parents pressed her. After a few months passed and her pickiness persisted, Adams talked to Lily's pediatrician, who connected the family with a psychologist and a dietitian. The dietitian calculated that Lily was eating only 700 calories a day—less than a third of what she needed. Adams supervised mealtime more closely, but when she managed to force her daughter to eat more than a few bites of vegetables or bread, Lily would ramp up her activity, racing her bike up and down their street, or sneaking in extra laps after swim practice. "It was like Lily suddenly had an uncontrollable urge to move," says Adams, who requested that we not use her or her daughter's real name for this story.

Within a year, Lily had grown 3 inches, but had not gained a single pound. She dropped from the 80th percentile to the 40th percentile on the growth chart. Previously a muscular little girl, she now had a jutting collarbone, prominent ribs, and a new layer of fine hair on her arms—lanugo, which the body grows as a way to help regulate its temperature. Barely out of third grade, she was diagnosed as having anorexia.

Lily's story is becoming increasingly familiar, as more and more young kids are developing anorexia, government statistics reveal. They're limiting their food intake so dramatically that they drop to a weight that's 85 percent or less of what it should be for their height, according to American Academy of Pediatrics' diagnostic criteria. Or, as they get older and more independent, they become bulimic, vomiting or using laxatives after eating an unusually large quantity of food in one sitting.

Left unchecked, bulimia may cause serious digestive and dental problems, while anorexia can lead to brittle bones, an abnormally slow heart rate, and, in 10 percent of cases, death. In fact, the National Eating Disorders Association (NEDA) says that eating disorders have the highest fatality rate of any mental illness, including depression.

It's estimated that up to 10 million Americans have an eating disorder, according to the National Association of Anorexia Nervosa and Associated Disorders, but hard data on the prevalence of these conditions in children are scarce. The number of children under 12 who were hospitalized with eating disorders more than doubled between 1999 and 2006, the biggest increase for any age group, according to the Agency for Healthcare Research and Quality. "The typical onset of anorexia used to be 13 to 17—but now it's dropped to 9 to 13," says psychotherapist Abigail Natenshon, author of *When Your Child Has an Eating Disorder,* and director of Eating Disorders Specialists of Illinois, a clinic in Highland Park. And the very youngest patients are getting younger: "We're treating 6- and 7-year-olds with anorexia, and 11- and 12-year-olds with bulimia—a problem that used to be almost nonexistent in children," says Ovidio Bermudez, M.D., medical director of child and adolescent services at the Eating Recovery Center, in Denver. "It baffles the mind." The pressure is also growing for boys, who make up 5 to 15 percent of anorexia and bulimia cases.

Unfortunately, these cases may be the tip of the iceberg. The number of children dieting or complaining about their body—considered "gateway" behaviors to anorexia and bulimia—is rising too, says Lynn Grefe, CEO of NEDA. "We're hearing about first- and second-graders who ask, 'Mommy, do I look fat in this?'" she says. "More children are displaying an unhealthy concern about food and body image. And parents are at a crossroads: They don't want their children to have eating disorders, but they don't want them to be overweight either."

Cultural Consequences

With obesity rates climbing, health experts have been pushing for the past decade for more nutrition education in schools and less fat and sugar in kids' foods. "The problem is, some kids are interpreting the message to be 'food is fattening' or 'food is the enemy,'" says Natenshon. "They'll say they don't need to eat breakfast, or think they can't eat a big meal unless they'll be burning those calories later." She describes an 11-year-old patient whose friends eat a smaller lunch on days when they don't have soccer practice. "These children are mimicking what they're seeing adults do," says Natenshon. "But kids' nutritional needs are different from those of adults. They need enough calories and fats to fuel their body, grow their bones, enter puberty, and create neuronal pathways in their developing brain."

It's hard to know how big a role the anti-obesity movement has played in the rise of eating disorders in younger kids. "The teasing that goes along with early-childhood obesity can become a trigger for food restriction and eating disorders as well," explains Natenshon. "In fact, a child's actual body weight has little or no bearing on the development of an eating disorder. The child's distorted self-perception leads to the sensation of feeling fat, even though she might be painfully thin." But obesity-prevention efforts are almost certainly contributing to delayed diagnoses, says Julie O'Toole, M.D., medical director of Portland, Oregon's Kartini Clinic for pediatric eating disorders. "Many pediatricians are so focused on curbing obesity that they'll miss an eating disorder that's right in front of them. If a child is declining rapidly on the growth chart, even if he was in a too-high percentile before, that's a red flag." Overweight kids are at special risk, because they may—out of pressure from parents or concerns about teasing—go on a diet severe enough to cause their heart to fall into a dangerously slow rhythm (a response to extreme caloric restriction, common in anorexia) before they drop enough weight to get the attention of parents and doctors, says Dr. O'Toole.

It doesn't help that celebrities aren't just thinner than ever, but younger too. "When I was a child, most of the big stars were in their late teens or older, so my friends and I didn't really compare ourselves to them," says Susan Deemer, 37, a teacher at an all-girls primary school in San Francisco and mother of a 7-year-old girl. "Now, kids have idols closer to their own age. This makes them concerned about their body at a much younger age."

The Eating-Disordered Brain

Though cultural forces may contribute to eating issues, experts now think that these disorders stem from abnormalities in the brain—and genes may be responsible. A study of twins conducted at Michigan State University found that eating disorders are 59 to 82 percent heritable. A child who has a close relative with anorexia is up to ten times more likely to get it herself.

More research is needed to find out which genes put a child at high risk. Until then, parents can recognize personality traits in their children that tend to go hand in hand with eating disorders—most often, anxiety, obsessive-compulsive disorder,

---

6 Signs of Trouble

1. **She's constantly looking in the mirror or running her hands over her body.** Sometimes referred to as "body checking," it's a way for children to monitor their weight-loss progress without stepping on the scale.
2. **He is frequently constipated.** Gut function slows down with your metabolism when you starve your body, says Dr. Ovidio Bermudez.
3. **She won't stop moving.** This can range from compulsive exercise to simply fidgeting in a chair. The child's goal is to burn calories at all times.
4. **She suddenly becomes a vegetarian.** Many anorexic children will use this as an excuse to restrict themselves from certain food groups.
5. **She doesn't get her period.** You may chalk this up to your child being an athlete. But if your daughter enters her teen years without a period or has an irregular cycle, be sure to monitor her growth on the weight chart closely with your pediatrician. Most girls start to menstruate between ages 10 and 15, with 12 being the average age.
6. **She checks out "thinspiration" or "pro-ana" websites.** The sites continue to crop up, despite advocates' efforts to ban them, and have tips for starvation plus photos of scary-thin celebs.

Nurturing a Healthy Eater

While parents don't cause eating disorders, moms and dads can push a vulnerable kid into the danger zone—or out of it, says Dr. Ovidio Bermudez. Many of the strategies for discouraging anorexia and bulimia are actually the same as those that curb overeating, he adds.

- **Model moderation.** You can help prevent hang-ups about "good" and "bad" foods by serving well-rounded meals—fruits, veggies, whole grains, lean meats—*and* treats. "There is nothing wrong with sweets in moderation," says eating-disorders expert Lynn Grefe. "Don't use a 'treat' as a reward or take it away as a punishment. It's just a food to be enjoyed."
- **Avoid the "D" word.** Talk of diets can lead to trouble. "When a mother says something as seemingly innocuous as, 'I'm skipping lunch today—my clothes are too tight,' it can have a powerful effect on her daughter's own body image," says Andrea Vazzana, Ph.D., a clinical psychologist at New York University's Child Study Center. Likewise, talk about how the right foods give you energy and keep you healthy, says Dr. Vazzana.
- **Cook for your kids and with your kids.** Keep a variety of healthy foods readily available at home, serve nutritious and well-balanced meals, and eat those meals together as often as possible, advises author Abigail Natenshon. Research shows that kids who regularly dine with their family are less likely to develop an eating disorder. Involving children in meal prep—measuring flour, pounding dough, topping a pizza—can help them learn to respect and appreciate what they're eating.

and perfectionism—and then watch for signs of eating-disorder behaviors, such as restricting certain food groups or obsessing over body size. "A child who tends to put a lot of pressure on herself might find that restricting what she eats helps her gain a sense of control over something in a satisfying way," says Dr. Bermudez.

An Intense Treatment

Today, Maria Adams credits a lot of home cooking and focused family meals for helping her anorexic daughter learn to enjoy food again. From the psychologist recommended by Lily's pediatrician, she learned about the Maudsley Method, a treatment approach that top specialists and advocacy organizations (including NEDA) consider to be especially successful in helping children, particularly those who have at least one parent who's able to be with them all day long. It required Adams, who also has a younger son, to prepare and oversee all of Lily's meals and forbid her daughter to leave the table unless she consumed a set number of calories that had been determined by her pediatrician, who weighed Lily weekly to track her progress.

The theory behind Maudsley: Malnourishment triggers illogical thinking, leading to more starvation and frenzied exercise; it's only when a child returns to a normal weight that she'll be able to respond to her natural hunger cues and reflect on her quest for thinness. Says Adams, "My mantra became, 'Food is your medicine.'"

When Lily's psychologist helped Adams realize that her own determination to eat only healthy foods might have been counterproductive in her daughter's recovery, she began to relax her rules and serve a greater variety of foods to the entire family. The early weeks were excruciating: Lily cried constantly and would often scream, "You're making me fat!" Her mom had to lock the door during meals to prevent her from running out of the house. "One day, I put a bowl of ice cream in front of her for dessert," she recalls. Six hours later, Lily downed the last soupy drop.

Within three months, Lily gained 25 pounds, returning to the 70th percentile for her age. "As soon as she hit the point where her body was naturally supposed to be, it was as if all those crazy behaviors started melting away," says Adams. During that school year, Lily got permission to eat all her meals

Early Eating Disorders

Talk to a doctor if your young child is showing signs of the following food issues.

Problem	Age of onset	What it is	Get help
Feeding disorder of infancy	Birth to 12 months	An infant refuses to eat or is unable to eat, leading to poor weight gain or significant weight loss over at least a one-month period. The cause is often an undeveloped sphincter muscle between the stomach and esophagus, or developmental delays, sensory processing disorders, or celiac disease (an autoimmune disorder that leads to an intolerance to the gluten in wheat and other grains).	Schedule regular doctors' visits to track your child's growth. A pediatric gastroenterologist can diagnose acid reflux and prescribe medication until your baby outgrows it. Occupational and speech therapists can work with children for whom eating is unpleasant or difficult.
Pica	2 to 3 years	As many as 30 percent of children at some point have pica, a compulsive tendency to eat nonfood items (such as dirt, paint chips, or laundry detergent) for one month or longer, beyond the baby years. Pica usually passes with age but can persist in developmentally delayed kids, who are also at higher risk for it.	Pica can cause lead poisoning, so keep nonfood items out of reach with high shelves and childproof locks. You may want to talk to your pediatrician or a child psychologist who specializes in eating disorders.
Selective eating disorder	3 to 10 years	A selective eater will progressively limit his diet to only a few foods. Most common in boys for reasons that remain unclear, selective eating doesn't lead to growth or health problems in most cases. There's no strong research showing that selective eaters are at risk for other eating disorders later.	Some experts say that if your child is growing normally, it's best not to make an issue of it—but find out whether your child should take a multivitamin and calcium supplement. A child psychologist can help teach him how to try new things.

at home—including lunch—but gradually, she needed less and less coaxing to eat.

Now a healthy eighth-grader, Lily plays soccer, swims competitively, and talks openly with her mother about body-image hang-ups when they arise. While Adams knows that anorexia is a chronic illness, she's grateful that she—and Lily—can now deal with a potential relapse and fight it. "Am I sad that my child had to deal with such a grown-up problem at such a young age? Yes," she says. "But I'm glad we caught it when we did."

Critical Thinking

1. Identify the six signs that a child or adolescent may exhibit if he or she is developing an eating disorder.

2. Describe steps that parents/caregivers can take to prevent the development of eating disorders in their children.

3. Define lanugo.

4. Identify the personality traits that are often linked to the development of eating disorders.

Healthy Food Looks Serious: How Children Interpret Packaged Food Products

CHARLENE D. ELLIOTT

"The fun starts here." Such was the promise—and the slogan—of Kraft Foods' 1999 campaign to promote its sweetened Post cereals to children. The campaign included, among other things, television and Internet advertising, coupon promotions, retail displays, redesigned packaging with greater "shelf impact," and cartoon stickers included in Post cereal boxes. Post's marketing push sought to capitalize on the 8.5% growth seen in its cereals from the previous year while the company affirmed its "commitment to innovation with its kid-targeted cereal brands" (Thompson, 1999b, p. 19).

This "commitment to innovation" in child-oriented food products was not unique to Kraft. The trend, which formally began in the 1950s with the sugar-laden cereals targeted at children (McNeal, 1992, p. 8), had significantly advanced by the 1999 campaign. Indeed, the fun *had* started by 1999, for in that year alone: Quaker Oats allocated U.S.$15 million just to market Cap'n Crunch Cereal (Thompson, 1999a, p. 8); Yoplait launched its enormously successful[1] GoGurt kids' yogurt tubes (Thompson, 2000, p. 30); Kellogg announced it was "bringing fun" into the cereal aisle by putting Sesame Street mini bean-bag toys into specially marked cereal boxes (Kellogg Company, 1999); and marketer James McNeal devoted an entire chapter of *The Kids Market* to careful instructions on how to "kidize" packaging. Specifically, McNeal (1999) explained how marketers could shift from the "A to K" (adult to kid) in package design, so as to better serve the "end user" (that is, the child) (p. 88).

The "fun start" promised by Post's campaign threads throughout contemporary children's food marketing. In 2001, Kraft Foods extended its "fun cereal" motif to the snack food category, with the U.S.$25 million launch of Lunchables Fun Snacks. "Some snacks have all the fun" was the slogan for these cookie or brownie snacks, which children could frost and decorate with sprinkles (Thompson, 2001, p. 45). Innovation, joined with theme of fun, is now standard in contemporary child-targeted foods. Kidized packaging is commonplace, and *fun* represents an entire category of food products. In today's supermarket, *fun foods* can be found in every food category. They populate the dry goods, dairy, meat, and refrigerated and frozen foods sections (Elliott, 2008b), and equally target every major meal. Such children's foods are not

junk or confectionary products; instead, they are regular foods whose packaging and contents specifically and unambiguously target children.

In the supermarket, children's foods are cued by their unusual product names and unconventional flavours or colours, by their cartoon images and (child-related) merchandizing tie-ins, and by their direct reference or allusion to fun/play on the package. Fun foods rest on the key themes that food is fun and eating is entertainment—these products emphasize foods' play factor, interactivity, artificiality, and general distance from ordinary or "adult" food (Elliott, 2008a; Elliott, 2008b). Yet no data has been collected on how this U.S.$15 billion industry (Gates, 2006, p. 38)[2] is influencing children's food preferences and dietary habits, or, more specifically, how children interpret the packaged food messages that are directly targeted at them. Although the childhood obesity epidemic has prompted sustained, critical scrutiny of food marketing to children (Federal Trade Commission, 2008; Harris, Pomeranz, Lobstein, & Brownell, 2009; Hastings, Stead, McDermott, Forsyth, MacKintosh, Rayner, Godfrey, Caraher, & Angus, 2003; Hawkes, 2004; Horgan, Choate, & Brownell, 2001; IOM, 2006) the focus has been predominantly on television advertising to children.[3] Even though recent studies have expanded in scope to probe online food marketing to children, such as advergaming (Alvy & Calvert, 2008; Moore, 2006) or product placement (Moore, 2004; Auty & Lewis, 2004; Tiwsakul, Hackley, & Szmigin, 2005), the powerful communicator of *food packaging* is routinely overlooked. Indeed, it appears that the only people dealing seriously and primarily with children's food packaging are the marketers themselves.[4]

Along with the tendency to overlook children's food packaging (and the types of supermarket products targeted at children), a clear gap also exists when it comes to asking children what this kid friendly food communicates to them. This reality is underscored by a recent Canadian policy consensus conference examining "Obesity and the impact of marketing on children." Hosted by the Chronic Disease Prevention Alliance of Canada (CDPAC) in March 2008, the conference assembled leading national and international experts to present the most current sociocultural, legal, and scientific evidence on the problem of marketing and childhood obesity. The panel of assessors, in developing their consensus statement, observed that:

> Advertising is but one component of marketing. Today's marketing is much more. We were not presented with any thorough research on the many dimensions of marketing in today's world, including but not limited to: pricing . . . labelling; branding, packaging; in-store displays . . . character creation and celebrity endorsements; and many other platforms that marketing now employs. (CDPAC, 2008)

The panel further remarked, "The health of Canadian children and the reduction of childhood obesity are at the centre of this discussion. In our view, the voices of children and youth themselves are missing in this process and they must be heard" (CDPAC, 2008).

It is within this context that the current research project was designed. The goal of this study extends beyond simply observing that food is marketed to children using child-friendly appeals (Elliott, 2008b; Linn & Novosat, 2008; Page, Montgomery & Ponder, 2008; Schor & Ford, 2007). Instead, it investigates how children interpret food packaging and, heeding the panel's call at CDPAC, seeks to bring children's voices into the discussion. Specifically, this project explores:

1. how children understand and respond to child-oriented foods—both in terms of packaging and the foods themselves;
2. how this understanding and response varies by age and/or gender; and
3. how children determine and classify what is healthy (both in general, and in relation to packaged goods).

Drawing from a series of focus groups of children from grades 1 to 6, separated according to age and gender, the project aims to provide some introductory probes into an overlooked topic. The question was *not* about whether fun foods contribute to childhood obesity (which is a complex, multi-factorial problem), but rather to probe the meaning and appeal of these packaged foods to children. To this end, the article first contextualizes the research on children and marketing and then outlines the research design and methodology. The research findings, along with the concluding section titled "Making sense of fun food," suggest some of the substantial implications of this type of symbolic marketing. Fun in food absolutely matters to these children, who fully appreciate the aesthetic, gustatory, tactile, and/or interactive features that these foodstuffs offer. However, although the children reveal extensive knowledge about the packaging cues they deem relevant to them, there is a remarkably limited literacy when it comes to health or nutrition. One unintended consequence of symbolically framing kids food as fun is that healthy food is seen as plain—and drab.

Contextualizing Research on Children and Food Marketing

The childhood obesity epidemic has fueled much of the recent scholarly and policy interest in food marketing to children. With 26 percent of children being over-weight or obese, Canada has one of the highest rates of childhood obesity in the developed world (Standing Committee, 2007). This problem of childhood obesity has pulled the food industry and its marketing practices into the spotlight. Food marketing is critiqued for establishing an "obesogenic" (Swinburn, Egger, & Raza, 1999) or "toxic environment" (Brownell & Horgen, 2004)—one where food is symbolically overvalued and always available (Ulijaszek, 2007). Referring specifically to childhood obesity, Schwartz and Brownell argue that the food industry makes "relentless efforts to market their brands to children" in a food environment that "promotes over-consumption of calorie-dense, nutrient-poor foods" (Schwartz & Brownell, 2007). Their critique is warranted: the Federal Trade Commission's (July 2008) report summarizing industry expenditures on marketing food to children revealed that 44 food and beverage companies spent over $1.6 billion in 2006 advertising foodstuffs directly to youth using the "full spectrum of promotional techniques and formats" (FTC, 2008). Most of these expenditures were used to promote precisely the types of poorly nutritious products that contribute to childhood obesity, including carbonated beverages, fast foods, and sugar-laden cereals.

Obesity aside, other interesting issues pertain to the relationship between food and children's perspectives, although (as previously noted) children's voices receive significantly less airtime. Even though academic research about children's culture and consumer practices/preferences has "grown at what seems to be an exponential rate" over the past two decades (Cook, 2008b, p. 220), critical studies on children's perspectives on food—especially supermarket foods—are rare. Marketing literature, however, provides some insight. Charles Atkin provided one approach in his 1978 study conducted in the supermarket, which observed parent-child "decision-making in the selection of breakfast cereals" (1978, p. 41). His study design called for unobtrusive observations of the parent-child negotiation over cereals, where a researcher (impersonating a store clerk carrying a clipboard) recorded "a verbatim description of the sequence of parent-child exchanges on a standardized form" (Atkin, 1978, p. 42). Basically, the children's voices were recorded, even though their opinions were not asked. Marketer James McNeal (1992) attempted to assess children's perspectives through a different method, using drawing exercises. McNeal asked a sample of 1,330 children (aged 4 to 12) to draw "what comes to your mind when you think about going shopping" (p. 60). A good percentage of the children (40.2%) thought of the supermarket first and crayoned supermarket carts filled with packaged goods and some produce. More recent studies (Cooke & Wardle, 2005; Wardle, Sanderson, Gibson, & Rapoport, 2001) have used food preference questionnaires to determine what foods children like—although these studies tend to focus on single foods (e.g., apples), mixed foods (e.g., lasagna), and condiments (e.g., jam) instead of packaged foods (see Cooke & Wardle, 2005).

In short, children's thoughts on supermarket packaged foods are not the subject of academic inquiry. Even Martin Lindstrom's BRANDchild, promoted as "the world's most extensive study of tween attitudes and brand relationships" (Lindstrom, 2004, p. 311),[5] does not address branded/packaged foods (with the exception of a cursory nod to branded colas). In Canada, some insight into the topic of children's preference was provided by Health Canada's Nutrition Programs Unit, which, in 1995, published the results of a national study on children's broad perceptions of healthy eating concepts (Nutrition Programs Unit, 1995). The report documented children's views about their own eating behaviours and the factors influencing their food choices. While this study proves helpful in detailing children's observations about healthy eating in general, it is now extremely dated and provides no guidance with regard to the category of packaged foods or children's interpretation of the foods (and food labels) targeted specifically at them.

Research Design and Methods

Assessing children's perspectives on packaged foods is perfectly suited to qualitative research methodology and principles. Qualitative research methods are an excellent choice when:

1. a concept or phenomenon is immature because of a lack of previous research in the area (Kitzinger, 1995);
2. the research problem fits well with the insistence in qualitative research that interpretations include the perspectives and voices of the people being studied (Lunt & Livingstone, 1996); and
3. when the nature of the concept (because of its seminal connection to the context in which it occurs) is not well suited to quantitative measures (Lunt & Livingstone, 1996).

All of these criteria apply to a study on child-responses to fun food.

In light of this, a series of focus groups were conducted with children from grades 1 to 6. Focus group research is designed to help understand what people think and why; as such, it provides an ideal research method for exploratory work on children's responses to fun food (Deacon, Pickering, Golding, & Murdock, 1999; Heary & Hennessy, 2002; Morgan, Gibbs, Maxwell, & Britten, 2002). Using a blend of random sampling and convenience sampling, a total of 36 children were recruited for 6 separate focus groups held in Ottawa in February 2007.[6] The groups were divided so that three separate focus groups were held for girls (grades 1/2, 3/4, and 5/6), and three separate focus groups were held for boys (with the same grade segmentation). This allowed the researchers to note differences in perspective according to both gender and age. (Participants were not screened specifically for family income or ethnic background.) The study was conducted in facilities where researchers could view and listen in on the groups via a two-way mirror and closed-circuit audio in an adjacent room. Heeding recommendations regarding the optimal size and length of children's focus groups (Deacon et al., 1999; Levine & Zimmerman, 1996; Morgan et al., 2002) the research design aimed for 4–6 children per group, with each session lasting approximately 60 minutes.

The focus groups were led using a customized moderator's guide that asked participants to select from and discuss various child-oriented foods and food packages. Questions probed children's food preferences, how they categorize different types of food (i.e., what they like and what they feel is healthy), and how they make sense of nutrition information/claims on fun food packaging. Specifically, children were asked to: draw their favourite dinner, conduct mock shopping trips (where they selected from an array of packages and discussed packaging appeals), sample and discuss their preferred selections of fun foods, and explain their thoughts on nutrition and nutrition information. Responses were audio-taped and subsequently transcribed (with pseudonyms used for all participants); field notes were also recorded by the researchers during and after each session. A provisional list of codes was created from the conceptual framework and the overarching

research questions outlined in the project objectives (described above), and inductive coding techniques (see Strauss & Corbin, 1998) were used to create a content analysis of particular topics. Salient themes were identified and coded following a grounded theory approach. For the purposes of this article, the goal is less to quantify the focus group findings than to provide a more nuanced exposition of children's perceptions and perspectives.

Please note that in the following discussion on the focus groups findings, for ease of readability, the term "children" refers *specifically* and solely to the children interviewed in the focus groups. As a small, exploratory study, it does not presume to speak for the preferences of all children.

What Would You Pick as Your Favourite Dinner?

At the outset of each focus group, the children were given a sheet of paper containing the image of an empty dinner plate. They were invited to draw their favourite meal and to explain why they chose the foods they did. Regardless of age or gender, children consistently drew a similar selection of foods. Pizza, fries, and "junk food" were top choices, with 84 percent of the participants selecting one (or more) of these items as constituting a favourite meal. Specific fruits and vegetables were infrequently mentioned—only 25 percent of children identified a fruit or vegetable as part of their meal. Likely this is unremarkable, since favourite meals may not contain the types of foodstuffs that children think they *ought* to eat. Yet the reasons children gave to explain *why* these foods were their favourite are worth noting. Several participants revealed that they love foods precisely because they are not "healthy" foods. In children's classification of foods, it appears junk food is enticing because it is junk (and perhaps in opposition to adult foods).

John (Grade 1) (G1): I like fries because it's junk food.

This same theme is elaborated on in the Moderator's (M) discussion with Kim (G2):

M: Can you tell us what you put on your dinner plate?
Kim (G2): Chips and treats.
M: And, why did you pick those for dinner?
Kim (G2): I like treats.
M: You like treats. What do you like the most about treats?
Kim (G2): Because they're junky.

Notions of junk were underscored by the general sense of imbalance characterizing some of the children's meals. Children were asked to draw their favourite meal, but the moderator was clear that the meal was dinner.[7] Several of the responses revealed complete indifference to balance in this meal:

M: Okay, do you want to tell us what you put for your dinner?
Shannon (G1): Pizza . . . and chicken nuggets. And, I was going to put fries. And, a spring roll.
James (G1): Donuts, fries, and chocolate. . . . I like the donut because it tastes like chocolate, and the fries are so good.
Olivia (G3): I made a pizza with a chocolate crust, caramel as a sauce, and then . . . no, wait. With chocolate sauce and caramel for the cheese.

Yet, as previously noted, the majority of children identified some variant of the "pizza/fries and something sweet/junky" (often ice cream) combination. Branded foods were notably absent from this dinnertime discussion, with the exception of four mentions (Coke [twice], Caramilk chocolate, and Rice Krispies Squares). Children in this study clearly did not associate their favourite meals with either branded food or fast foods.

Selecting from Child-Oriented Packaged Foods

At this point in the focus group, participants were asked to go on pretend shopping trips and to select the package they found most appealing. Two shopping stations were set up, displaying various fun and regular food packages of products in the same food category. To ensure participants were not influenced by the selections of others in the group, children went to each station one-by-one with a clipboard and recorded their choices in secret. They then returned to the table and explained the reasons for their selections.

Shopping Station 1 contained the same options for all of the focus groups, three boxes of chicken nuggets: a box of President's Choice® (PC) Mini Chefs™ Jungle Buddies™ breaded chicken nuggets, a box of Janes Kids© Disney© Pixar Buzz Lightyear "fun-shaped breaded" chicken nuggets, and a box of President's Choice® breaded chicken nuggets.

Shopping Station 2 contained a selection of either six children's breakfast cereals or nine fruit snacks. Breakfast cereal or fruit snack packages were rotated between groups, so as to provide a broader scope of perspectives.

It was in this pretend shopping that differences in perspectives according to age started to emerge. The youngest children (G1/2) unanimously selected the fun shaped nuggets—either PC® Mini Chefs Jungle Buddies™ or Janes Kids© Disney© Pixar Buzz Lightyear. Their focus was on the shape of the nuggets (50 percent of participants noted this) and the merchandizing tie-in with Buzz Lightyear (33%). Some children (17%) observed that the fun nuggets looked like they would taste better. The older children (G3/4 and G5/6) were less likely to indicate that they selected a package because of its fun shapes (11 percent and 13 percent, respectively), and none of them mentioned the merchandizing tie-in as a reason for their choice. For grades 3/4, all of the boys and half of the girls selected the regular chicken nuggets as their top choice—which was also the choice for all of the girls and 4 out of 6 boys in grades 5/6. The reasons provided were considerably more focused on the aesthetics of the package and/or a focus on taste: almost 56 percent of grade 3/4 participants and 67 percent of grade 5/6 participants made some direct reference to package aesthetics or the product "looking tastier" as the reason for their selection. The girls were more attuned to the package attractiveness, colour, and overall design:

Kristen (G5): I picked number 3 [the regular nuggets] because it looks pretty and, I don't know, I just like it.
M: You find the food looks pretty?
Kristen (G5): The whole box looks pretty.
Susan (G5): I liked number 3 as well; I think it looks a bit more perfect to me. It also just, looking at the way it is displayed, it looks more appetizing. The other ones just don't look as good tasting.

Kristen (G5): I also notice that it looks like it is from a restaurant because it's in a small basket with the cloth and the little vegetables in the background. That makes it look prettier.

At first blush, it appears that these children's preferences matured from a focus on fun and shapes (G1/2) to an appreciation of aesthetics and taste (G3/4 & 5/6). However, the older children's responses were deeply informed by a concern about how their selections might appear to the rest of their peer group. When it came to the chicken nuggets, the older children were resistant to selecting packages that were "too young for them."

Carly (G5): I like number 3 because I look at number 1 [Jungle Buddies] and I saw it was in animal shapes and I had that when I was four. And with the little persons [Buzz Lightyear package], I thought it looked like for little kids . . .
Hailey (G6): I had the same one as Carly. I think it is maybe because sometimes, depending on what age you are, you don't necessarily like certain shapes that maybe younger kids would like. . . . If you were to have younger kids in the group, they would have probably gone for those [the other selections].
Susan (G5): [PC nuggets] It's just more appropriate for me.

Again, this appeared to be driven solely by the children's desire to be perceived by their peers as mature. When they were asked which product they thought *their friends* might like, half of the older children selected the fun shaped nuggets instead of the plain ones, and provided rather enthusiastic explanations as to why.[8]

Children's Cereals and Fruit Snacks

Shopping Station 2 provided a greater array of packaged products, yet the children's selections (and their explanations) generally mirrored the trends observed in their first shopping venture. Grade 1/2 children were more likely to cite cross-merchandizing as a reason for choosing a product (although it was not a dominant reason), whereas older children were more likely—far more likely—to specifically comment on the packaging or package aesthetics. None of the children in grades 1 to 4 referred to packaging to explain why they selected particular cereals or fruit snacks, whereas 50 percent of the girls and 43 percent of the boys in grades 5/6 made mention of it.

Mavis (G5): [Explaining why she liked one package over the other choices] It's yeah, the colour. It makes it stand out. I think if you go to a store and you were to walk by, you wouldn't see C since the colours, well they don't pop out to you as much as the other ones do. If you have a better package for it, then someone may look at it more than people usually would.
Kristen (G5): I agree. If you had like highlighters, you would say "oh it's highlighters" . . . your eyes are attracted to it. And with the colours, why I chose B is because of the colours . . . the green and the yellow, and that's why . . .

Aesthetic reasons were also provided for why a product was not chosen:

Simon (G5): I hate the box, the box is ugly. . . . The other ones probably taste better and have a little bit more flavour.

Daniel (G5): It doesn't really stand out as much, and it [the cereal] is small, and people don't want to pick small things. It's not that interesting because there's just this bowl standing still with a bunch of cereal.

Daniel's comment reveals the degree to which fun matters to children, irrespective of the older children's desire to distance themselves from little kids' food. In fact, concerns over selecting packages that were too young were largely absent in the children's discussion of cereals and fruit snacks. It is important to emphasize that older children do *not* associate fun with little kids. (They have no problem with the concept of fun!) Moreover, all of the children showed considerable interest in the unique product claims or play aspects the packages trumpeted, as well as their surface appearance.

Shawn (G3): [Discussing Betty Crocker Tongue Talk Tattoo fruit snacks] You can get a tattoo from it and you can roll it up into a ball and suck on it. I like to put it around my finger.

James (G1): [Discussing Sun-Ripe Squiggles fruit snacks] It's junk food and I love it. It's very long and they squiggle like a worm.

Lindsay (G2): The Polly Pockets [fruit snacks] look fun because they have sparkles and everything.

Tyler (G2): [Discussing General Mills Chocolate Lucky Charms] The marshmallows are magical and each one has a power. And I like the colours on the box.

Simon (G5): [Discussing Chocolate Lucky Charms] It looks delicious.

M: What makes it look tastier than the other ones?

Simon (G5): Because of the rainbow things. And, it's in a pot of gold.

Jake (G6): It looks kinda cool. The box looks cool with streaks of colour coming out.

The Appeal of Fun Foods

Interest in surface appearance and play extended, not surprisingly, to the foods themselves. Children were asked to select their top choice from a tray containing samples of nine child-oriented cereals or fruit snacks. Selections were rotated in each session so that the children who examined cereal packages during their shopping trip sampled fruit snacks, and vice versa. (Children were able to taste/eat the snacks they selected.) Then all of the children had the opportunity to choose from an array of child-oriented yogurts or pudding snacks (and taste their choice). No packages or identifying material accompanied the samples; children selected them based on the look of the foodstuff alone. (An exception is the yogurts/puddings, which were individually packaged in tubes or cups.)

Again, the theme of play factored strongly; children were intrigued by the foods' unusual colours and shapes and often indicated that they selected a sample because of these unique characteristics. The more unusual the colour or unique the feature, the better. Ryan (G5) selected pudding because "the [blue] colour stood out, and it looked good"; Jake (G6) picked pink pudding for the same reason ("the pink stood out"). Some participants were drawn to Yogo's fruit snacks because of their "neat" multi-colours, but also because "you can throw them up in the air" (Kim, G2) or because "they look like you can roll them" (Brendan, G2). In short,

a general feeling expressed in all the focus groups is that fun or play remains an important variable.

Interactivity versus Aesthetics

Differences in gender emerged in the discussion of why certain products were chosen over others. Interest in a food's interactivity was substantially more pronounced for boys, whereas girls (particularly the older ones [G5/6]) generally focused on the aesthetic qualities of food. In the case of the yogurt/pudding samples, all children were invited to select from nine products. This included yogurt in brightly coloured portable tubes (Babang and Kaboum flavours), as well as Squeeze N Go pudding (also in a tube). A number of portable pudding snacks (in clear plastic) were offered, including bubblegum and cotton candy flavours (coloured bright pink and robin blue, respectively), Chocolate Splat! pudding (brown), and layered parfait-style puddings (one chocolate and vanilla, and the other, Oreo cookie layered puddings). Gendered differences to these options were remarkable. All of the boys (except two) chose the yogurt or pudding *tubes*— packages that allowed kids to squirt its contents into their mouths (often holding the tubes far up in the air with head tilted back to catch it), or squeeze the product onto their lips, or suck it up all in at once, as if through as straw. Although the boys did not usually articulate that the tube motivated their choice, they were absolutely drawn to this form of packaging.[9]

In contrast, all of the girls selected the parfait-style puddings. Unlike Eric's (G4) observation that "when things look fancier, they taste worse," the girls appreciated the "pretty" components of the product, and the fact that (unlike the squirtable tubes) they could be savoured:

Gwen (G4): [Discussing the chocolate/vanilla parfait pudding] I can enjoy it more and I can save it for later, but with the tubes, it finishes very fast.

Isabella (G6): I thought it was a pretty package.

M: So, you like the colour? Why did you pick it over the tube things?

Isabella (G6): I like the stripes.

Mavis (G5): I thought it was interesting how it had stripes. . . . It looked the most appetizing.

The girls also were more likely to discuss the associational values evoked by the food/package, noting it reminded them of something (be it a movie, family outing, feeling, et cetera). This did not happen with the boys, who provided more concrete explanations or focused on what they could do with the product (i.e., squeeze it, stretch it, twist it, play with it).

Vivienne (G1): [Discussing Oreo striped parfait pudding] I picked it because me and my friend went to a farm of cows, and it reminded me of the cow. Sometimes they are black and white.

Kristen (G5): [Discussing Jungle Buddies chicken nuggets] It looks funner because I like animals. And because, well actually, for the other box [of Buzz Lightyear shaped nuggets] in class we are doing space and it makes me think of homework.

Melissa (G2): [Discussing Froot Loops cereal] At school we made a necklace with Froot Loops, and at the end we got to eat it.

Classifying Healthy: In General, and for Packaged Foods

Classifying healthy is another important question when it comes to probing children's interpretations of packaged food—and food in general. Cereals, fruit snacks, yogurts, cheeses, canned pasta, frozen meals, packaged lunches—all offer fun food for sale. Yet no published research assesses how children classify what is healthy and not healthy in this vast array of consumables. Given this, the focus groups also probed what children consider to be healthy food and how they make sense of the healthfulness of packaged goods.

Without question, Canadians are concerned about food's health qualities. The latest *Tracking Nutrition Trends* surveyed over 2,000 Canadians (18 years and older) and reported that 91% of those polled deemed a food's "healthfulness" either "somewhat important" or "very important" when choosing what to eat (CCFN, 2008, p. 3). But healthfulness is a nebulous concept, both for adults (see CCFN, 2008, p. 2) and for children. Indeed, the children in this study showed a limited understanding of the health qualities of food. When asked to name a healthy food and explain why it was healthy, 67% of the children named a fruit or a vegetable, 17% named bread or pasta, and 7% named yogurt or cheese. Fifteen percent of children said "they didn't know"—comments made more interesting given that the focus group setting allows children to echo another child's response, should they desire.[10]

With 67% of participants naming a fruit or vegetable as a healthy food, it perhaps seems odd to argue that they have limited understanding of the health qualities of food. Yet this logic becomes clear when one considers the range of foods identified: specific fruits and vegetables were mentioned, but dairy, whole grains, lean meats, and fish were rarely given as examples of healthy foods. Consider, too, children's explanations of *why* the food is healthy.

Stuart (G3): Carrots, because it's a vegetable.

Melissa (G2): Apples. . . because, fruits are good for you.

Ryan (G5): I would say fruits and vegetables, because everybody says they're healthier for you.

Mavis (G5): Broccoli. It's a green vegetable, and I heard they are healthy.

Simon (G5): Pasta, because it's good for you . . . I think.

While a number of children (starting from grades 3 up) observed that fruits or vegetables are healthy because they have "vitamins" (and two children identified calcium as the reason cheese/yogurt is healthy), 70% of the children either did not know why the item they selected was healthy or provided a self-evident answer (i.e., oranges because they're fruit). This lack of knowledge over healthy extended to children's evaluation of packages and nutritional claims as well.

"The Box Looks Serious": Children Discuss How to Tell If a Packaged Product Is Good for You

When asked what they looked for on packaging to help them determine whether the food is healthy or not, children pointed to a number of important clues. They mentioned the ingredient list (22%) or the presence of a "smart check" or symbol (17%). Some children conflated the absence of (allergy-inducing) ingredients with product healthfulness, with 14% saying that "a peanut with a circle and a line" on a package is a clue that a food is healthy.

Zack (G5): One of the rules that I always was taught is if there's big words, like really big words that you can't pronounce, it's probably another way to say sugar.

Awareness of the nutrition facts table was remarkably low: only 8% of children (all from grades 5/6) named the nutrition facts table as means of evaluating whether a product is "good for you." While this suggestion was well received by the other participants in the grades 5/6 focus group (some nodded agreement or verbally called out in affirmation), the children could not actually explain what the nutrition facts table "meant." They simply knew to look for it on packages, because they had learned it at school (and for some, at home).

This said, children provided remarkably sophisticated—although not necessarily accurate—explanations about how to tell if a packaged food is healthy. Some of the answers (from 16% of the children, mostly grades 1/2) were completely wrong headed:

Christine (G1): You can tell [it's healthy] by the front cover. If [the food] is shaped, then it may have been cut with a dirty knife.

Yet most of the statements demonstrated a savvy reasoning, even if the answers were incorrect. Kim (G6) used calories as the sole indicator of health ("it has only 130 calories per serving, which makes it really healthy"), whereas 20% of the children relied on some aspect of the package *image* to determine healthy:

Katie (G3): If the box looks serious [it's a healthy food].

Christine (G1): Green means it's healthy.

Brendan (G2): When there is green on the box, it means it's healthy.

Joshua (G3): [Explaining why Honeycomb cereal was a healthy choice] It has honey on the box.

Several children suggested that they can simply tell by looking.

Susan (G5): Usually I know what's healthy; even if you look at the picture you can tell.

Travis (G3): [The box] *looks* really good and healthy.

This reliance on the visual assessments and associational indicators of health also played out in the children's selection of foods. If a serious package or its colour could indicate healthfulness for some children, then so could look of the foodstuff itself. Jake (G6) picked the Kellogg's Fruit Winders fruit snack to eat because, even though he thought the Froot Loops fruit snack "probably tasted better," the Fruit Winders "*looked better for you.*"[11] Zack (G5) explained that Honeycomb cereal was healthy because it was brown. The flipside also held true. Gwen (G4) explained that Lucky Charms cereal probably was *not* healthy "because they have covered the marshmallows in food colouring."

"It Says Fat Free, So You Won't Get Fat": Children's Understanding of Nutrition Claims

Front-of-package labelling has become ubiquitous in recent years, as food manufacturers strive to position their products to capitalize on consumers' interest in health. Canada's decade-old Health Check program (governed by the Heart and Stroke Foundation) exists to "help consumers make healthy food choices within food categories, at the point of purchase, across all eligible food categories" (Heart and Stroke Foundation, 2008, pp. 3–4). Numerous other front-of-pack "nutrition symbols" or food rating systems also exist, since food manufacturers have each created their own logos, slogans, or symbols—as well as their own criteria—as a strategy to communicate a food's health-fulness to consumers.

While certain scholars have criticized the validity of nutrition claims in general (see Elliott, 2008a; Nestle, 2002; Pollan, 2008; Smith, Stephen, Dombrow, & MacQuarrie, 2002), they are also promoted as a strategy for improving people's diets. Even the Standing Committee on Health, which issued the *Healthy Weights for Healthy Kids* report in 2007, suggests that "Increas[ing] Awareness Through Front of Package Labelling" can help to promote healthy weights in children (Standing Committee on Health, 2007, p. 22) and is something that "must be done" to "tackle the issue of childhood obesity" (p. 18).

But this imperative seems wrong-headed, since children in this study revealed little understanding of the meaning of nutrition claims. First, (as earlier noted) they rarely referred to nutrition symbols in explaining the *clues* to use in evaluating whether a packaged food was healthy (17%). When directly asked about particular symbols found on the packaged foods being examined, children were rarely able to demonstrate a comprehension of what it *means* for food to be fat free, organic, or made with whole grains, etc. Children would literally read the claim ("it says fat free") and then come up with their own, reasonable, explanations. Discussing a round, orange symbol that proclaimed *FAT FREE,* participants observed:

Matthew (G1): It says fat free so you won't get fat.
Abigail (G3): You won't get any fatter if you're already very fat.
Geoff (G4): It means you won't get fat.

Regarding a green *CERTIFIED ORGANIC* logo:

Zack (G5): I've not seen it before, but I can tell that it is a sponsor saying that something about this is true. Like for that it means it is good quality food. That company probably has taste testers.
Daniel (G5): I'm not 100% sure what it is. But it says certified organic. So that means organic food and it was tested and looked at to make sure that it actually is organic and it's not just flavours that make it look organic or taste organic.
Kristen (G5): The label is green so it's not mass produced in some greenhouse.

There was also the tendency to assume the symbols cued other diet or health-related qualities. Jake (G6) interpreted the *FAT FREE*

symbol to mean "low in calories, [so] it's good for you." Vivienne (G1), and many others, equated the symbol with healthy ("it means it is really healthy"). Judging from the discussion in these focus groups, it appears that front-of-package labelling is of little help to children in accurately assessing the health of a product. Most of the children did not notice the claims on their own. It is worth noting, however, that some of the older female participants (G5/6) engaged in a lengthy, critical discussion over the use of several nutrition claims on the front of a particular box of sugared cereal. They dismissed the claims as lacking in credibility.

Susan (G5): No one's going to believe it.
Hailey (G6): I don't believe it since chocolate is unhealthy and marshmallows are unhealthy. The only thing healthy is the milk. It's just to get you to buy it.

Yet this was the *only* group to discuss the credibility of package claims. Remarkably, no such skepticism was voiced regarding any of the other semiotic elements on the package.

Making Sense of Fun Food: Discussion and Implications

Although a small-scale study, these focus groups provide fascinating insight into how children make sense of fun food and its packaging. As the sales figures attest, parents and care-givers are certainly purchasing these supermarket products for their children. Children, in turn, show deep appreciation for the aesthetic, gusta-tory, tactile and/or interactive features that these foodstuffs offer. The focus groups consistently revealed how passionate children can be about food; they spoke enthusiastically and extensively about their favourite edibles and about why they selected particular packages. "Loving" food was articulated repeatedly (e.g., "I *love* chocolate," "I *love* the cheese [on pizza]," "It's junk food, and I *love* it," "They're yummy, and I'm in *love* with them").

These children were equally interested in taste, primarily explaining their selections in light of personal taste preferences (i.e., appreciation for chocolate, marshmallows, sweetness, sour-ness). The food package's *look* factored strongly in the children's comments about taste, and they were very clear about what *looked* tastier. This said, a discernable evolution was present in terms of the appreciation of the aesthetic qualities of packaging. While younger children were more likely to be attracted to cross-merchandizing techniques (i.e., Buzz Lightyear, Spiderman, or Polly Pocket) and fun shapes, older children contemplated the over-all look of the package—its colours, design, and their appreciation (or not!) of its images. The oldest girls in particular demonstrated a fairly sophisticated aesthetic sense, commenting on whether products looked tasty and selecting items based on overall display—be it the "pretty" package or "appetizing" nature of the parfait puddings "with the stripes."

Although a clear progression existed with regard to aesthetic appreciation, this study did not reveal any discernable evolution in terms of actual taste. Children, regardless of age, showed, and said, that they *loved* chocolate, junk food, and sugary cereals/fruit snacks/puddings. They did not grow out of chocolate Lucky Charms cereal by Grade 6, for example—virtually every child in the study (92%) selected it as their top choice.

Of course, the central interest in this study pivoted on children's interpretation of and responses to fun food—and the focus groups revealed that fun *absolutely* matters to children. Food holds a special position in children's lives, and not for nutritive reasons. As Newton (1992) argues in her discussion of popular culture foodways:

> Playing with food—by learning the 'rules' for eating Oreo cookies or spaghetti or Jell-O—quickly becomes part of a child's repertoire of play behaviour. Although this food play is not approved of in most households, often adults and children have a tacit understanding about Jell-O: Jell-O for dessert is license to play. (p. 253)

Yet as the proliferation of fun food underscores, no longer is a "license to play" reserved for Oreos or Jell-O. Scholars such as Buckingham (2000), Seiter (1993), and others have long emphasized that cultural constructions of childhood are defined in opposition to adulthood. This opposition also unfolds with regard to food, and is reinforced by child-oriented food marketing. As Schor and Ford (2007) observe, the symbolic marketing characterizing children's food persuades children "to eat particular foods, not on the basis of their tastiness, or other benefits, but because of their place in a social matrix of meaning" (p. 16). This "place," I suggest, resides squarely within the theme of fun. Food marketers design and offer up fun food for consumption, and in many ways children are merely acting out the scripts provided for them. But these scripts clearly resonate with children.

Researchers probing the relationship between food advertising and childhood obesity affirm that "today, children opt for their own preferred food and drink rather than acquiescing to parental preferences" (Eagle, Bulmer, de Bruin, & Kitchen, 2004, p. 52), and the focus group participants patently demonstrated that these foods were of utmost appeal. Boys were particularly drawn to the interactivity (and transgressive eating practices) promised by the food products; they also liked foods because of their strange colours and "cool" shapes. Girls were more likely to choose products because of their pretty colours and general aesthetic appeal. The fun resided in the colours, "in the sparkles" and the associational elements the food presented—be it a memory, a personal experience with family/friends/at school, or a link to a movie. As a whole, the children were highly attuned to the range of cues that made food fun, quickly identifying the Polly Pocket or SpongeBob Squarepants fruit snacks, the "gushing" quality of Betty Crocker's Fruit Gushers, or the fun tattoo feature of Betty Crocker's Tongue Talk Tattoo Fruit Roll-Ups. Many could (and would spontaneously) identify the special "power" represented by each marshmallow in Lucky Charms. These responses reveal the degree to which young children are embedded in a world of commercial marketing/media—but the children's interest in the packages and products themselves (e.g., colours, interactivity, aesthetics, et cetera) did not stem solely from cross-merchandising or advertising appeals.

While the children discussed the fun aspects of food at length, their understanding of health was quite limited. Their ideal meals certainly did not reflect Canada's Food Guide recommendations, and their discussion of healthy foods often comprised self-evident claims. But it is their evaluation of *how to determine if a packaged food is healthy* that is the most remarkable because, while the nutrition facts table or ingredient list was given a cursory nod, children favoured their own interpretive accounts. These accounts equally tended to conflate certain markers with "healthy"

(e.g., green = healthy, serious = healthy). Policy recommendations for more front-of-pack labelling (such as those suggested by the Standing Committee on Health, 2007) may influence adult food selections, but such labels certainly did not lead to more informed food choices with the children interviewed in these focus groups. Indeed, children's misunderstanding of nutrition (communicated through symbols/logos) also played out in their discussions of why they might pick certain products over another. For instance, Honeycomb cereal was identified as a healthier choice by several participants because of the honey pictured on the box or because it was coloured brown. Alpha Bits cereal was preferred by one participant *because,* she argued, "I don't really like sugared cereals." These kinds of responses underscore the opportunity for further education for children when it comes to determining healthy foods. As already mentioned, the children were highly literate when it came to deciphering packages—just not in the right arenas.

In fairness, the food industry has complicated the issue by putting front-of-pack nutrition claims on products that children do *not* identify as "good for you." So-called "goodness corners" on boxes of sugary, marshmallow-laden cereals are a case in point, and some older children rightfully observed that the presence of these claims worked to undermine the credibility of the product as a whole. But the bigger issue is that children do not associate fun—or fun food—with nutrition. The more fun the package and product appears to be, the less children correlate it with health or classify it as a healthy selection. This raises some interesting challenges for food manufacturers who have developed "fun *and* healthy" product lines for children, but use the exact same techniques (such as cartoon images, unusual shapes, fun product names, wild colours, et cetera) to cue children's food to children and their parents. To reiterate one of the more interesting claims made in the focus groups, some of the children observed that they could tell if a product was healthy simply by seeing whether the package looked serious or not. Serious packages, for children, are healthy food packages. Fun packages, regardless of the presence of nutrition claims, are not evaluated under the lens of health.

But the biggest issue underpinning this fun food marketing is the question of meaning. What are the implications of promising (as did Post's cereal campaign) that "the fun starts here"? There is certainly something problematic about positioning food mainly as fun. Eating for entertainment (or distraction) is one of the main drivers of the current obesity epidemic, and it leads to a distorted relationship with food. (Like food marketing in general, fun food marketing also does not address any notion of portion control.) The fact that children are being taught, through fun food messages, to value food strictly for its play factor is troubling; children learn taste preferences very early on, and they persist over time. When we teach children that "the fun starts" when they sit down in front of processed and pointedly artificial food—comprised of strange shapes, bizarre colours, or magical qualities—we are leading them down a dangerous path. Healthy food, as one child observed, *does* look serious, and (especially in light of the childhood obesity epidemic) it is critical that *serious* food be given prominence in the social matrix of meaning that defines children's fare.

Notes

1. Described as "kid-targeted slurpable yogurt in a tube," Yoplait's Go-Gurt captured $100 million in retail sales within eight months of its launch, "bolstering General Mills to No. 1 in

refrigerated yogurt ahead of Dannon Co." and "trigger[ing] a new growth phase for the category as a whole" (Thompson, 2000, p. 30).

2. Data are not available on the overall sales of fun foods in Canadian supermarkets. However, the sales of food individual brand lines are equally striking. Fun yogurts targeted at children—such as Yoplait's Go-Gurt and Dannon's D'animals line—had sales of U.S.$99.9 million and $94 million, respectively, for the 52-week period ending in March 2007 (Cultured products shine, 2007, p. 16). In Canada, the Toronto-based NDP group identified fruit snacks/rolls as one of the fastest growing snack foods (Cooper, 2006, p. 6). And Canada's President's Choice Mini Chefs brand—launched nationally in December 2004 and targeted specifically at children—has since tripled the number of products in the line.

3. See, for example, Batada, Seitz, Wootan, & Story, 2008; Botterill & Kline, 2006; Consumers International, 1996; Cook, 2008a; Harris, 2008; Gantz, Schwartz, Angelini, & Rideout, 2007; IOM, 2006; Kotz & Story, 1994; Livingstone, 2005; Powell, Szczypka, Chaloupka, & Braunschweig, 2007. As the U.S.-based Institute of Medicine *Committee on Food Marketing and the Diets of Children and Youth* reported "television advertising remains the dominant form of marketing reaching children . . . that is formally tracked" (IOM, 2006, p. 15).

4. In 2006, Palmer and Carpenter observed that marketers spend "over $3 billion annually to design food product packaging that children and youth will want to purchase" (2006, p. 167)—a figure that has undoubtedly increased, particularly in light of the number of supermarket food brands (or sub-brands) aimed exclusively at children. These include, for example, Loblaw's highly popular President's Choice Mini Chefs brand, Safeway's Eating Right Kids line, Nature's Path EnviroKidz brand and Earth's Best Sesame Street line of children's foods.

5. The BRANDchild study spanned seven countries and interviewed thousands of children.

6. Ethics approval and written parental consent was obtained prior to holding the focus groups. Recruits for the convenience sample comprised 32 of the 36 children and were drawn from acquaintances of the research company (Delta Media Inc.) that hosted and moderated the focus groups. To completely fill the groups, four children were recruited randomly using a standard telephone directory listing for Ottawa.

7. The moderator's instructions included: "So, if you could choose what you would have for dinner, what would it be? . . . Remember, there are no right or wrong answers, just do your best to draw your favourite dinner."

8. This enthusiasm over kids' food (despite what the older children might have said) was demonstrated throughout the focus groups. At points, the children were literally crawling on the table to get their first pick of the cereals.

9. The remaining two boys were drawn to the most unnatural shades of pudding—blue and pink.

10. The percentage breakdown (67% fruit/vegetable; 17% bread/pasta; 7% yogurt/cheese; and 15% "don't know") adds up to more than 100 because some children provided more than one example of a healthy food.

11. Neither product was a healthy choice, owing to the high proportion of calories coming from sugar and the fact that the fruit snack would be better classified as a fruit-flavoured snack.

References

Alvy, Lisa & Calvert, Sandra L. (2008). Food marketing on popular children's websites: A content analysis. *Journal of the American Dietetic Association, 108*(4), 710–713.

Atkin, Charles. (1978). Observation of parent-child interaction in supermarket decision-making. *Journal of Marketing, 42*(4), 41–45.

Auty, Susan & Lewis, Charlie. (2004). Exploring children's choice: The reminder effect of product placement. *Psychology & Marketing, 21*(9), 697–713.

Batada, Ameena, Seitz, M. D., Wootan, Margo, & Story, M. (2008). Nine out of 10 food advertisements shown during Saturday morning children's television programming are for foods high in fat, sodium, or added sugars, or low in nutrients. *Journal of the American Dietetic Association, 108*(4), 673–678.

Botterill, Jacqueline & Kline, Stephen. (2006). *Flow, branding and media saturation: Towards a critical analysis of promotional marketing in children's television.* Paper presented at Child and Teen Consumption, 2006, Copenhagen Business School.

Brownell, Kelly, & Horgen, Katherine Battle. (2004). *Food fight: The inside story of the food industry, America's obesity crisis and what we can do about it.* New York: Contemporary Books.

Buckingham, David. (2000). *After the death of childhood.* Cambridge: Polity Press.

CCFN (Canadian Council of Food and Nutrition). (2008). *Tracking nutrition trends VII.* Woodbridge, ON: CCFN.

CDPAC (Chronic Disease Prevention Alliance of Canada). (2008). *Obesity and the impact of marketing on children: Policy consensus statement.* Ottawa, ON. URL: www.cdpac.ca/media .php?mid=433 [August 2009].

Consumers International. (1996). *A spoonful of sugar: Television food advertising aimed at children—An international comparative study.* London: Consumers International.

Cook, Brian. (2008a). *Overview of television food advertising to children.* Championing Public Health Nutrition Conference, October 22–23, Ottawa, ON. URL: www.cspinet.org/ canada/2008conference/presentation/BCook.pdf [August 2009].

Cook, Daniel. (2008b). The missing child in consumption theory. *Journal of Consumer Culture, 8*(2), 219–243.

Cooke, Lucy & Wardle, Jane. (2005). Age and gender differences in children's food preferences. *British Journal of Nutrition, 93,* 741–746.

Cooper, Carolyn. (2006). Snack attack. *Food in Canada, 66*(1), 7.

Cultured products shine on. (2007). *Dairy Foods, 108*(7), 16.

Deacon, David, Pickering, Michael, Golding, Peter & Murdock, Graham. (1999). *Researching communications: A practical guide to methods in media and cultural analysis.* London: Arnold.

Eagle, Lynne, Bulmer, Sandy, de Bruin, Anne & Kitchen, Philip. (2004). Exploring the link between obesity and advertising in New Zealand. *Journal of Marketing Communications, 10*(1), 49–67.

Elliott, Charlene. (2008a). Assessing fun foods: Nutritional content and analysis of supermarket foods targeted at children. *Obesity Reviews, 9,* 368–377.

Elliott, Charlene. (2008b). Marketing fun food: A profile and analysis of supermarket food messages targeted at children. *Canadian Public Policy, 34*(2), 259–274.

(FTC) Federal Trade Commission. (2008). Marketing food to children and adolescents: A review of industry expenditures, activities, and self-regulation: A Federal Trade Commission Report to Congress. URL: www.ftc.gov/os/2008/07/ P064504foodmktingreport.pdf.

Gantz, Walter, Schwartz, Nancy, Angelini, James & Rideout, Victoria. (2007). *Food for thought: Television food advertising to children in the United States.* Menlo Park, CA: Kaiser Family Foundation. URL: www.kff.org/entmedia/upload /7618.pdf [August 2009].

Gates, Kelly. (2006, October 30). Tempting tummies. *Supermarket News, 54*(44), 39–48.

Harris, Jennifer. (2008). *Children and food advertising effects: When are they old enough to resist?* Championing Public Health Nutrition Conference, October 22–23, Ottawa, ON. URL: www.cspinet.org/canada/2008conference/presentation/Harris.pdf [August 2009].

Harris, Jennifer L., Pomeranz, Jennifer L., Lobstein, Tim & Brownell, Kelly D. (2009). A crisis in the marketplace: How food marketing contributes to childhood obesity and what can be done. *Annual Review of Public Health, 30,* 211–225.

Hastings, Gerard, Stead, Martine, McDermott, Laura, Forsyth, Alasdair, MacKintosh, Anne Marie, Rayner, Mike, Godfrey, Christine, Caraher, Martin, & Angus, Kathryn. (2003). *Review of Research on the Effects of Food Promotion to Children, Final Report.* [Prepared for the UK Food Standards Authority]. London: UK Food Standards Authority; Glasgow, Scotland: Centre for Social Marketing, University of Strathclyde. URL: www.food.gov.uk/multimedia/pdfs/foodpromotiontochildren1.pdf [August 2009].

Hawkes, Corinna. (2004). *Marketing foods to children: The global regulatory environment.* Geneva, Switzerland: World Health Organization.

Heart and Stroke Foundation. (2008). *Assessing the impact of the Health Check food information program.* URL: www.hsf.ca/research/images/PDF/final%20rfp%20sept%2025%2008%20eg.pdf [August 2009].

Heary, Caroline & Hennessy, Eilis. (2002). The use of focus group interviews in pediatric health care research. *Journal of Pediatric Psychology, 27*(1), 47–57.

Horgen, Katherine Battle, Choate, Molly, & Brownell, Kelly. (2001). Television food advertising: Targeting children in a toxic environment. In D.G. Singer & J.L. Singer (Eds.), *Handbook of children and the media.* Thousand Oaks, CA: Sage.

IOM (Institute of Medicine). (2006). *Food marketing to children and youth: Threat or opportunity?* Washington, DC: National Academies Press.

Kellogg Company brings fun back into the cereal aisle with Sesame Street Mini-Beans in-pack premium offer. (1999, December 8). *Business Wire.* URL: http://findarticles.com/p/articles/mi_m0EIN/is_1999_Dec_8/ai_58079654 [August 2009].

Kitzinger, Jenny. (1995). Qualitative research: Introducing focus groups. *British Medical Journal, 311,* 299–302.

Kotz, Krista & Story, Mary. (1994). Food advertisements during children's Saturday morning television programming: Are they consistent with dietary recommendations? *Journal of the American Dietetic Association, 94,* 1296–1300.

Levine, I. S., & Zimmerman, J. D. (1996). Using qualitative data to inform public policy: Evaluating Choose to De-Fuse. *American Journal of Orthopsychiatry, 66*(3), 363–377.

Lindstrom, Martin. (2004). *BRANDchild.* London: Kogan Page.

Linn, Susan & Novosat, Courtney. (2008). Calories for sale: Food marketing to children in the twenty-first century. *The Annals of the American Academy of Political and Social Science, 615,* 133–155.

Livingstone, Sonia. (2005). Assessing the research base for the policy debate over the effects of food advertising to children. *International Journal of Advertising, 24*(3), 273–296.

Lunt, Peter, & Livingstone, Sonia. (1996). Rethinking the focus group in media and communications research. *Journal of Communication, 46*(2), 79–98.

McNeal, James. (1992). *Kids as customers: A handbook of marketing to children.* New York: Lexington Books.

McNeal, James. (1999). *The kids market: Myths and realities.* Ithaca, NY: Paramount Market Publishing.

Moore, Elizabeth S. (2004). Children and the changing world of advertising. *Journal of Business Ethics, 52*(2), 161–167.

Moore, Elizabeth S. (2006). *It's child's play: Advergaming and the online marketing of foods to children.* Menlo Park, CA: Kaiser Family Foundation. URL: www.kff.org/entmedia/7536.cfm [August 2009].

Morgan, Myfanwy, Gibbs, Sara, Maxwell, Krista & Britten, Nicky. (2002). Hearing children's voices: Methodological issues in conducting focus groups with children aged 7–11 years. *Qualitative Research, 2*(1), 5–20.

Nestle, Marion. (2002). *Food politics: How the food industry influences nutrition and health.* Berkeley: University of California Press.

Newton, Sarah E. (1992). The Jell-O Syndrome: Investigating popular culture/foodways. *Western Folklore, 51*(3/4), 249–267.

Nutrition Programs Unit. (1995). Food for thought: Results of a national study on children and healthy eating. *Report.* Ottawa, ON: Nutrition Programs Unit, Health Canada.

Page, Randy, Montgomery, Katie, Ponder, Andrea & Richard, Amanda. (2008). Targeting children in the cereal aisle: Promotional techniques and content features on ready-to-eat cereal product packaging. *American Journal of Health Education, 39*(5), 272–282.

Palmer, Edward & Carpenter, Courtney. (2006). Food and beverage marketing to children and youth: Trends and issues. *Media Psychology, 8,* 165–190.

Pollan, Michael. (2008). *In defense of food.* New York: Penguin.

Powell, Lisa, Szczypka, Glen, Chaloupka, Frand J., & Braunschweig, Carol L. (2007). Nutritional content of television food advertisements seen by children and adolescents in the United States. *Pediatrics, 120,* 576–583.

Schor, Juliet & Ford, Margaret. (2007). From tastes great to cool: Children's food marketing and the rise of the symbolic. *Journal of Law, Medicine & Ethics, 35*(1), 10–21.

Schwartz, Marlene & Brownell, Kelly. (2007). Actions necessary to prevent childhood obesity: Creating the climate for change. *Journal of Law, Medicine & Ethics, 35*(1), 78–89.

Seiter, Ellen. (1993). Utopia or discrimination? Commercials for kids. In E. Seiter, *Sold separately: Children and parents in consumer culture* (pp.115–144). New Jersey: Rutgers University Press.

Smith, Shannon, Stephen, Alison M., Dombrow, Carol & MacQuarrie, Doug. (2002). Food information program. *Canadian Journal of Dietetic Practice and Research, 63*(2), 55–60.

Standing Committee on Health, House of Commons. (2007, March). Healthy weights for healthy kids. *Report.* Ottawa, ON: Rob Merrifield (Chair). URL: http://cmte.parl.gc.ca/Content/HOC/committee/391/hesa/reports/rp2795145/hesarp07/hesarp07-e.pdf [August 2009].

Strauss, Anselm & Corbin, Juliet. (1998). *Basics of qualitative research: Techniques and procedures for developing grounded theory* (2nd ed.). Thousand Oaks, CA: Sage.

Swinburn, B. A., Egger, G., & Raza, F. (1999). Dissecting the obesogenic environments: The development and application of a framework for identifying and prioritizing environmental interventions for obesity. *Preventative Medicine, 29,* 563–570.

Thompson, Stephanie. (1999a). Cap'n goes AWOL as sales flatten; Quaker redirects cereal brand's marketing budget to focus on kids. *Advertising Age, 70*(48), 8.

Thompson, Stephanie. (1999b). Kraft-y promo: Post gives coins for 'comb.' *Advertising Age, 70*(41), 19.

Thompson, Stephanie. (2000). Go-Gurt. *Advertising Age, 71*(27), 30.

Thompson, Stephanie. (2001). Kraft launches Lunchables for *snack* attacks. *Advertising Age, 72*(11), 45.

Tiwsakul, Rungpaka, Hackley, Chris, & Szmigin, Isabelle. (2005). Explicit, non-integrated product placement in British television programmes. *International Journal of Advertising, 24*(1), 95–111.

Ulijaszek, Stanley. (2007). Obesity: A disorder of convenience. *Obesity Reviews, 8*(1), 183–187.

Wardle, J., Sanderson, S., Gibson, E. L., & Rapoport, L. (2001). Factor-analytic structure of food preferences in four-year-old children in the UK. *Appetite, 37,* 217–223.

Critical Thinking

1. What are "fun foods"?

2. What are some marketing techniques that make foods interactive and concentrate on play rather than nutrition?

3. Explain why positioning "food as fun" and "eating as entertainment" to kids could have negative consequences to taste perceptions/preferences and long-term outcomes on their health.

CHARLENE D. ELLIOTT is Associate Professor of Communication Studies at the University of Calgary.

Acknowledgments—Funding for this research was generously provided by the Canadian Institutes of Health Research. The author would like to thank Bernie Gauthier for his assistance in coordinating and overseeing the focus groups.

UNIT 3
Nutrients

Unit Selections

Learning Outcomes

After reading this Unit, you will be able to:

- Describe the health benefits of potassium, vitamin D, magnesium, and B-12.

- Defend the concept that consuming certain nutrients from foods is better than consuming them from supplements or fortified foods.

- Critique the proposed negative effects of folic acid fortification of U.S. cereal grains with the positive effect.

- Explain why the type of research that is conducted is the most important consideration when reviewing information about research on nutrients.

- Compare and contrast epidemiological or observational studies with randomized intervention-based clinical trials.

- Identify the four groups that should pay particular attention to sodium content of foods and consume no more than 1,500 mg of sodium per day, as recommended in the Dietary Guidelines for Americans.

- Describe the health benefits of consuming monounsaturated and omega-3 fatty acids.

- List the benefits of consuming docosahexaenoic acid and identify the best food sources for this long-chain omega-3 fatty acid.

Student Website

www.mhhe.com/cls

Internet References

Dietary Supplement Fact Sheet: Vitamin D
http://ods.od.nih.gov/factsheets/vitamind.asp
Food and Nutrition Information Center
www.nal.usda.gov/fnic
Nutritionalsupplements.com
www.nutritionalsupplements.com
Office of Dietary Supplements: Health Information
http://ods.od.nih.gov/Health_Information/Health_Information.aspx
U.S. National Library of Medicine
www.nlm.nih.gov

Nutrition is a young and evolving science. Early research into nutrients began in the mid-18th century with investigations into how the body requires and uses calories from the macronutrients (carbohydrates, protein, and fats). It wasn't until the early 20th century that scientists began to discover, investigate, and identify the micronutrients and their affect on human health. The fundamentals of nutrition were discovered just over 100 years ago. From a perspective of scientifically confirming results, this is a short amount of time. A vast amount of knowledge about nutrients has been discovered, and scientists continue to investigate the best way for these nutrients to be provided—safely and in proper amounts to facilitate optimal functioning of the human body.

The articles of this unit have been selected to present current knowledge about macronutrients and micronutrients, with particular interest in the nutrients of concern as indicated in the 2010 U.S. Dietary Guidelines: vitamin D, calcium, potassium, sodium, and "good fats."

One of the current challenges in nutrition science is evaluating the scientific studies and how the results of the different types of studies can be translated and applied to improve human health. The golden standard for research by researchers is the randomized clinical trial; however, there are weaknesses in clinical trials designs with a nutrition focus. In the article "Which Pills Work?" Melinda Moyer discusses the current controversy over recommendations for vitamin D intake and supplementation.

Too often the resounding message about nutrition and our diets is that we eat too much of the "bad stuff." An important message that is underpublished is that our diets commonly lack certain vitamins and minerals that are beneficial. In the first article, "Getting Enough, What You Don't Eat Can Hurt You," Bonnie Liebman sheds light on the nutrients that are commonly deficient in the U.S. diet: potassium, vitamin D, magnesium, and vitamin B-12.

The USDA and HHS are now recommending that all American adults strive to consume 1,500 mg of sodium rather than the previously recommended 2,300 mg. The reasoning for lowering the recommended amount across the board is that over 70% of the population fits into groups that are at high risk for developing hypertension, stroke, and heart disease. The challenge with meeting this guideline is that it will be difficult to consume processed foods or eat in restaurants in the United States. "Keeping a Lid on Salt: Not So Easy" by Nanci Hellmich covers many of these challenges with restricting sodium in the current U.S. food environment.

Another topic of current interest is omega-3 fatty acids, especially the best and safest sources for these beneficial fats. A great deal of information has been published regarding the imbalance of the polyunsaturated fatty acids, omega-6 and omega-3, in the typical American diet. The vast use of corn, vegetable, and soybean oil in the Western diet has led to an unhealthy proportion of fats from omega-6 fatty acids. This imbalance of omega-6 to omega-3 fatty acids has been implicated in atherosclerosis, heart attack, and stroke. Demand for supplements and fortified

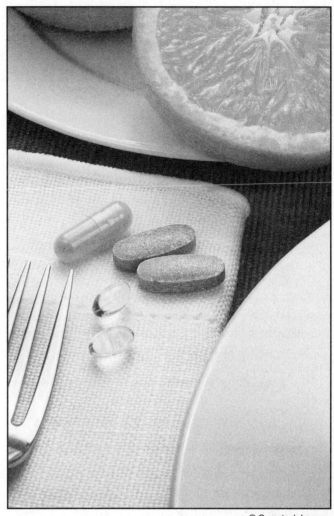

© Comstock Images

foods containing omega-3s has culminated in a number of products on the market. Since the metabolic pathways of these PUFAs are complex, there is a great deal of confusion when information is presented on the label and/or in the media. The most beneficial of these omega-3s is docosahexaenoic acid (DHA) found in coldwater fatty fish (salmon, halibut, swordfish, tilefish, shark, tuna), which are frequently high in heavy metals and other toxins. The current recommendation from the Dietary Guidelines for Americans is to vary types and sources of fish that you consume. The article by Julie Hanus will address how to balance the great fats in coldwater fish with the risk of consuming environmental toxins. Future research to address the problem of how to consume safe sources of DHA will strengthen, with particular attention to improving fish farming techniques.

The articles selected for Unit 3 will provide additional information to the vitamins, minerals, and fats sections of a general nutrition course. Several of the articles also address the challenges of interpreting and evaluating scientific nutrition research.

Getting Enough?

What You Don't Eat Can Hurt You

BONNIE LIEBMAN

Too much sugar. Too much salt. Too much saturated fat. We eat too much of all three. And we eat too much, period.

Yet we also eat too little.

Many Americans fall short of the recommended intakes of a handful of nutrients. Several key players—potassium, magnesium, vitamin D, and vitamin B-12—may make or break your risk of high blood pressure, diabetes, and brittle bones. For some of those nutrients, only foods—not pills—can make up the shortfall. For others, only a pill will do.

Here's why and how to get the nutrients you may be missing.

Here are four key nutrients you may lack—and where to get them.

Potassium

The numbers are staggering:

- One in three adults in the United States has high blood pressure, or hypertension. Among those over 65, it's two out of three. And another one out of four adults has pre-hypertension.

- Of the 74.5 million Americans with hypertension, 56 percent don't have it under control. That includes 22 percent who don't even know they have it.

- Roughly three out of four people who suffer a stroke, a heart attack, or congestive heart failure have hypertension.

Too much salt, too much weight, too little exercise, too much alcohol, and other risk factors can raise blood pressure. Potassium can trim it.

"It's absolutely clear that potassium can lower blood pressure," says Frank Sacks, professor of cardiovascular disease prevention at the Harvard School of Public Health in Boston.

In 1988, the INTERSALT study of 52 large populations reported that people with higher potassium intakes had lower blood pressures.[1] By 1997, a meta-analysis of 33 studies found that potassium supplements (2,300 milligrams a day) lowered systolic blood pressure by an average of 3.3 points.[2] (Systolic pressure is the higher of the two blood pressure numbers.)

"That meta-analysis conclusively showed that potassium supplements reduce blood pressure," says Lydia Bazzano, assistant professor of epidemiology at the Tulane School of Public Health in New Orleans.

In animal studies, potassium protects rats from stroke.[3] "And in human population studies, low potassium is a predictor for stroke," adds Sacks.

For example, in a study that tracked 43,000 men for eight years, those who consumed the most potassium (4,300 mg a day) were 38 percent less likely to suffer a stroke than those who consumed the least (2,400 mg a day).[4]

Potassium matters because it seems to counter the damage caused by sodium. "If people are eating high amounts of sodium, potassium will lower blood pressure more," explains Sacks. "The higher the sodium, the more potassium helps."

And when researchers tracked 2,275 participants in the Trials of Hypertension Prevention for 10 to 15 years, they found that the risk of heart attack or stroke depended more on potassium *and* sodium than on either one alone.[5]

Even without berries, half a cantaloupe has 16 percent of a day's potassium and only 90 calories. Mmm.

Scientists aren't sure exactly how potassium lowers blood pressure. Among the possibilities: it makes the larger blood vessels more flexible.[6]

"The flexibility of the big arteries like the aorta or carotid arteries is very important in maintaining a nice, lower, youthful blood pressure," explains Sacks. "In older people, arteries are less elastic." And that boosts blood pressure.

The Bottom Line

Whether it's blood pressure, stones, or bones you're worried about, the message is clear: "Eat potassium-rich fruits and vegetables like you'd get in a DASH diet," says Tulane's Lydia Bazzano.

Potassium may also lower blood pressure by dilating the small blood vessels.[6] "You don't want the tiny vessels clenched," says Sacks. "Resistance to blood flow will increase blood pressure."

What's clear is that a healthy, potassium-rich diet can revitalize arteries, big or small. "Conditions we thought were permanent with age can be reversed in four weeks," says Sacks. "Four weeks of a lower-sodium, potassium-rich DASH diet completely reverses the effect of age on blood pressure."

A DASH (Dietary Approaches to Stop Hypertension) diet is rich in potassium, thanks to 11 (modest) servings a day of fruits and vegetables, with two servings of low-fat dairy foods, and with low levels of saturated fat, added sugars, and refined flour.

"Potassium may account for half of the effect of the overall DASH diet," says Sacks.

The citrate that's usually bound to the potassium in fruits and vegetables could also help. Potassium citrate lowers blood pressure more than the potassium chloride that is in some salt substitutes, supplements, and potassium-fortified foods.[7]

Another reason to get potassium from food: high-dose potassium supplements—far more than the amounts that occur naturally in food—can be hazardous.

"If you have kidney disease and don't know it, you could potentially end up with too much potassium in your blood, and that's life-threatening," explains Bazzano. "It can stop your heart."

Bonus: getting potassium citrate from fruits and vegetables may prevent kidney stones.

In the Health Professionals Follow-Up Study of more than 45,000 men, those who consumed the most potassium (about 4,300 mg a day) had roughly half the risk of kidney stones over 14 years of those who ate the least (roughly 2,700 mg).[8]

"If you eat more fruits and vegetables, your urine citrate goes up, and that should reduce the risk of kidney stones," says study coauthor Gary Curhan, associate professor of epidemiology at the Harvard School of Public Health.

"But it's probably the citrate or some other alkali, not the potassium."

How does citrate prevent kidney stones?

"It forms soluble complexes with calcium, so it keeps the calcium from sticking to oxalate or phosphate," says

Potassium on Tap

If you're like 90 percent of men and 99 percent of women, you get less potassium than experts recommend (4,700 mg a day). Go for fruits and vegetables so you can eat bigger servings—these are small—without piling on calories.

Potassium	Calories	% IOM*
Clams (4 oz. cooked)	170	15
Beet greens (½ cup cooked)	20	14
Yellowfin tuna or Halibut (4 oz. cooked)	160	14
Pacific cod (4 oz. cooked)	120	12
Non-fat or Low-fat plain yogurt (8 oz.)	135	12
Swiss chard (½ cup cooked)	20	10
Acorn squash (½ cup cooked)	55	10
Sweet potato with skin (½ cup cooked)	90	10
Lima beans (½ cup cooked)	110	10
Edamame, shelled (½ cup cooked)	130	10
Wild Coho salmon (4 oz. cooked)	160	10
Spinach (½ cup cooked)	20	9
Tomato sauce (½ cup)	30	9
Banana (1)	105	9
Orange juice (1 cup)	120	9
Low-fat fruit yogurt (8 oz.)	225	9
Farmed Atlantic salmon (4 oz. cooked)	235	9
Cantaloupe (¼)	45	8
Dried apricots (¼ cup)	80	8
Non-fat or Low-fat milk (1 cup)	90	8
Kidney beans or Lentils (½ cup cooked)	115	8
Avocado (½ cup)	120	8
Navy or Pinto beans (½ cup cooked)	125	8
Tomato paste (2 Tbs.)	25	7
Baked potato with skin (½ cup cooked)	55	7
Great Northern beans (½ cup cooked)	105	7
Prunes (¼ cup)	105	7
Pistachios (¼ cup)	180	7
Tomato (1)	20	6
Beets (½ cup cooked)	35	6
Butternut squash (½ cup cooked)	40	6
Peach or Nectarine (1)	60	6
Raisins (¼ cup)	110	6
Brussels sprouts (½ cup cooked)	30	5
Artichoke hearts (½ cup cooked)	45	5
Spinach (¼ cup raw)	5	4
Grapes (1 cup)	60	4
Apple (1)	95	4
Boston or Romaine lettuce (1 cup raw)	10	3

*Percent of the daily intake (4,700 milligrams) recommended by the Institute of Medicine (IOM).

Sources: USDA and manufacturers. Chart compiled by Amy Ramsay, Danielle Hazard, and Melissa Pryputniewicz.

Curhan. "So it's less likely that oxalate or phosphate crystals will form."

Preventing calcium oxalate crystals is key. "More than 80 percent of kidney stones are made of calcium oxalate," says Curhan.

And there may be a bonus for bones, he adds. "Citrate should reduce urine calcium excretion as well."

Scientists used to think that potassium could lower the risk of osteoporosis, but no longer.

"Potassium isn't the key to bone health," says Bess Dawson-Hughes, director of the Bone Metabolism Laboratory at the Jean Mayer U.S. Department of Agriculture Human Nutrition Research Center on Aging at Tufts University in Boston. "It's the alkaline accompaniment of potassium that's good."

Vitamin D

Osteoporosis, or brittle bones, takes a huge toll on the public's health:

- One in two women and one in four men over age 50 will break a bone because of osteoporosis.[9]
- Osteoporosis caused more than 2 million fractures in 2005, including roughly 297,000 hip fractures, 547,000 spine fractures, 397,000 wrist fractures, 135,000 pelvic fractures, and 675,000 fractures at other sites.
- Half of all women and 30 percent of all men over 50 have osteopenia (low bone mass) in their hips, which often leads to osteoporosis.[10]
- Six months after a hip fracture, only 15 percent of patients can walk across a room without help.

If you ask people how to strengthen bones, the nutrient they're most likely to mention is calcium. But, in fact, average calcium intakes are now close to the recommended levels, in part because 43 percent of Americans get some calcium from a supplement.[11]

What many people don't know is that calcium may not prevent fractures if you don't get enough vitamin D, which helps the body absorb calcium.

"It's looking like the combination of calcium and vitamin D is effective," says Tufts' Bess Dawson-Hughes.

In a 2007 meta-analysis, calcium supplements alone didn't lower the risk of fractures.[12]

"But when you look at calcium plus vitamin D, the risk reduction was significant," says Dawson-Hughes. "So we should absolutely aim for the recommended levels of both."

Calcium plus D could also protect young bones. In a study of 3,700 young female U.S. Navy recruits, those who were given calcium (2,000 mg a day) and vitamin D (800 IU a day) were 20 percent less likely to be diagnosed with stress fractures during eight weeks of training than those who got a placebo.[13]

How much vitamin D is enough?

The Bottom Line

Shoot for 800 to 1,000 IU of vitamin D a day from foods and supplements if you're over 60, and 400 IU a day if you're younger. Shoot for 1,200 mg of calcium a day from food and supplements if you're over 50, and 1,000 mg a day if you're a younger adult.

"My interpretation of current evidence is that our blood levels should not be lower than 30 nanograms per milliliter," says Dawson-Hughes. "If you look at data from the National Health and Nutrition Examination Survey, about 70 percent of older adult men and women were lower than that."

To reach adequate blood levels, most older people need more vitamin D than is now recommended (400 IU a day from age 51 to 70, and 600 IU over 70).

"The vast majority of the older global population would need 800 to 1,000 units of vitamin D a day," from food or a supplement, explains Dawson-Hughes. She led a group of experts who came up with new guidelines for the International Osteoporosis Foundation.[14]

"And high-risk older people—those who have no effective sun exposure or don't absorb vitamin D well or who have very dark skin or osteoporosis—would need more than 800 to 1,000 units a day to get to desired serum levels," she adds.

It's tough to get even 800 IU of vitamin D from foods. A cup of milk is fortified with only 100 IU, and a tablespoon of fortified margarine has 60 IU. Unless you eat fish like red salmon (800 IU per 3 oz. of cooked fish) almost every day, you won't reach those levels.

Getting enough vitamin D may protect more than bones. Evidence suggests that it may lower the risk of colon cancer, heart attacks, stroke, Type 2 diabetes, falls, and some autoimmune diseases.

And a 2007 meta-analysis of 18 trials found a 7 percent lower risk of dying over six months to seven years when people were given vitamin D (usually to reduce the risk of bone fractures).[15]

However, a recent study raised the possibility that high blood levels of vitamin D could increase the risk of pancreatic cancer.[16] The higher risk was only seen in people from states with low sun exposure (Michigan, Minnesota, and Wisconsin, in this study), and it wasn't linked to how much vitamin D people were getting from supplements, so it's somewhat of a mystery.

"The government has funded a huge vitamin D intervention trial giving people 2,000 IU a day or a placebo," says Dawson-Hughes. "So that will give us more information."

(Most women over 65 or men over 60 are eligible to join the VITAL trial, which is also testing fish oil. If you're interested, call 1-800-388-3963 or go to vitalstudy.org.)

"We're looking at cancer, heart disease, stroke, diabetes, high blood pressure, vision, bone density, memory loss, depression, and autoimmune outcomes," says JoAnn Manson, a professor of medicine at the Harvard Medical School who is leading the trial.

Too much calcium without vitamin D may also pose a risk. In July, British researchers reported that high doses of calcium from supplements—1,000 mg a day in most cases—*without* vitamin D raised the risk of heart attacks, but only in people who were already getting more than 800 mg of calcium from food.[17] (The average adult gets 1,000 to 1,200 mg of calcium a day from foods and supplements combined.[11])

Beans are rich in magnesium, not to mention fiber, folate, protein, and potassium. Such a bargain!

"I would not go a whole lot above the recommended intake because it adds no value and could be adding risk," says Dawson-Hughes. (The researchers didn't look at people who were given calcium plus vitamin D, citing evidence that vitamin D would lower death rates.)

Magnesium

An estimated 23.6 million Americans—including one out of four people aged 60 or older—have Type 2 diabetes. Roughly 5.7 million of them don't know it. And 57 million others have pre-diabetes.

The disease takes a heavy toll:

- Adults with diabetes are two to four times more likely than others to have a stroke or to die of heart disease.

- Diabetes is the leading cause of new cases of blindness among people 20 to 74 and the leading cause of kidney failure.

- More than 60 percent of people with diabetes have nervous system damage.

- Each year, about 70,000 Americans with diabetes have a foot or leg amputated.[18]

Type I diabetes, which typically strikes in childhood, occurs when the body's immune system destroys beta-cells in the pancreas that make insulin, the hormone that controls blood sugar levels. Type 1 accounts for 5 to 10 percent of diabetes cases.

In Type 2 diabetes (which this article will refer to simply as "diabetes"), the body's cells don't use insulin properly. As the need for insulin rises, the pancreas gradually loses its ability to make enough, and blood sugar levels climb.

What causes diabetes?

Extra pounds are by far the biggest risk factor. Genes, lack of exercise, and diet also play a role. Whole grains,

A Mouthful of Magnesium

A typical woman gets 250 milligrams of magnesium a day, but should get 320 mg. A typical man gets 335 mg, but should get 420 mg. The Daily Value (DV) is 400 mg. Here's how to get more magnesium without overdoing the calories.

Magnesium	Calories	% DV*
Pumpkin seed kernels (¼ cup)	170	41
Brazil nuts (¼ cup)	220	31
Halibut (4 oz. cooked)	160	30
Kellogg's Original All-Bran cereal (½ cup)	80	25
Almonds (¼ cup)	205	25
Cashews (¼ cup)	195	22
Spinach (½ cup cooked)	20	20
Swiss chard (½ cup cooked)	20	19
Soybeans (½ cup cooked)	150	19
Yellowfin tuna (4 oz. cooked)	160	18
Lima beans (½ cup cooked)	105	16
Quinoa (½ cup cooked)	110	15
Black beans (½ cup cooked)	115	15
Dark chocolate (1.4 oz.)	220	15
Haddock (4 oz. cooked)	125	14
Peanuts (¼ cup) or Peanut butter (2 Tbs.)	195	14
Hazelnuts (¼ cup)	210	14
Beet greens (½ cup cooked)	20	12
Okra (½ cup cooked)	25	12
Black-eyed peas (½ cup cooked)	100	12
Navy beans (½ cup cooked)	125	12
Semisweet chocolate (1.4 oz.)	190	12
Walnuts (½ cup)	195	12
Oat bran (½ cup cooked)	45	11
Great Northern beans (½ cup cooked)	105	11
Kidney or Pinto beans (½ cup cooked)	115	11
Non-fat plain yogurt (8 oz.)	125	11
Brown rice or Lentils (¼ cup cooked)	110	10
Garbanzo beans (¼ cup cooked)	135	10
Low-fat plain yogurt (8 oz.)	145	10
Sunflower seed kernels (¼ cup)	190	10
Tofu (½ cup raw)	95	9
Pistachios (¼ cup)	175	9
Oatmeal (½ cup cooked)	85	8
Post Original Shredded Wheat (½ cup)	85	8
Canned light tuna in water (4 oz.)	130	8
Low-fat fruit yogurt (8 oz.)	225	8
Bulgur (½ cup cooked)	75	7
Non-fat milk (1 cup)	85	7
Spinach (1 cup raw)	5	6
Whole wheat bread (1 slice, 1 oz.)	70	6

*Percent of the Daily Value (400 milligrams).

Sources: USDA and manufacturers. Chart compiled by Amy Ramsay, Danielle Hazard, and Melissa Pryputniewicz.

The Bottom Line

"I would recommend consuming high levels of magnesium-rich foods," says Song. "Fruits, vegetables, whole grains, nuts, beans. It's very safe to get more magnesium in your diet."

fiber-rich foods, and coffee (decal or regular) seem to lower the risk. Sugar-sweetened beverages, processed meats, and white potatoes seem to raise it.

One nutrient that often gets overlooked: magnesium.

"We have a lot of evidence from observational studies that magnesium is beneficial for preventing Type 2 diabetes," says Yiqing Song, an associate epidemiologist at Brigham & Women's Hospital in Boston.

For example, when researchers tracked more than 85,000 women in the Nurses' Health Study for 18 years and 42,000 men in the Health Professionals Follow-Up Study for 12 years, those who consumed the most magnesium (about 375 mg a day for women and 450 mg a day for men) had a 27 percent lower risk of diabetes than those who consumed the least magnesium (about 200 mg a day for women and 270 mg a day for men).[19]

The Iowa Women's Health Study and the Women's Health Study came up with similar results.[20,21]

"In the Women's Health Study, we found an association between a low magnesium intake and an increased risk of diabetes only among overweight women," says Song.

"Magnesium may be more beneficial for overweight women because they are more likely to be at high risk for diabetes," he notes.

In some studies, women with higher magnesium intakes—no matter what their weight—had lower fasting insulin levels.[21,22] That may mean a lower risk of diabetes.

What's more, in the Nurses' Health Study and the Women's Health Initiative Observational Study, those who consumed more magnesium had lower levels of c-reactive protein and other signs of chronic low-level inflammation.[23,24]

"Chronic inflammation may be the link between obesity and Type 2 diabetes," explains Song. "Obesity can cause chronic inflammation.

"The two major features of diabetes are insulin resistance and beta-cell dysfunction," he notes.

"Chronic inflammation may cause insulin resistance in peripheral tissues, and it may damage the beta-cells in the pancreas that secrete insulin."

Still, adds Song, "Observational studies can't show cause and effect. We need direct evidence from a large, long-term clinical trial before we can make any conclusive statements for magnesium and Type 2 diabetes."

The first step: a small pilot trial giving magnesium to people for a few months. "We're going to assess the direct effects of oral magnesium supplements on insulin sensitivity and insulin secretion in obese individuals because they are at high risk for diabetes," says Song.

A trial is critical because it could be something other than the magnesium in magnesium-rich foods that protects against the disease.

"Fiber, folic acid, potassium, and magnesium are all correlated together," says Song. "But for magnesium, we also have evidence from animal studies. There's no evidence from animal studies that fiber, potassium, or folic acid reduces the risk of diabetes. So if you consider all the evidence, we think magnesium is an important factor."

Vitamin B-12

"Low vitamin B-12 status is very common in older people," notes Martha Morris of the USDA Human Nutrition Research Center on Aging at Tufts University.

Vitamin B-12 is found in animal foods, including dairy, eggs, fish, poultry, and meat. But most people with low B-12 don't run short because they lack those foods.

"Low B-12 status occurs because of how our digestive systems age," says Morris. "Some people lose the ability to extract vitamin B-12 from food protein."

In about 30 percent of older people, the lining of the stomach starts to wither, so it doesn't secrete enough gastric acid to release vitamin B-12 from food.

That's why the Institute of Medicine recommends that anyone over age 50 get at least 2.4 micrograms of B-12 a day from a fortified food or supplement. Even without stomach acid, you can still absorb the crystalline form of B-12 they contain.

Roughly one out of five Americans aged 60 or older has low B-12 status.[25] "These people don't feel like they have anything wrong with them," notes Morris. But they're more likely to do poorly on tests of memory and mental ability.[26]

"We found cognitive impairment was almost twice as common in people with low B-12 status," she adds.

And in the Chicago Health and Aging Project and the Oxford Healthy Ageing Project in England, seniors who entered the studies with low B-12 status were more likely to show a drop in cognitive test scores six to ten years later.[27,28]

"This association suggests that low B-12 status contributes to cognitive impairment in the elderly," says Morris. She uses the word "suggests" because these types of studies can't prove cause and effect.

So far, studies that have given people high doses of vitamin B-12 (often with other B vitamins) for up to six months haven't found improved test scores.[29] (And B vitamins don't slow memory loss in people who already have Alzheimer's disease.[30])

However, in the Women's Antioxidant and Folic Acid Cardiovascular Study, which tested high doses of B vitamins on 2,000 women aged 65 or older who were at high risk

The Bottom Line

If you're over 50, make sure your multivitamin contains at least 100 percent of the Daily Value (DV) for vitamin B-12 (6 micrograms).

If you don't take a multi, take a B-12 supplement (the lowest dose available may be 100 mcg, which is okay). A month's supply of a store brand shouldn't cost more than about $1.50.

To play it safe, don't take a daily multivitamin with 100 percent of the DV for folic acid *and* eat a breakfast cereal (or other food) every day that contains more than 25 percent of the DV. Don't worry about fruits, vegetables, or other foods that are rich in naturally occurring folate.

for heart disease, the vitamins seemed to help women who entered the trial with low B-vitamin intakes. Those women were less likely to decline on memory and other cognitive tests over five years if they got B vitamins than if they got a placebo.[31]

But if too little B-12 is a problem, simply getting more from a multivitamin or breakfast cereal may not be the answer.

"Among people with low B-12 status, high folic acid status is strongly associated with cognitive impairment," says Morris.

The folate that occurs naturally in food isn't a problem. "The normal circulating form of folate—methylfolate—was not related to cognitive impairment at all," says Morris. "Only unmetabolized folic acid was."[32]

Unmetabolized folic acid comes from vitamin supplements or from grain foods—breads, cereals, pasta, rice, and tortillas—that are made with "enriched" flour. In 1998, the Food and Drug Administration added folic acid to the other B vitamins and iron that companies are required to add to refined flour and white rice. The folic acid lowered rates of spina bifida and other neural tube birth defects by 26 percent.[33]

If you're taking a multi with 100 percent of a day's folic acid, look for a cereal with no more than 25 percent of a day's worth. Unsweetened shredded wheat has no added folic acid.

But no one expected fortification to lead to unmetabolized folic acid.

"When the FDA decided to fortify the food supply with folic acid, scientists assumed that all the folic acid would be converted to natural folate on the way through the digestive tract," says Morris.

"But we're finding folic acid in body tissues. In a recent paper, we found that a third of seniors have circulating unmetabolized folic acid."

Older people with unmetabolized folic acid are more likely to take supplements and eat fortified foods, but that doesn't completely explain why they have higher levels than others.[34] Genetics may affect what happens to folic acid once it's in your body.

But the link with cognitive decline in people with too little B-12 and too much folic acid is worrisome. "Something is going on in the brain with unmetabolized folic acid, and we don't know what it is," says Morris.

And that makes it tricky to get more B-12. "I can't say take a multivitamin or fortified breakfast cereal because it would also give you a lot of folic acid," she adds. "If you're taking a multi, you're getting a full day's supply." That's 400 micrograms.

"Then you may be getting 100 mcg from fortified grain foods. And if you eat certain breakfast cereals, you'll get another 400 mcg, so you're getting more than two full days' supply. You really have to read cereal boxes."

To complicate matters, getting a blood test for vitamin B-12 may not tell you much. "The test is very insensitive," says Morris.

A more sensitive test is for methylmalonic acid, which goes up when you get too little B-12. (Levels over 210 mmol/L can mean low B-12 status.) But it's more expensive.

References

1. *BMJ 297:* 319, 1988.
2. *JAMA 277:* 1624, 1997.
3. *Hypertension 7:* 110, 1985.
4. *Circulation 98:* 1198, 1998.
5. *Arch. Intern. Med. 169:* 32, 2009.
6. *Hypertension 55:* 681, 2010.
7. *Hypertension 45:* 571, 2005.
8. *J. Am. Soc. Nephrol. 15:* 3225, 2004.
9. nof.org/osteoporosis/diseasefacts.htm
10. *J. Bone Miner. Res. 25:* 64, 2010.
11. *J. Nutr. 140:* 817, 2010.
12. *Lancet 370:* 657, 2007.
13. *J. Bone Min. Res. 23:* 741, 2008.
14. *Osteoporosis Internal. 21:* 1151, 2010.
15. *Arch. Intern. Med. 167:* 1730, 2007.
16. *Cancer Res. 69:* 1439, 2009.
17. *BMJ 341:* c3691, 2010.
18. cdc.gov/diabetes/pubs/factsheet07.htm
19. *Diabetes Care 27:* 134, 2004.
20. *Am. J. Clin. Nutr. 71:* 921, 2000.
21. *Diabetes Care 27:* 59, 2004.
22. *J. Am. Coll. Nutr. 22:* 533, 2003.
23. *Am. J. Clin. Nutr. 85:* 1068, 2007.
24. *Diabetes Care 33:* 304, 2010.
25. *Am. J. Clin. Nutr. 89:* 693S, 2009.
26. *Am. J. Clin. Nutr. 89:* 702S, 2009.
27. *Neurology 72:* 361, 2009.

28. *Am. J. Clin. Nutr. 86:* 1384, 2007.
29. *Arch. Intern. Med. 167:* 21, 2007.
30. *JAMA 300:* 1774, 2008.
31. *Am. J. Clin. Nutr. 88:* 1602, 2008.
32. *Am. J. Clin. Nutr. 91:* 1733, 2010.
33. *MMWR 53:* 362, 2004.
34. *Am. J. Clin. Nutr. 92:* 383, 2010.

Critical Thinking

1. Describe the health benefits of potassium, vitamin D, magnesium, and vitamin B-12

2. Compare the amount of potassium recommended by the Institutes of Medicine with the RDA for potassium.

3. Defend the premise that it is better to consume potassium-rich foods than to take potassium chloride in supplements.

4. Explain why researchers cannot definitively say that magnesium intake is linked to type 2 diabetes even though there are several epidemiological studies that support the claim.

From *Nutrition Action HealthLetter,* September 2010, pp. 2–8. Copyright © 2010 by Center for Science in the Public Interest. Reprinted by permission.

Vitamins, Supplements

New Evidence Shows They Can't Compete with Mother Nature

Americans want to believe in vitamin and mineral pills: We spent an estimated $10 billion on them in 2008, according to the Nutrition Business Journal. But recent studies undertaken to assess their benefits have delivered a flurry of disappointing results. The supplements failed to prevent Alzheimer's disease, cancer, heart attacks, strokes, type 2 diabetes, and premature death.

"We have yet to see well-conducted research that categorically supports the use of vitamin and mineral supplements," says Linda Van Horn, PhD, a professor of preventive medicine at Northwestern University's Feinberg School of Medicine in Chicago. "Most studies show no benefit, or actual harm."

The Power of Food

While some people may need supplements at certain stages of their lives, nutritional deficiencies are uncommon in the U.S. "Almost all of us get or can get the vitamins and minerals we need from our diet," says Paul M. Coates, PhD., director of the Office of Dietary Supplements at the National Institutes of Health (NIH).

Major health organizations for cancer, diabetes, and heart disease all advise against supplements in favor of a healthful diet rich in fruits, vegetables, whole grains, and legumes. Unlike pills, those foods contain fiber plus thousands of health-protective substances that seem to work together more powerfully than any single ingredient can work alone. "That's why it's dangerous to say, 'I know I don't eat well, but if I pop my vitamins, I'm covered,'" says Karen Collins, RD, nutrition adviser to the American Institute for Cancer Research. "We now know that you're not covered."

Too Much Can Harm

Another concern is that some vitamin pills can be toxic if taken in high doses for a long time. Studies show that beta-carotene pills, for example, can increase the risk of lung cancer in smokers, and a 2008 review suggests that the pills, plus supplemental doses of the vitamins A and E, may increase the risk of premature death. In addition, a government survey found that more than 11 percent of adults take at least 400 international units of vitamin E a day, a dose that has been linked to heart failure, strokes, and an increased risk of death.

People are also apt to combine vitamin tablets and fortified foods, which can cause problems. For instance, too much folic acid—added to wheat products in this country—can mask vitamin B12 deficiency. Untreated, that can lead to irreversible nerve damage. In addition, high doses of folic acid may be associated with an increased risk of precancerous colon polyps, according to a trial of some 1,000 people at risk for them. "We're getting several alarming signals that more may not be better," says Susan T. Mayne, PhD., a professor of epidemiology at the Yale School of Public Health.

Yet despite the unfavorable results, vitamin and mineral pills are widely used to fend off diseases. Read on to find our review of the latest evidence on their effects.

Critical Thinking

1. If people choose to consume their nutrient requirements by taking supplements, what nutrients are they not consuming?

2. What type of cancer has been linked to excess intake of folic acid?

3. What nutrient in supplement form has been shown to increase the risk for smokers developing lung cancer?

Which Pills Work?

The recent finding that vitamin D supplements are largely unnecessary exposes a rift among nutrition researchers.

MELINDA WENNER MOYER

Physicians have recommended vitamin D supplements to their patients for a decade, with good reason: dozens of studies have shown a correlation between high intake of vitamin D—far higher than most people would get in a typical diet and from exposure to the sun—and lower rates of chronic diseases, such as cancer and type 1 diabetes. So when the Institute of Medicine, which advises the government on health policy, concluded in November that vitamin D supplements were unnecessary for most Americans and potentially harmful, patients were understandably confused.

The issue exposes a rift among experts over what constitutes valid proof when it comes to nutrition and could affect medical advice on many other supplements. On the one hand are scientists who insist that the only acceptable standard is the randomized clinical trial, which often compares the effects of a medical intervention, such as high intake of vitamin D, with those of a placebo. The scientists who reviewed the vitamin D findings fall heavily into this camp: trials "typically provide the highest level of scientific evidence relevant for dietary reference intake development," they wrote. Their report set intake levels based only on clinical trial data.

The institute panel, however, discarded a raft of observational studies, in which researchers compare the health of populations who take vitamin D supplements with those who do not. In theory, such epidemiological studies are inferior to clinical studies because they rely on observations out in the real world, where it is impossible to control for the variables scientists seek to understand. Researchers compensate for the lack of control by using large sample sizes—some vitamin D studies track 50,000 people—and applying statistical techniques. According to these studies, high levels of vitamin D are generally beneficial.

In the aftermath of the institute report, some physicians are now taking potshots at clinical studies. In nutrition, they say, true placebo groups are hard to maintain—how do you prevent people in a control group from, say, picking up extra vitamin D from sunlight and food, which can lead to underestimating the vitamin's benefits? It is also tough to single out the effect of one vitamin or mineral from others, because many work in tandem. "It is wrong-headed thinking that the only kind of evidence that is reliable is a randomized controlled trial," says Jeffrey Blumberg, a Tufts University pharmacologist.

The next chapter in this debate may come in the spring, when the Endocrine Society releases its own vitamin D guidelines. The organization now recommends higher blood levels of the vitamin than the institute suggested—30 nanograms per milliliter as opposed to 20—which would require supplements. Stay tuned.

Critical Thinking

1. Explain why the IOM concluded that vitamin D supplements are unnecessary and possibly harmful for most Americans.

2. Defend the position of physicians who are opposed to the IOM excluding results from the large observational research studies in favor for the randomized clinical trials only.

3. Differentiate observational research and intervention research.

4. Compare and contrast epidemiological, laboratory, clinical trials, and case study research designs.

Keeping a Lid on Salt: Not So Easy

Known as a silent killer, it's part of how we live.

NANCI HELLMICH

For years, Americans have been advised to consume less sodium, and they've taken that advice with a grain of salt.

Even many health-conscious consumers figured it was the least of their worries, especially compared with limiting their intake of calories, saturated fat, trans fat, cholesterol and sugar.

All that changed last week when a report from the Institute of Medicine urged the government to gradually reduce the maximum amount of sodium that manufacturers and restaurants can add to foods, beverages and meals. The report put a spotlight on what doctors and nutritionists have argued is a major contributor to heart disease and stroke.

More than half of Americans have either high blood pressure or pre-hypertension, says cardiologist Clyde Yancy, president of the American Heart Association and medical director at the Baylor Heart and Vascular Institute in Dallas.

"That puts a lot of us in the bucket of people who need to be on a lower sodium diet. Sodium contributes to most people's high blood pressure, and for some it may be the primary driver."

Cutting back on sodium could save thousands of people from early deaths caused by heart attacks and strokes each year, and it could save billions of dollars in health care costs, he says.

Others second that. "Salt is the single most harmful element in our food supply, silently killing about 100,000 people each year," says Michael Jacobson, executive director of the Washington, D.C.-based Center for Science in the Public Interest. "That's like a crowded jetliner crashing every single day. But the food industry has fended off government action for more than three decades."

Now salt has our attention.

But reducing it in the American diet is easier said than done. "We have, in essence, ignored the advice because we are driven by convenience, and sodium makes a fast-food lifestyle very easy," Yancy says. "To change, we would need to live and eat differently."

Very differently.

Americans now consume an average of about 3,400 milligrams of sodium a day, or about 1½ teaspoons, government data show. Men consume more than women.

But most adults—including those with high blood pressure, African Americans, the middle-aged and the elderly—should consume no more than 1,500 milligrams a day, according to the dietary guidelines from the U.S. Department of Agriculture. Others should consume less than 2,300 milligrams, or less than a teaspoon, the guidelines say.

And yet it's virtually impossible to limit yourself to such amounts if you often eat processed foods, prepared foods or restaurant fare, including fast food. Most Americans' sodium intake comes from those sources, not the salt shaker on the table.

Some restaurant entrees have 2,000 milligrams or more in one dish. Fast-food burgers can have more than 1,000 milligrams. Many soups are chock-full of sodium. So are many spaghetti sauces, broths, lunch meats, salad dressings, cheeses, crackers and frozen foods.

Can't see it, can't taste it.

Salt serves many functions in products. Besides adding to a food's taste, it is a preservative. "You can't see it," Yancy says. "You can't even taste it because you are so accustomed to it. If you want the freedom to make healthy choices, you are limited by today's foods. That's a problem."

To change that, food companies and restaurants will have to come up with new ways to formulate products and recipes to help consumers gradually lower their salt levels, which would wean them off the taste.

That's a huge challenge, but nutritionists and public health specialists say it can be done and will be worth it. "There is no health benefit to a high-sodium diet, and there is considerable risk," says Linda Van Horn, a professor of preventive medicine at Northwestern University Feinberg School of Medicine.

Even those whose blood pressure is in the normal range should watch their intake, Yancy says. "Here's a wake-up call: Every American who is age 50 or older has a 90% chance of developing hypertension. That increases the risk of heart disease and stroke. This is a preventable process, and it's preventable with sodium reduction, weight control and physical activity."

Why It Can Be Harmful

There are several theories for why sodium increases blood pressure, Yancy says, "but the most obvious one is that it makes us retain fluids, and that retention elevates blood pressure," which injures blood vessels and leads to heart disease and stroke. "It's a connect-the-dots phenomenon."

Some people, especially some African Americans, are more salt-sensitive than others, Yancy says.

"When they are exposed to sodium, they retain more fluid, and because of the way their kidneys handle sodium, they may have a greater proportional rise in blood pressure," he says.

The cost of this damage? An analysis by the Rand Corp. found that if the average sodium intake of Americans was reduced to 2,300 milligrams a day, it might decrease the cases of high blood pressure by 11 million, improve quality of life for millions of people and save about $18 billion in annual health care costs.

The estimated value of improved quality of life and living healthier longer: $32 billion a year. Greater reductions in sodium consumption in the population would save more lives and money, says Roland Sturm, a senior economist with Rand.

Yancy says the country doesn't just need health care reform, "we need health reform. If we don't adjust the demand part of the equation, no system will work. Remarkably, people might be overall healthier by simply reducing sodium."

But Yancy says people need to keep in mind that sodium is just one of the factors that increase the risk of heart disease and stroke. Others include obesity, consuming too much sugar and too few fruits and vegetables, lack of physical activity and smoking.

Salt Industry Disagrees

Leaders in the salt industry say their product is being unfairly maligned. The Institute of Medicine report and the government "are focusing on one small aspect of health, which is a small increase in blood pressure in a small segment of population," says Lori Roman, president of the Salt Institute, an industry group.

Some of the research that ties salt to health risks is based on faulty assumptions and extrapolations, Roman says. She says a recent worldwide study indicated there is no country where people eat an average of less than 1,500 milligrams a day. "That's way below the normal range," Roman says. The Italians eat more sodium than Americans, but their cardiovascular health is better than Americans', and the reason is they eat a lot of fruits and vegetables, she says.

"This is the real story that the government is missing," Roman says. "It is the secret to good health."

She says people may end up following a less healthy diet if they cut back on sodium. "Have you ever bought a can of low-sodium string beans and then tried to season it to taste good? It's impossible," Roman says. "Here's one of the unintended consequences of this recommendation: People will eat fewer vegetables, and by eating fewer vegetables, they will be less healthy."

Yancy says the first step for many people is making the decision to cut back on salt intake. He knows from experience that it can be done.

An African American, Yancy, 52, has high blood pressure and a family history of heart disease and stroke. He's lean and exercises for an hour a day, but still he has to take medication for hypertension. Before he started watching his sodium intake a few years ago, Yancy says, he was consuming more than 4,000 milligrams a day, partly because he grew up in southern Louisiana and was used to a salty, high-fat diet.

But he has weaned himself off the taste. He doesn't have a salt shaker in his house, and he reads the labels on grocery store items and doesn't buy any that have more than 100 milligrams of sodium in a serving.

"I taste the salt in items and put them aside. I find it difficult to enjoy prepared soups. I can taste the salt in prepared meals. I've learned to make my own soups."

When he eats out, he orders salads and asks for his fish and meat to be grilled. "Typically, I eat fish with lemon juice and pepper."

Even so, he believes his sodium intake is probably higher than it should be because he often eats in restaurants and cafeterias, and many foods have hidden sodium.

Changes in food products need to be made over time as the Institute of Medicine report suggests, says Van Horn, a research nutritionist at Northwestern. "If we drop the sodium overnight, people will be desperately seeking salt shakers."

So how hard is it going to be to reduce the salt in processed and prepared foods?

"We've been trying to reduce the sodium in foods for more than 30 years. If this were easy, it would have been accomplished," says Roger Clemens, a professor of pharmacology at the University of Southern California and a spokesman for the Institute of Food Technologists.

The primary dietary source of sodium is sodium chloride, also known as table salt, he says. There are other sodium salts, such as sodium bicarbonate (baking soda) in baking and sodium benzoate (preservative) in bread and beverages. And there are potassium salts that are used in foods—as emulsifiers in cheese and buffers in beverages, he says.

"Salt is a natural preservative. It has been used in the food supply to ensure food safety for centuries," Clemens says. "It's critical for preserving bacon, olives, lunch meats, fish and poultry."

"Some foods, such as cheese, can only be produced with salt. No other compound allows the proteins to knit together to become cheese."

If It Doesn't Taste Good...

To make cheese that is lower in sodium, foodmakers must put the cheese through a special procedure that basically extracts some of the sodium. "It's a very long, tedious process," he says.

Salt also is crucial for making most breads. To get dough to rise, manufacturers use sodium chloride and sodium bicarbonate, Clemens says. "If you were to eat a sodium-free product, the texture and flavor would be markedly different. It would be more compressed. I don't think you'd like it at first."

He says some manufacturers have experimented with low-sodium items, and in some cases consumers have turned up their noses. "If it doesn't taste good, consumers won't buy it."

Melissa Musiker, a nutrition spokeswoman for the Grocery Manufacturers Association, agrees. "You can't get ahead of consumers," she says. "You work on the recipes, test them, see how consumers respond and go back and tweak."

There is no one single alternative for replacing it in various foods, she says. "It has to be replaced on an ingredient-by-ingredient basis."

Clemens says food companies will continue to try to develop new technologies to lower the sodium.

"It has taken us 30 years to get this far, and it will probably take us another decade to get a significant difference in the intake. If we can lower sodium in our diet, we'll have a huge health impact on generations to come."

Critical Thinking

1. Identify the four groups of people who should consume less than 1,500 mg of sodium per day, as recommended in the Dietary Guidelines for Americans.

2. What is the largest source of sodium in the typical western diet?

3. How does dietary sodium increase blood pressure in someone who is salt sensitive?

Seafood Showdown: Fatty Acids vs. Heavy Metals

Julie Hanus

Ever feel like we've just totally screwed ourselves with the oceans? I'm not even talking about BP's gushing well: It's this recent report from the *Telegraph* that U.K. nutritionists are now advising pregnant women to eat more fish.

Fish, of course, contains mercury, a heavy metal pollutant that comes from human industry (and, to be fair, from some natural sources like volcano eruptions). Pregnant women, children, the elderly—nutritional convention has been to watch how much you eat. Except seafood also is a rich source of omega-3s, and nutritionists now say that the fatty-acid benefits, especially for pregnant women, could outweigh the heavy-metal risks.

What benefits, you say? The star of the omega-3 cast is docosahexaenoic acid (DHA), and as *The Economist* tidily explains: DHA is a component of brains, particularly the synaptic junctions between nerve cells, and its displacement from modern diets by the omega-6 acids in cooking oils such as soya, maize and rape is a cause of worry.

Many researchers think this shift—and the change in brain chemistry that it causes—explains the growth in recent times of depression, manic-depression, memory loss, schizophrenia and attention-deficit disorder. It may also be responsible for rising levels of obesity and thus the heart disease which often accompanies being overweight.

Stateside nutritionists are also changing their minds. A group has petitioned the Food and Drug Administration to adjust its stance on pregnant women's diets, and the Department of Defense plans to launch a program to augment soldiers' diets with omega-3s, *The Economist* reports. Low levels of DHA are a suicide risk factor for people in the service.

So here's the positive take-away, if there is one: Should you wish to get more fish-based omega-3s into your diet, eating lower on the fish food chain is the best way to make that happen, keep mercury levels low, and, oh yeah, stop straining the ocean's ecosystems by gobbling up big predators like tuna, swordfish, and grouper. (For what it's worth, there are also plant-based sources of omega-3s, although there have been studies that shed doubt on whether they are as beneficial as the fish-based ones.)

For some excellent reading about eating lower on the fish food chain, follow the link to an excerpt from Taras Grescoe's book *Bottomfeeder,* which is one of the most illuminating studies I've read on how to eat fish ethically. (And he's a big fan of the omega-3s.)

Critical Thinking

1. What type of fatty acid is docosahexaenoic acid (DHA)? Identify the fish that are the best sources of DHA.

2. What are the health benefits of consuming DHA?

3. Soybean oil, corn oil, and rapeseed (canola) oil are examples of what type of fat?

UNIT 4
Diet and Disease

Unit Selections

Learning Outcomes

After reading this Unit, you will be able to:

- Summarize the relationship of type 2 diabetes and obesity, insulin resistance, and fatty liver disease.

- Compare and contrast the physiological actions of glucose vs. fructose in the body.

- Explain why the results from the majority of research on fructose, diabetes, and obesity are rarely conclusive.

- Summarize the immune response to a pathogen and the type of nutrients involved at each phase.

- Identify nutrients needed to maintain a strong immune system.

- Illustrate the link between the consumption of high-fructose corn sweeteners and increased risk for heart disease, metabolic syndrome, type 2 diabetes, gout, and accumulation of visceral fat.

- Define discretionary calories. Identify the recommended amount of discretionary calories for an average male and female.

- Discuss why it is more challenging for older adults to lose or maintain their body weight.

- Describe the DASH diet. Identify how many servings of fruits and vegetables and how much sodium is recommended per day with the DASH diet.

Student Website
www.mhhe.com/cls

Internet References

American Cancer Society
www.cancer.org
American Diabetes Association
www.diabetes.org
American Heart Association (AHA)
www.americanheart.org
Medline Plus
www.nlm.nih.gov/medlineplus
National Eating Disorders Association
www.nationaleatingdisorders.org

Research that focuses on the connection between diet and disease has unraveled the role of many nutrients in the delay of onset of certain diseases, prevention of diseases, and in some instances disease reversal. The challenging aspect of releasing results from nutrition research is communicating this information in a manner that is not controversial or contradictory to previously released messages. With the increasing interest in health and disease prevention among Americans, media outlets publish scientific findings prematurely and without the physiological context in which the message should be conveyed. Scientific research takes time to answer the questions about health, nutrition, disease, and medicine, whereas consumers want answers to these questions much quicker than scientifically possible.

Medical and nutrition research has changed since the mapping of the human genome. We have come to better understand the role of genetics in the expression of disease and its role in how we respond to dietary change. In addition, research about diet and disease has enabled us to understand the importance and uniqueness of the individual (age, gender, ethnicity, and genetics) and his or her particular response to dietary interventions. Individualizing one's diet to prevent disease and promote health is a concept that we will see developing in the future.

The prevalence of diet and lifestyle related diseases in the United States is astronomical. Heart disease, type 2 diabetes, obesity, stroke, high blood pressure, osteoporosis, and certain cancers are diet- and lifestyle-related conditions that affect millions of Americans. Proper nutrition plays a vital role in these diseases. Components of foods such as saturated fats, trans fats, sodium, and added sugars continue to be highlighted as the premier culprits of these diseases.

The American Institute for Cancer Research estimates that 45 percent of colon cancers, 38 percent of breast cancers, and 69 percent of esophageal cancers would be prevented if Americans ate better, weighed less, and exercised more. One of the articles in this unit describes why a Western diet, obesity, and physical inactivity all contribute to a higher risk for cancer and discusses the importance of lifestyle changes on decreasing the incidence of these diseases.

The number one concern of the health of the United States is the prevalence of overweight and obesity. Although much of the attention is centered on childhood obesity and tactics to prevent or curtail it, there is also an ongoing problem with overweight or obesity as our population ages. On average, Americans in their sixties are 10 pounds heavier than they were just a decade ago. A typical woman in her 40s weighs 168 pounds, compared to 143 pounds in the 1960s. People used to start midlife at a lower weight and lose weight when they reached their 50s. Humans need fewer calories as they age because of slower metabolism and the tendency to lose muscle mass and gain fat, especially abdominal fat. Since muscle burns more calories than fat, it is challenging to lose weight in older years and maintain weight while eating the usual intake. Staying lean and eating right can delay onset or prevent certain diseases that plague older Americans, such as osteoporosis, heart disease, hypertension, insulin resistance, memory loss, arthritis, and some cancers.

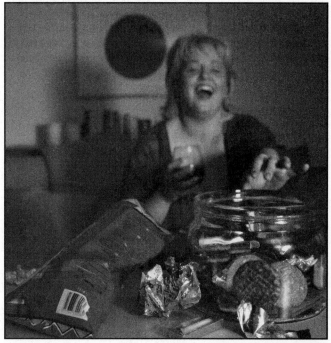

© BananaStock/PunchStock

One of the latest areas of concern is the degree of added sugars that are consumed by Americans. The average American consumes 350 to 475 grams of added sugars each day. The most commonly consumed form of added sugars is high-fructose corn syrup, but other forms of sugar such as table sugar, honey, and cane juice are considered to be "added sugar" too. As more research explores the negative effects of high-fructose corn syrup on human health, food companies are developing products using other forms of sugar. These "natural sugars" still provide empty calories in the diet that may lead to weight gain if consumed in excess and not balanced by physical activity. Discretionary calories (calories consumed after nutrient needs are met from healthy food and beverage sources) are an effective way to think about the calories that you consume in relation to the calories needed to provide adequate nutrient intakes. The USDA recommends discretionary calories of approximately 100 calories for women and 150 calories for men. Individual recommendations for discretionary calorie allowances can be calculated using mypyramid.gov.

High-fructose sweeteners have been linked to greater risk for heart disease, metabolic syndrome, type 2 diabetes, gout, and accumulation of visceral fat. The link may be secondary to increased triglycerides and uric acid in the bloodstream secondary to the way fructose is metabolized. Epidemiological data supports that there may be a relationship between fructose sweeteners and heart attacks. The Nurse's Health Study found that drinking 12 oz of regular soda correlates with increased risk of heart attack by 24 percent, and 24 or more ounces correlates to a risk of greater than 35 percent. Liquid calories from sugar sweetened beverages are not only empty calories, but also promote increased calorie intake at meals, possibly through suppression of leptin, a hormone that triggers you to stop eating.

The links between diet and lifestyle to certain chronic diseases are becoming common knowledge due to the amount of research conducted on the topics and the public health messages that attempt to translate the science into easily understood health messages. One disease that is not commonly listed among the diet/lifestyle related diseases is non-alcoholic liver disease. Research on this type of liver disease is fairly new and the incidence of non-alcoholic liver disease is increasing due to the prevalence of obesity and diabetes. Obesity and diabetes can cause excessive fat deposits in the liver. Non-alcoholic fatty liver disease affects an estimated 70–90 percent of obese people with type 2 diabetes. The article published in the *Harvard* *Health Letter* describes non-alcoholic liver disease, its diagnosis, and possible treatments.

The immune system is commonly taken for granted; however, it is a fascinating system of defense that is essential to our existence and optimal health. Proper nutrition and balanced nutrient intake is required for our immune system to function optimally. The article by Susan Percival describes the complex immune response and how nutrient deficiencies impair our immune system.

The articles in Unit 4 will be useful as a supplement to diet and chronic disease sections of general nutrition courses. The article topics add a slightly different view of the commonly known diet-related diseases and other diseases that are not publicized as often.

We Will Be What We Eat

When it comes to staving off the problems of aging, from bone and muscle loss to high blood pressure and heart disease, your diet is your friend—or enemy.

Meryl Davids Landau

If your mental image of an older person is someone frail and thin, it may be time for an update. For the generation currently moving through middle age and beyond, a new concern is, well, growing: obesity. "We're already seeing a large number of obese elderly, and if we don't do something, that figure is sure to rise," laments David Kessler, former commissioner of the Food and Drug Administration and author of *The End of Overeating*. Government figures show that Americans in their 60s today are about 10 pounds heavier than their counterparts of just a decade ago. And an even more worrisome bulge is coming: A typical woman in her 40s now weighs 168 pounds, versus 143 pounds in the 1960s. "People used to start midlife [at a lower weight] and then lose weight when they got into their 50s, but that doesn't happen as much anymore," Kessler says.

People used to start midlife at a lower weight than they do now and then lose weight in their 50s, but not anymore.

If you're entering that danger zone now, be aware that it's not going to get any easier to lose weight, because people need fewer calories as they age. Blame slowing metabolism and the body's tendency starting in midlife to lose muscle mass—a process known as sarcopenia—and gain fat, especially around the abdomen. (Fat burns fewer calories than does muscle.) "All that conspires to make it harder for people to maintain the same body weight when they eat their usual diets," says Alice Lichtenstein, director of the Cardiovascular Nutrition Laboratory at Tufts University. "People have fewer discretionary calories to play with, so they need to make better food choices."

Why do those choices matter? First, carrying an extra 20 or 30 pounds with you into old age doesn't bode well for attempts to head off the myriad diseases that strike in midlife and later and are linked to weight—including diabetes, arthritis, heart disease, and some forms of cancer. (It's probably not a coincidence that one recent study finds that people in their 60s have more disabilities than in years past.)

But paying attention to what you eat isn't only about controlling weight; the need for certain vitamins and minerals increases with age. One is calcium, necessary to protect bones. Another is B_{12}, since some older adults make less of the stomach acid required to absorb the vitamin. More vitamin D also is required. "The skin gets less efficient at converting sunlight into this vitamin, so more is needed from other sources," Lichtenstein says. Fewer than 7 percent of Americans between 50 and 70 get enough vitamin D from the foods they eat, and fewer than 26 percent get enough calcium.

Staying lean and eating right are both crucial for maintaining health through the years. (Kessler recalls a fellow researcher at Yale who, upon realizing the panoply of diseases linked to body weight, promptly lost 30 pounds.) If weight is a problem, it is especially important to cut back on the processed foods that combine sugar and fat. Studies with rats indicate that when the two are added to chow, animals can't easily stop eating, says Kessler. This happens in humans, too, he says, and food manufacturers have taken note and added sugar and fat to many products.

So what should people eat? A healthful diet at midlife is the same as for younger adults—it's just that the stakes may be higher. The focus should be on fruit, vegetables, whole grains, low- and nonfat dairy, legumes, lean meats, and fish. For someone whose current diet is far from this ideal, Lichtenstein suggests starting small: Swap dark-green lettuce for iceberg, load more veggies on the dinner plate, eat more skinless chicken or beans in place of hamburger. And exercise. Walking briskly for at least 30 minutes every day makes it easier to get away with the occasional cookie. With some further fine-tuning of that basic healthful eating plan, you can greatly improve your odds of staving off the major barriers to a vital old age.

Bone Loss

No nutrient can stop bones from losing mass over time, but consuming sufficient calcium and vitamin D can slow the deterioration, says Felicia Cosman, an osteoporosis specialist at Helen Hayes Hospital in West Haverstraw, N.Y., and clinical director of the National Osteoporosis Foundation. Once a person reaches age 50, calcium requirements jump from 1,000 mg to 1,200 mg per day. Cosman recommends adding up the number of servings consumed in a typical day of dairy products and foods that are highly calcium-fortified, such as orange juice and cereal, and multiplying that by the 300 mg each most likely supplies. Add 200 to 300 mg for the combined trace amounts in leafy green vegetables, nuts, and other sources. Then get the remainder in a supplement. By midlife, adults also need at least 800 to 1,000 IU of vitamin D to help the body absorb calcium and, possibly, prevent other diseases, according to the NOF. Sources include fatty fish such as salmon (also important for heart health), egg yolks, and fortified foods, but most people need to supplement.

Heart Disease

By now, every American surely knows the roll call of foods that affect your heart, for better and for worse. Good for the ticker: monounsaturated fats like olive oil and the omega-3 fatty acids found in such cold-water fish as salmon and herring and in flaxseed and walnuts. Harmful: too much red meat and full-fat dairy, because of their saturated fat content, and margarine and baked goods, because of the trans fats they contain.

But expunging troublesome foods from your daily fare can be surprisingly difficult. "Although many supermarket products have removed the trans fats, they're hardly history. Restaurants, especially, continue to use them," cautions Robert Eckel, former president of the American Heart Association and a professor at the University of Colorado-Denver. Some food manufacturers, moreover, have simply swapped out their trans fats for saturated fat, which is equally problematic, Eckel says. Saturated fat should total no more than 7 percent of daily energy intake—about 16 grams for the average 2,000-calorie diet.

Recent research points to another potential heart danger. It's not fat; it's high-fructose corn syrup, commonly found in soda. The decades-long, 88,000-woman Nurses' Health Study found that, even controlling for weight and other unhealthful habits, drinking one 12-ounce can of regular soda daily boosts a woman's risk of later having a heart attack by 24 percent; two or more servings raise the risk by 35 percent. "We don't know exactly why this is, but fructose does increase uric acid and triglycerides in the blood, which are known contributors to hypertension and heart disease," says study coauthor Teresa Fung, associate professor of nutrition at Simmons College in Boston.

Hypertension

Lowering high blood pressure before it contributes to the development of heart disease is vital for people in midlife. It can be accomplished with an eating plan known as the DASH (Dietary Approaches to Stop Hypertension) diet. "The DASH diet has the same effect as taking a blood-pressure-lowering medication," Eckel says. The DASH-Sodium version, which subtracts salt, works as well as up to two medications. The plan is rich in fruits and vegetables (eight to 10 servings a day for someone on a 2,000-calorie diet), grains (six to eight servings daily, with most being whole grains), and low-fat protein sources. And it's low in saturated fats and added sugars. The biggest difference from standard healthful eating advice is DASH's focus on lowering

sodium, which can damage artery walls in people sensitive to the nutrient. The diet limits sodium to 2,300 mg a day, while DASH-Sodium slashes it to 1,500 mg—just two thirds of a teaspoon. It's not enough to go easier on the salt shaker; the National Institutes of Health recommends looking for low- or no-salt labels, limiting high-sodium foods like bacon and sauerkraut, and rinsing canned foods. (A one-day sample menu of a DASH eating plan is available on the *U.S. News* website at www.usnews.com/dash.)

Insulin Resistance

Research has repeatedly demonstrated that type 2 diabetes and insulin resistance (a precursor to the disease in which the body begins to respond less well to the hormone that clears glucose from the blood stream) can often be prevented or postponed with a healthful diet, exercise, and weight loss. That three-part combination, in fact, actually has been shown to be more effective than medication. An eating plan aimed at minimizing the risk of insulin resistance does not have to be complex. "I coach people to mentally divide their lunch and dinner plate into thirds, with one third protein, one third nonstarchy vegetables, and the final third a starch like brown rice, whole-wheat pasta, potatoes, or corn," says Nora Saul, a dietitian and diabetes educator at Harvard's Joslin Diabetes Center in Boston. It's also a good idea to get serious about cutting back on sugar and white flour, both of which have a high glycemic index and can spike blood glucose levels.

Memory Problems

Alas, there's no magic bullet that will guarantee protection from dementia. But researchers are finding that a Mediterranean diet—similar to a conventional healthful diet but with an emphasis on fish and olive oil—seems to lower the odds of developing cognitive problems. Scientists at Columbia University followed more than 1,300 people for up to 16 years; those most closely adhering to this diet developed Alzheimer's at half the rate of those who didn't. One caveat: Alcohol (particularly in the form of wine), one element of the Mediterranean Diet that has been suggested to enhance memory function, has not been proved to do so, says Gary Kennedy, director of geriatric psychiatry at Montefiore Medical Center in New York.

Joint Disease

Although age is a risk factor for arthritis, the breakdown of cartilage in the joints is not inevitable. Minimizing weight gain goes a long way toward avoiding this problem, because every extra pound translates to 3 pounds of pressure on the knees while walking. It is also a good idea to limit foods that encourage inflammation in the body, particularly omega-6 fatty acids (found in corn and soybean oils and many snack and fried foods), the Arthritis Foundation says.

Cancer

Some 45 percent of colon cancers, 38 percent of breast cancers, and 69 percent of esophageal cancers would never occur if Americans ate better, weighed less, and exercised more, estimates the American Institute for Cancer Research. "It's not just cancers of the digestive tract. What you eat and what you weigh affect certain other cancer types as well," says Alice Bender, AICR's nutrition communications manager. The organization recommends limiting red meat to 18 (cooked) ounces per week and loading up on plant-based foods, which are high in the phytochemicals and antioxidants known to inhibit cancer cell growth in lab animals. Those with the deepest colors—like purple grapes, blueberries, and leafy green vegetables—tend to have the most beneficial compounds. One recent study, for example, showed that eating foods such as broccoli and kale that have lots of sulforaphane, an antioxidant, suppresses a bacterium linked to stomach cancer.

It looks as if food is the best source of healthful nutrients. "Numerous studies on supplements—of vitamin C, lycopene, beta carotene, and even fiber—have all proved disappointing," Bender says. Yet another reason to swap that cookie for a carrot.

Critical Thinking

1. Why is it more difficult for people over the age of 50 to lose or maintain their weight?

2. Which nutrients are needed in higher quantities by older adults?

3. What is the DASH diet? How many servings of fruits and vegetables and how much sodium is recommended per day on the DASH diet?

Sugar Overload
Curbing America's Sweet Tooth

What led the American Heart Association to issue its new scientific statement on "Dietary Sugars Intake and Cardiovascular Health"?

The association cited the "worldwide pandemic of obesity and cardiovascular disease" in explaining its "heightened concerns about the adverse effects of excessive consumption of sugars."[1]

"Added sugars have become such a predominant feature of the American diet that we can't help but recognize their major contribution to excess calories," explains Van Horn. The average American swallows 350 to 475 calories' worth of added sugars each day (depending on the type of data used to estimate intakes).

Exactly what *are* added sugars? They include high-fructose corn syrup, ordinary table sugar, honey, agave syrup, and all other sweeteners with calories. (In this article, the word "sugars" refers to them all.)

To hear some critics talk, high-fructose corn syrup is the real villain. Table sugar gets a free pass. (See "Fear of Fructose".)

In fact, high-fructose corn syrup is roughly half fructose and half glucose, as is table sugar (sucrose) once it breaks down in the body. And although the fructose half may cause some problems, the glucose half causes others. So if there's a villain, it's *all* sugars.

"Added sugars are added sugars," says Rachel Johnson, a professor of nutrition at the University of Vermont who chaired the heart association panel that issued the new sugars advice.

Who can afford the roughly 400 calories' worth of added sugars that the typical American consumes each day?

"No adults, except those who are extremely physically active—we're talking about the Michael Phelpses of the world," says Linda Van Horn, a professor of preventive medicine at the Northwestern University Feinberg School of Medicine in Chicago. "The rest of us have no business consuming that many calories from sugars."

There's new evidence that added sugars—or sugar-sweetened beverages—may raise the risk of obesity, heart disease, diabetes, and gout.

What's wrong with sugars? For starters, they're not good for your teeth, especially if they come in sticky foods. Here are 10 reasons to cut back.

1. **You can't afford the empty calories.** The American Heart Association based its advice on what scientists call "discretionary calories"—that is, how much room you have for empty calories once you've eaten all the vegetables, fruit, lean protein, low-fat dairy, whole grains, and other foods you need to stay healthy. (It's like discretionary income that people can spend on luxuries once they've paid their bills.)

"There's no question that sugars are a major culprit in obesity, because they're a source of empty calories that most Americans don't need," says Van Horn. "They have no nutritional benefit whatsoever."

The fact is that most people simply can't afford a 500-calorie scone or a 600-calorie Venti White Chocolate Mocha when they stop at Starbucks.

"Added sugars either crowd out healthy foods, or they make you fat if you eat them in addition to healthy foods," explains Frank Sacks, a professor of cardiovascular disease prevention at the Harvard School of Public Health in Boston.

So the heart association turned to the discretionary calorie allowances calculated by the U.S. Department of Agriculture. (To find yours, go to mypyramid.gov.)

A typical woman, who should shoot for 1,800 calories a day, for example, would need about 1,600 calories a day from vegetables, fruits, lean protein, dairy foods, and whole grains to get the nutrients she needs.

That leaves about 200 calories to spend (like discretionary income) on whatever she wants. "We said, okay, half of that discretionary calorie allowance can come from solid fats and half can come from added sugars," explains Johnson. That's about 100 calories each.

A typical man should shoot for 2,200 calories a day. He gets about 150 calories to spend on each.

"Solid fats" include not just butter or margarine, but the extra fat you get if you choose dairy foods (milk, cheese, yogurt, ice cream) that aren't fat-free, poultry with skin, and cakes, cookies, pies, and other sweets that aren't fat-free. So unless you eat mostly fat-free foods, your 100-calorie solid-fat allowance is going to disappear quickly.

Sucrose

Sucrose (table sugar) is broken down—in the body and (to some extent) in foods—to half fructose and half glucose. At that point it is essentially identical to high-fructose corn syrup.

Sugar by Any Other Name

Here's the scoop on some popular sugars. Sucrose (table sugar) breaks down into 50% fructose, 50% glucose in the body.

Agave syrup or nectar *(84% fructose, 8% glucose, 8% sucrose).* From the Mexican Agave cactus.

Apple juice concentrate *(60% fructose, 27% glucose, 13% sucrose).* Made by cooking down apple juice.

Brown sugar *(97% sucrose, 1% fructose, 1% glucose).* Granulated white sugar mixed with a small amount of molasses.

Corn syrup *(8% to 96% glucose, 0% fructose, 0% sucrose).* A liquid made from cornstarch.

Evaporated cane juice *(100% sucrose).* Crystals made by evaporating liquid that has been pressed from sugarcane.

Fructose *(100% fructose).* Found naturally in fruits and vegetables. We get most of our fructose from high-fructose corn syrup.

Glucose or Dextrose *(100% glucose).* Small amounts are found naturally in fruit and vegetables, but most is made from cornstarch. It's also found in honey and most other sugars.

Grape juice concentrate *(52% fructose, 48% glucose).* Made by cooking down grape juice.

High-fructose corn syrup (HFCS) *(typically 55% fructose, 45% glucose or 58% glucose, 42% fructose).* Corn syrup with some of its glucose converted into fructose.

Honey *(50% fructose, 44% glucose, 1% sucrose).* Made by honeybees from plant nectar.

Maple syrup *(95% sucrose, 4% glucose, 1% fructose).* Boiled down tree sap from the sugar maple tree.

Molasses *(53% sucrose, 23% fructose, 21% glucose).* By-product of sugarcane refining. Blackstrap molasses is a good source of iron and calcium.

Orange juice concentrate *(46% sucrose, 28% fructose, 26% glucose).* Made by cooking down orange juice.

Raw sugar *(100% sucrose).* Partially refined sugar with some molasses left.

Table sugar, Confectioner's sugar, Baker's sugar, Powdered sugar *(100% sucrose).* Most is refined from sugarcane or beets.

Note: If percentages don't add up to 100, other sugars account for the difference.

Sources: USDA Nutrient Database and company information.

And guess what happens to your added sugars allowance if you want a glass of wine or beer.

"It's been shocking to some people when I've said that we've been fairly conservative, because if you're consuming alcohol regularly, you should be having even less added sugar," notes Johnson.

If you want more sugar, you can always burn more calories.

"What I tell people who can't live with the added-sugars recommendation is that they need to move more," says Johnson. "Then you can have more sugar."

2. **Sugar-sweetened beverages promote obesity.** We're eating 20 percent more added sugars now than we did in 1970. What's largely responsible for the leap in sugars intake?

"Soft drinks, soft drinks, soft drinks," says Johnson. In 1965, Americans got an average of 12 percent of their calories from beverages. In 2001, beverages accounted for 21 percent.[1]

"Soft drinks are the number-one source of added sugars in Americans' diets," says Johnson. And sugary liquids may make us fatter because they don't curb our appetite for more food.[2]

"When you give people liquid calories before a meal, they don't compensate by eating less at the meal or later, in the same way they do for calories from solid food," notes Johnson.

In a classic study at Purdue University, researchers gave 15 young adults 450 calories of sugars each day as either a liquid (a soft drink) or a solid (jelly beans).[3] After one month on the jelly beans, the volunteers compensated by eating less of other foods, so they gained no weight. But on the soft drinks, they actually ate slightly *more* food than before. That plus the calories in the soft drinks led them to gain weight.

Where's the Added Sugar?

Coke. Pepsi. Sprite. Regular sodas add the most sugar to a typical American's diet. But don't forget about coffee drinks, teas, sports drinks, and fruit drinks that have a health halo.

And in a recent trial that lasted 1½ years, people who cut back on liquid calories lost more weight than those who cut the same number of solid calories.[4]

"I keep telling people, 'If you're trying to cut back on added sugars, look at what you're drinking,' " says Johnson.

What's more, in a study of 51,000 women, those who went from drinking regular soda no more than once a week to at least once a day gained the most weight over four years.[5]

It's not just soda pop.

"If you look at consumption data, soft drinks are leveling off, but other sugar-sweetened beverages—sports drinks, energy drinks, sweetened teas—are taking off," Johnson notes.

"Just walk down the supermarket aisles. An entire one is filled with soft drinks and another is filled with other sugar-sweetened beverages that have a health halo."

3. **Sugar-sweetened drinks may raise the risk of heart disease.** "Sugars have for many years been considered neutral in their impact on cardiovascular disease," says Northwestern University's Linda Van Horn. "But in an obese environment like ours, we can't turn a blind eye to added sugars that contribute to excess calorie intake."

Fear of Fructose

"Made with no high-fructose corn syrup," brags the label of Thomas' Original English Muffins and dozens of other foods. What's wrong with high-fructose corn syrup (HFCS)?

Here's what the popular website run by Dr. Joseph Mercola (mercola.com) claims: "Part of what makes HFCS such an unhealthy product is that it is metabolized to fat in your body far more rapidly than any other sugar, and, because most fructose is consumed in liquid form (soda), its negative metabolic effects are significantly magnified."

"Among them: diabetes, obesity, metabolic syndrome, an increase in triglycerides and LDL (bad) cholesterol levels, liver disease."

There's some truth to some of those claims, but Mercola makes a common mistake: he seems to confuse high-fructose corn syrup with fructose, as though high-fructose corn syrup were mostly fructose. It's not.

"High-fructose corn syrup is typically 55 percent fructose, explains Kimber Stanhope, who conducts research on sugars at the University of California, Davis." "But sucrose, or table sugar, is 50 percent fructose."

Glucose makes up the rest of both HFCS and sucrose. So it's not surprising that researchers find few differences—in blood sugar, insulin, ghrelin (which stimulates appetite), or leptin (which curbs appetite)—when they pit high-fructose corn syrup against table sugar.[1]

"We still have no comparative data showing that HFCS or sucrose is better or worse than the other," says Stanhope.

What's the harm in minimizing high-fructose corn syrup? Nothing. "But people become so conscious of avoiding high-fructose corn syrup that they forget about avoiding other sweeteners," says University of Vermont researcher Rachel Johnson.

"I ate a granola bar the other day that listed brown rice syrup on the ingredient list. Doesn't that sound healthy? It's just a sweetener. Added sugars all add empty calories."

[1]Am. J. Clin. Nutr. 87: 1194, 2008.

Clearly, excess weight isn't good for the heart. A big belly is one part of the metabolic syndrome, which raises the risk of heart disease (and diabetes). But sugar-sweetened beverages may promote heart disease whether or not they make you gain weight.

When Harvard researchers tracked more than 88,000 women for 24 years, they found that—regardless of weight—those who drank at least two sugar-sweetened beverages a day had a 20 percent higher risk of heart disease than those who drank less than one sugar-sweetened beverage a month.[6]

"Our data suggest that soft drinks increase the risk above and beyond their impact on weight," notes study coauthor JoAnn Manson, a professor of medicine at Harvard Medical School.

And when scientists tracked 4,000 men and women in the Framingham Heart Study for four years, those who drank at least one soft drink a day had a 44 percent higher risk of being diagnosed with the metabolic syndrome than those who drank less than one soft drink a day, regardless of how much they weighed.[7]

Why else would sugar-sweetened drinks raise the risk of heart attacks? One possibility: the fructose in added sugars (like high-fructose corn syrup and table sugar) raises levels of fats called triglycerides. Higher-than-normal triglycerides are another sign of the metabolic syndrome.

4. **Fructose raises triglycerides.** Cholesterol isn't the only thing in blood that's linked to heart attacks. People with higher-than-normal triglycerides (at least 150) are also at risk, especially if their triglycerides soar after a meal.[8]
   And fructose raises triglycerides after meals.

For example, researchers at the University of Minnesota fed 24 men and women a diet that got 17 percent of its calories from either glucose or fructose.[9]

(That's a high dose, since Americans average 16 percent of their calories from added sugars, roughly half of it from fructose and half of it from glucose.)

After six weeks, triglyceride levels throughout the day were 32 percent higher when the men (but not the women) ate the high-fructose diet.

Peter Havel and colleagues at the University of California, Davis, got similar results when they studied 32 over-weight or obese men and women over 40. Participants got a hefty 25 percent of their calories from beverages sweetened with either fructose or glucose for 10 weeks.[10]

Once again, blood levels of triglycerides after a meal were higher on fructose than on glucose. "It's a strong and consistent effect," says researcher Kimber Stanhope, who works with Havel.

Triglycerides rose more in men, but they also rose in women, notes Stanhope, "possibly because the women in our study were older and heavier" than those in the earlier study.

Why would people on a high-fructose diet have higher triglycerides than people on a high-glucose diet?

When you consume a large dose of glucose, the liver doesn't pull much of it in if you don't need the calories. In contrast, fructose ends up in the liver whether you need the calories or not.

"The liver will take up nearly the entire amount of fructose," says Stanhope. "Very little of the fructose stays in the bloodstream."

What does the liver do with all that fructose? "It starts converting some of the fructose into fat," Stanhope explains. "Much of this fat gets sent into the bloodstream, resulting in higher levels of triglycerides."

That would explain why large doses of fructose boost triglyceride levels in the bloodstream and possibly in the liver. Would smaller doses do the same?

"We're testing lower doses right now," says Stanhope. "We're studying over 200 younger people, so it will take a while."

5. **Sugar-sweetened beverages may promote diabetes.**
   When researchers tracked roughly 91,000 women for eight years, those who drank at least one sugar-sweetened soft drink a day had an 83 percent higher risk of type 2 diabetes than those who drank less than one a month.[5]

When the scientists took weight out of the equation, soda drinkers had a 40 percent higher risk.

Tout de Sweet

A typical woman should get no more than 100 calories (about 6½ teaspoons) a day from added sugars, says the American Heart Association. A typical man should get no more than 150 calories (about 9½ teaspoons)—roughly what's in a 12 oz. can of Coke.

Here's how much added sugars you'd get in a sampling of popular foods. (The numbers don't include the naturally occurring sugars in fruit or milk.) To convert teaspoons to grams of sugar, multiply by 4. To convert teaspoons to calories from sugar, multiply by 16.

Food	Added Sugars (teaspoons)
Dairy	
Ice cream, vanilla *(½ cup)*	3
Chocolate milk, reduced fat 2% *(8 fl oz.)*	3½
Yogurt, low-fat vanilla *(6 oz.)*	3½
Yogurt, low-fat fruit *(6 oz.)*	4½
Silk Chocolate Soymilk *(8 fl oz.)*	5
TCBY Old Fashioned Vanilla Frozen Yogurt *(regular cup, 8.7 oz.)*	6*
Baskin-Robbins Vanilla Ice Cream Cone *(double scoop, 8.4 oz.)*	11½*
Chocolate shake, fast food *(16 fl oz.)*	13
Dairy Queen Heath Blizzard *(medium, 14.5 oz.)*	26*
Baskin-Robbins Oreo Outrageous Sundae *(12.6 oz.)*	27*
Coldstone Creamery Founders Favorite *(Gotta Have It, 14.6 oz.)*	30½*
Beverages	
Propel Lemon *(24 fl oz.)*	1½
Starbucks Caffè Mocha *(grande, 16 fl oz.)*	3*
Starbucks Caramel Macchiato *(grande, 16 fl oz.)*	4*
Starbucks Vanilla Latte *(grande, 16 fl oz.)*	4*
Hawaiian Punch Fruit Juicy Red *(8 fl oz.)*	4½*
SunnyD Tangy Original *(8 fl oz.)*	4½*
Starbucks Cinnamon Dolce Latte *(grande, 16 fl oz.)*	5*
Starbucks Tazo Shaken Iced Tea, any flavor *(grande, 16 fl oz.)*	5
Gatorade Lemon-Lime *(20 fl oz.)*	8½
Glacéau Vitamin Water Revive *(20 fl oz.)*	8½
Starbucks Tazo Passion Shaken Iced Tea Lemonade *(grande, 16 fl oz.)*	8½
Coca-Cola *(12 fl oz. can)*	10
Snapple Lemon Tea *(16 fl oz.)*	10½
Nestea Iced Tea Sweetened Lemon *(16.9 fl oz.)*	12
Schweppes Tonic Water *(20 fl oz.)*	14
SoBe Green Tea *(20 fl oz.)*	15½
Sprite *(20 fl oz.)*	16
Arizona Southern Style Sweet Tea *(23 fl oz.)*	16½
Coca-Cola *(20 fl oz.)*	16½
Minute Maid Lemonade *(20 fl oz.)*	17
Pepsi *(20 fl oz.)*	17½
Sunkist Orange Soda *(20 fl oz.)*	21

Candy, Chocolate, etc.	Added Sugars (teaspoons)
Werther's Original Hard Candies *(3 pieces, 0.6 oz.)*	2½
Lindt Excellence 70% Cocoa Dark Chocolate *(4 squares, 1.4 oz.)*	3
Dove Dark Chocolate Promises *(5 pieces, 1.4 oz.)*	5
Hershey's Milk Chocolate Bar *(1.6 oz.)*	5½*
York Peppermint Patties *(1 patty, 1.4 oz.)*	6½
Jelly Belly Jelly Beans *(35 pieces, 1.4 oz.)*	7
M&M's Milk Chocolate *(56 pieces, 1.7 oz.)*	8
Maple syrup *(¼ cup, 2.9 oz.)*	12

Sweets *(1 item, unless otherwise noted)*	
Pepperidge Farm Milano, original *(3 cookies, 1.2 oz.)*	3
Entenmann's Crumb Coffee Cake *(1/10 cake, 2 oz.)*	3½
Mrs. Fields semi-sweet Chocolate Chip Cookie *(1.2 oz.)*	3½
Nabisco Oreo *(3 cookies, 1.2 oz.)*	3½
Pepperidge Farm Double Chocolate Milano *(3 cookies, 1.4 oz.)*	4
Entenmann's Rich Frosted Donut *(2.1 oz.)*	4½
Jell-O Strawberry *(1 snack cup, 3.5 oz.)*	4½
Sara Lee All Butter Pound Cake *(1 slice, 2.7 oz.)*	5
Entenmann's Glazed Buttermilk Donut *(2.1 oz.)*	5½
Krispy Kreme Chocolate Iced Kreme Filled Doughnut *(3.1 oz.)*	6
Entenmann's Chocolate Fudge Cake *(⅙ cake, 2.3 oz.)*	7
Krispy Kreme Glazed Chocolate Doughnut *(2.8 oz.)*	7
Starbucks Chocolate Chunk Cookie *(3 oz.)*	8
Starbucks Marble Loaf *(1 slice, 3.8 oz.)*	8
Panera Chocolate Chipper Cookie *(3.3 oz.)*	8½
Panera Chocolate Fudge Brownie *(3.5 oz.)*	8½
Starbucks Classic Coffee Cake *(4 oz.)*	8½
Hostess Twinkies *(2 cakes, 3 oz.)*	9
Starbucks Pumpkin Scone *(4.2 oz.)*	11
Entenmann's Super Cinnamon Buns *(6 oz.)*	11½
Hostess Sno Balls *(2 cakes, 3.5 oz.)*	11½
Panera Pecan Roll *(5.5 oz.)*	12
Panera Pumpkin Muffin *(6 oz.)*	12
Cinnabon Classic Cinnamon Roll *(7.8 oz.)*	14
Denny's Hershey's Chocolate Cake *(1 slice, 5 oz.)*	14
Dunkin' Donuts Coffee Cake Muffin *(5.8 oz.)*	14½
Uno Chicago Grill Chocolate Chocolate Malt Layer Cake *(1 slice, 9.5 oz.)*	25

Cereals & Cereal Bars	
Kashi TLC Trail Mix Chewy Granola Bar *(1 bar, 1.2 oz.)*	1½
General Mills Cinnamon Toast Crunch *(¾ cup, 1.1 oz.)*	2½
General Mills Honey Nut Cheerios *(¾ cup, 1 oz.)*	2½
Kellogg's Bite Size Frosted Mini-Wheats *(24 biscuits, 2.1 oz.)*	3
Kashi GoLean Crunch! Original *(1 cup, 1.9 oz.)*	3½
Kellogg's Cracklin' Oat Bran *(¾ cup, 1.8 oz.)*	4
Kashi GoLean Cookies 'N Cream Chewy Bar *(1 bar, 2.8 oz.)*	9

Miscellaneous	
Bush's Homestyle Baked Beans *(½ cup, 4.5 oz.)*	3
Cracker Jack *(½ cup, 1 oz.)*	4
Häagen-Dazs Chocolate Sorbet *(½ cup, 3.7 oz.)*	5

*CSPI estimate. Note: Added sugars are rounded to the nearest half teaspoon.

Sources: Company information and U.S. Department of Agriculture Nutrient Database. Chart compiled by Amy Ramsay.

Sweet Nothings

When researchers gave people either regular or diet soft drinks for several weeks, the participants gained weight only on the regular sodas.[1,2] But all non-caloric sweeteners are not created equal. Here's our take on their safety:

- **Acesulfame-potassium.** Tests conducted in the 1970s were of mediocre quality. One suggested an increased cancer risk in female rats.
- **Aspartame (NutraSweet, Equal).** Judging by two recent rat studies, it may slightly increase cancer risk. At the very least, new studies should be conducted.
- **Saccharin (Sweet'N Low).** In animal studies, it has caused cancer of the urinary bladder, uterus, ovaries, skin, blood vessels, and other organs.
- **Stevia.** Coke and Pepsi have started to use it to sweeten some beverages. It appears to be safe, though there should be more independent testing.
- **Sucralose (Splenda).** It appears to be safe, though there hasn't been much independent testing. (Sucralose isn't as natural as ads have implied. It's made by chlorinating sugar molecules.)

[1]*Am. J. Clin. Nutr. 76:* 721, 2002.

[2]*Am. J. Clin. Nutr. 51:* 963, 1990.

"Weight gain appears to account for half of the increased risk," says Manson.

What could explain the other half? "Sugar-sweetened soft drinks might also increase the risk of type 2 diabetes because they're high in rapidly absorbable carbohydrates," she suggests.

High-fructose corn syrup is roughly half fructose, which goes largely to the liver, so it doesn't raise blood sugar. But the glucose half of high-fructose corn syrup heads straight to the bloodstream.

"Consumption of sugar-sweetened soft drinks causes a fast and dramatic increase in blood sugar levels," says Manson. "In our studies, people who eat foods that raise blood sugar levels have a higher risk of diabetes."

6. **Fructose may boost visceral fat.** In the University of California, Davis, study, the 32 men and women gained about the same weight (roughly three pounds) after 10 weeks whether they drank beverages sweetened with fructose or glucose.[10] But there were differences.

The fructose eaters (especially the men) gained more deep abdominal—or visceral—fat than the glucose eaters. That's critical because visceral fat is linked to a higher risk of heart disease and diabetes.

In contrast, the glucose eaters gained more subcutaneous fat, which is just below the skin and is less likely to raise the risk of diabetes and heart disease.

Since this study was the first to see fructose's effect on visceral fat, Stanhope notes, "it would be good to see the result confirmed in other studies."

Another new finding: the fructose drinkers had a drop in insulin sensitivity. Reduced sensitivity to insulin is linked to a higher risk of heart disease and diabetes. But it's too early to know if Stanhope's results will hold up in future studies.

If fructose makes insulin less efficient, no one knows how. "It may be due to an increase in the amount of triglyceride stored in the liver," speculates Stanhope, "which could then lead to a chain of events that causes insulin receptors to perform less effectively."

7. **Fructose may raise the risk of gout.** Gout hurts. If your blood has too much uric acid, the excess ends up in joints (especially those of the big toe), where it can cause excruciating pain.

"Obesity is the major risk factor for gout because it's so common and it substantially increases the risk," says Gary Curhan, an associate professor of medicine at the Harvard Medical School.

But fructose is also a culprit. "We know that fructose increases uric acid, and that uric acid causes gout," says Curhan.

In a study of roughly 46,000 men, those who got at least 12 percent of their calories from fructose were nearly twice as likely to be diagnosed with gout over the next 12 years as those who got less than 7 percent of their calories from fructose.[11]

"After we adjusted for weight and all the other risk factors for gout that we know about, people with higher intakes of fructose had a substantially higher risk of gout," Curhan explains.

At least that's true in men, who are far more likely to get the disease. "We're just starting to look at women," says Curhan.

8. **Fructose may promote over-eating.** Leptin is a hormone made by fat cells. It's supposed to make you stop eating.

"Leptin tells your brain that you've got enough calories on board," says Robert Lustig, a professor of clinical pediatrics at the University of California, San Francisco, who served on the heart association sugar panel. "When you don't get that signal, you're still hungry."

When researchers fed rats a huge dose of fructose (60 percent of their diet) for six months, the animals became resistant to leptin—that is, leptin injections failed to curb their appetite.[12]

(Obese people can also be leptin-resistant. "They have lots of leptin, but it doesn't work," explains Lustig.)

Over time, a high-fructose diet blocks the leptin signal in the brain, notes Lustig. "So leptin can't extinguish hunger and can't extinguish reward." The result: you keep eating.

In fact, when the rats were allowed to eat as much palatable food as they wanted, they gained nearly twice as much weight as rats that got no fructose.

But so far, it's not clear what happens when people eat fructose in less-excessive amounts.

The Bottom Line

- Shoot for 100 calories (6½ teaspoons, or 25 grams) a day of added sugars if you're a woman and 150 calories (9½ teaspoons, or 38 grams) a day if you're a man. Even less may be better for your heart (see "What Should I Eat?" *Nutrition Action,* Oct. 2009).
- Don't drink sugar-sweetened beverages. Limit fruit juices to no more than 1 cup a day.
- Limit *all* added sugars, including high-fructose corn syrup, cane or beet sugar, evaporated cane juice, brown rice syrup, agave syrup, and honey.
- Don't worry about the naturally occurring sugar in fruit, milk, and plain yogurt.
- To estimate your calorie needs and get a more precise added-sugars limit, go to mypyramid.gov and click on "Get a personalized plan" in the "I Want To . . ." box.
- If a food contains little or no milk or fruit (which have natural sugars), the "Sugars" number on the package's Nutrition Facts panel will tell you how much added sugars are in each serving.

In two preliminary studies, 17 obese men and women and 12 normal-weight women had higher leptin levels over a 24-hour period when they consumed 30 percent of their calories from glucose-sweetened beverages with meals than when they consumed the same amount of fructose-sweetened beverages with meals.[13,14] Few other studies have been done.

Does that mean we should be eating foods sweetened with glucose, which is what's in ordinary corn syrup?

"Why do we need corn syrup anyway?" asks Lustig. "We're better off getting carbs from foods that are packaged naturally with their own fiber. If we got carbs from whole grains, vegetables, fruit, and beans, we wouldn't overeat."

Fruit contains fructose (as well as sucrose and glucose). Do we need to limit apples and oranges? "I'm not concerned about fructose from fruit," says Lustig. "How many oranges can you eat in one sitting?"

9. **Minimizing added sugars keeps a lid on blood pressure.** "There's a possibility that sugar raises blood pressure," says Frank Sacks of the Harvard School of Public Health. "But it's far from definitive."

However, what *is* clear is that there's little place for sugar in a diet that's designed to lower blood pressure (see *Nutrition Action,* Oct. 2009, cover story).

The OmniHeart Study tested three diets on people with hypertension (blood pressure at least 140 over 90) or pre-hyper-tension (blood pressure at least 120 over 80).[15] Each diet was rich in fruits, vegetables, low-fat dairy foods, beans, nuts, and other foods that supply potassium, magnesium, and other key nutrients.

"The higher-carb OmniHeart diet did a great job of lowering blood pressure," says Sacks. It had just five teaspoons (80 calories) of added sugars a day. In people with hypertension, it trimmed systolic blood pressure (the top number) by an impressive 13 points.

But, adds Sacks, "the other two Omni-Heart diets—which were higher in either protein or unsaturated fat—did better." Those diets, which contained only two or three teaspoons (30 to 50 calories) of added sugars a day, cut systolic blood pressure by 16 points in people with hypertension.

"There's not much room for added sugars in most people's diets," concludes Sacks. "And certainly not if you're trying to optimize your diet to lower blood pressure."

His advice: "I never drink liquid calories, and I keep sweets and snacks out of the house. It's okay to indulge once in a while, but if I get hungry at night and there are no sweets around, I eat nuts or an apple."

10. **Most sugary foods are junk.** Coca-Cola, Pepsi, Cinnabon, Krispy Kreme, Dunkin' Donuts, Snapple, Entenmann's, Hostess, Sara Lee, Little Debbie.

Just about any sweets made by those and similar companies are high in sugars and low in nutrients. Many are also packed with virtually worthless white flour. And many are now supersized. Do you need a Cinnabon that's the size of a boxed lunch?

To stick to the heart association's new recommendations, you'll need to use your added sugars calorie allowance wisely. (To find out how much added sugar is in popular foods, see "Tout de Sweet").

"Be discriminating," suggests the University of Vermont's Rachel Johnson. "People enjoy sweet taste, and if you're discriminating, it has a role in a healthy diet. We're not all going to eat non-fat plain yogurt."

But "they're called discretionary calories for a reason," she adds. "Use them to enhance the palatability of already nutritious foods."

"I'd rather see someone consume added sugars in a flavored yogurt or a whole-grain breakfast cereal or by putting maple syrup on oatmeal than consume them in a doughnut or soft drink."

Notes

1. *Circulation 120:* 1011, 2009.
2. *Physiol. Behav. 59:* 179, 1996.
3. *Int. J. Obesity 24:* 794, 2000.
4. *Am. J. Clin. Nutr. 89:* 1299, 2009.
5. *JAMA 292:* 927, 2004.
6. *Am. J. Clin. Nutr. 89:* 1037, 2009.
7. *Circulation 116:* 480, 2007.
8. *JAMA 298:* 309, 2007.
9. *Am. J. Clin. Nutr. 72:* 1128, 2000.
10. *J. Clin. Invest. 119:* 1322, 2009.
11. *BMJ 336:* 309, 2008.
12. *Am. J. Physiol. Regul. Integr. Comp. Physiol. 295:* 1370, 2008.
13. *J. Clin. Endocrinol. Metab. 89:* 2963, 2004.
14. *J. Clin. Endocrinol. Metab. 94:* 1562, 2009.
15. *JAMA 294:* 2455, 2005.

Critical Thinking

1. Describe the concept of discretionary calories. What are the recommended amount of discretionary calories for an average male and female?

2. Explain why consuming high-fructose corn sweeteners increases the risk for heart disease, metabolic syndrome, type 2 diabetes, gout, and accumulation of visceral (abdominal) fat.

3. Why do fructose sweeteners promote overeating? Identify the hormone that is involved.

From *Nutrition Action HealthLetter,* January/February 2010, pp. 3–8. Copyright © 2010 by Center for Science in the Public Interest. Reprinted by permission.

Fructose Sweeteners May Hike Blood Pressure

Human study confirms trend seen earlier in animals.

JANET RALOFF

The more fructose American adults add to their diets, the higher their blood pressure tends to be. The new finding adds fuel to a simmering controversy about whether this simple sugar—found in fruits, table sugar, soft drinks and many baked goods—poses a health hazard that goes beyond simply consuming too many empty calories.

If the new data are confirmed, they might go a long way toward explaining a more than tripling in hypertension rates over the past century—a period when "fructose consumption has increased dramatically in industrialized nations including the United States," the authors say.

The idea that fructose might play a role in hypertension is not new. In 2008, an international team of researchers found that among mice, "Fructose feeding decreased salt excretion by the kidney and resulted in hypertension." The scientists also homed in on a potential mechanism: the activity of a gene responsible for helping the small intestine absorb salt and secrete bicarbonate. When these researchers fed fructose to mice without the functioning gene or to animals eating a salt-free diet, the animals' blood pressure remained unaltered.

But that was in rodents.

Diana Jalal and fellow nephrologists at the University of Colorado Denver Health Sciences Center in Aurora decided to look for evidence that fructose might have a similar effect in people. So they pulled data collected from a representative cross-section of Americans as part of the National Health and Nutrition Examination Survey. Conducted every few years, the new study's data came from the 2003 to 2006 survey and included more than 4,500 adults with no prior diagnosis of hypertension.

Sure enough, when Jalal's group stratified the participants by blood pressure—and many had undiagnosed prehypertension or outright vascular disease characterized by significantly elevated blood pressure—mean intake of added dietary fructose climbed by group. Their findings appear in the *Journal of the American Society of Nephrology,* published online July 1 ahead of print.

Their focus was "added" fructose. The qualifier refers to fructose intake other than that occurring as a natural constituent of any fruits or other produce. And the reason: Americans are not renowned for downing even the recommended daily servings of fruits and vegetables, much less an excess.

So these nephrologists—kidney specialists—concentrated on the fructose present as a sweetener in processed foods and beverages. Although fructose constitutes half of table sugar, it's actually sweeter than the other constituent (glucose), so manufacturers have taken to sweetening most products with a high-fructose corn syrup. This somewhat increases the fructose content of the diet.

The new paper shows a barely significant trend toward increasing blood pressure with increasing fructose intake—until its authors applied a statistical technique (logistic regression analysis) to investigate the likelihood of blood pressure increasing as fructose consumption rises. Then they found a statistically significant link—but just for people with bonafide hypertension and only for systolic blood pressure (the higher of the two numbers in a blood-pressure reading).

Explains Jalal, her team's new data indicate that "High fructose intake is a strong predictor of a greater risk of hypertension." The average intake for people proved to be about 74 grams of added fructose per day, an amount equivalent to 2.5 soft drinks. People who ingest more than that "are at increased risk of high blood pressure when compared to the ones that ingest low fructose within each blood-pressure category," she says.

While the Denver group was working on this study, another came out last year focusing on "sugar-sweetened beverage consumption, a significant source of dietary fructose." It too focused on NHANES data—in this case, on almost 4,900 U.S. adolescents during the previous survey period: 1999 to 2004. And here, drinking sugary soda pop was again linked with elevated systolic blood pressure.

Of course, there are caveats. NHANES participants report their own dietary intake. The data are collected on diet the day before, not what each individual typically eats most days. And some people may be more sensitive to fructose impacts, whatever they might be.

Expect push back from the sweetener industry, especially the Washington, D.C.-based Corn Refiners Association, which has been defending high fructose corn syrup. Its website says: "Research confirms that high fructose corn syrup is safe and no different from other common sweeteners like table sugar and honey."

I asked Michel Conchol, another of the Denver authors, about what's next for his group: Will you conduct a feeding trial to control for differences in fructose contributions to the diet? Yes, he said: "We are already planning such a study."

Critical Thinking

1. The two studies cited in this article were analyses of National Health and Examination Survey (NHANES) data. What is NHANES?

2. What component of blood pressure (systolic or diastolic) is elevated in these two studies?

3. Do these two studies prove (show a cause and effect) that drinking added fructose sweeteners causes increased blood pressure? Explain your answer.

Role of Sugar Intake in Beverages on Overweight and Health

Max Lafontan, PhD

The present overview will be limited to the analysis of the putative impact of sugar inclusion in beverages on health, obesity, and diabetes risk. Mechanisms of action and physiological end points will be highlighted to clarify the differences existing in the health impact of various kinds of sugars.

Sugars, Heterogeneity, Basic Biology, Major Metabolic Impacts and Health-Related Questions

The term *sugars* (carbohydrates) includes a large family of monosaccharides and disaccharides, which are naturally present in (or added to) food or beverages. Sugar is the most common word for saccharose (sucrose); it represents 75 percent of added sugars, whereas glucose syrup represents only 25 percent in France. The most commonly used sweetener in the United States is high-fructose corn syrup (55 percent fructose and 45 percent glucose). The mean sugar content of sugar-sweetened beverages (SSBs) commonly used in the United States is 10 g/100 g (ranging from 4.5 to 16 g/100 g). Sugar-sweetened beverages represent the major source of dietary fructose, as provided in various forms including carbonated soft drinks, juice-based beverages, 100 percent juices, flavored milk, gourmet coffees, and liquid meal replacement mixtures for weight loss. Fructose is also included in solid foods (pastries, desserts, and a number of processed foods). The introduction of high-fructose corn syrup in the 1970s in the United States has resulted in a 30 percent increase in total fructose intake in the last 20 years. It is associated with a remarkable increase in the rates of obesity and diabetes.[1–3]

Glycemic Index, Glycemic Load, and Feeding

The glycemic index (GI) is the method of indexing the glycemic response to a fixed amount of available carbohydrate from a test food, to the same amount of available carbohydrate from a standard food consumed by the same subject. Initially, the standard "food" was glucose, now it is white bread. The glycemic load (GL) is a ranking system integrating sugar content and portion size; it is the product of the GI and total carbohydrates in the food portion. Detailed data on GI and GL are reported by Foster-Powell et al.[4] Foods with high GI are suspected to be the dietary factor that promotes repeated insulin release and contributes to the settlement of chronic diseases in patients at risk. Drinking SSBs when eating food contributes to a high GI of the overall diet.

Glucose and Fructose Possess Strikingly Different Metabolic Fates

Main alimentary polysaccharide hydrolysis generates glucose, fructose, and galactose, which are absorbed by the intestinal cells and delivered into circulation. Glucose and fructose have different metabolic fates in terms of absorptive processes, metabolic effects, and actions on leptin, ghrelin, and insulin secretion. Growing evidence suggests direct and opposite actions of glucose and fructose on hypothalamic neurons and food intake.

The site, rate, and extent of carbohydrate digestion and absorption from the gut are keys to understanding the many roles of carbohydrates. Glucose and galactose are absorbed via a Na^+/glucose cotransporter (SGLT1), whereas fructose is absorbed further down the duodenum by a non–Na^+-dependent process (Glut 5 transporter). The gastrointestinal system plays an important role in the neuroendocrine regulation of food intake. Recent mechanisms governing sugars and other nutrient sensing and peptide secretion by enteroendocrine cells have been discovered. Novel taste-like pathways exist in the enteroendocrine cells, which express several G protein–coupled receptors identified as taste receptors similar to those previously found in the taste buds on the tongue.[5] Several enteroendocrine cell types throughout the gut express T1R2/3 sweet taste G protein—coupled receptors, T2R-family bitter receptors, and/or the taste-specific G protein $G\alpha_{gustducin}$.[6] The combination of T1R2+3 recognizes natural sugars such as sucrose and glucose and also artificial sweeteners such as saccharin and acesulfame K.[7]

Glucose is an energy-providing substrate; glucose consumption by muscle considerably increases during physical exercise. Glucose oxidized during physical activity comes from glycogen stores in the liver and muscles and from ingested carbohydrates. Oxidation of other hexoses (eg, fructose and galactose) is lower than that of glucose. They must be transformed into glucose by the liver before utilization by skeletal muscle. Glucose need depends on the type of exercise, its intensity and duration, age, sex, and the level of physical training of the subjects. Nutrition recommendations for men and women performing exercise must be adapted to their individual needs according to the exercise performed.

Outside its role as an energy-providing substrate in numerous tissues, glucose is also an important signaling molecule. Glucose is involved in the regulation of the expression of genes regulating glycolysis and lipogenesis via a pathway involving a new transcription factor (ie, carbohydrate regulatory element binding protein).[8] Fructose metabolism has unique characteristics; it is largely metabolized in the liver (50 percent–70 percent), with the rest being metabolized by the kidneys and adipocytes. Fructose possesses beneficial effects at low concentrations (hepatic glucose uptake) while exerting a number of deleterious effects when chronically consumed in excess (hepatic steatosis, insulin resistance, inflammation, and hyperuricemia).[9]

Glucose sensing is an important function of the brain.[10] Two populations of glucose-sensing neurons have been identified in hypothalamic areas: those that are excited (ie, increased electrical activity) and those that are inhibited (ie, decreased activity). They are triggered at different glucose concentrations. Unlike glucose, which suppresses food intake, fructose increases food intake when metabolized by the central nervous system. Fructose has the opposite effect of glucose on the AMP activated kinase/malonyl–CoA signaling system and thereby feeding behavior. Thus, increased fructose metabolism within the brain increases food intake and obesity risk.[11]

Sugars and Sweetness Are Important in Establishing Lifelong Food Habits

It is important to understand the early factors that determine choice and ingestion, when designing strategies to enhance the health of infants, children, and adults. Early experiences set the stage for later food choices, and they are important in establishing lifelong food habits.[12] Different brain regions are responsive to sweetness intensity and pleasantness perceptions in humans.[13] Psychological and behavioral components of sweetness are very complex. Full development of this question is considered to be outside the present review.

Glucose, Insulin Secretion, and Glucotoxicity

High dietary GI and GL have been associated with an increased risk of developing type 2 diabetes mellitus in large prospective studies.[14] The foods that were the most consistently associated with increased risk of type 2 diabetes are white rice, white bread, potatoes, and SSBs. Type 2 diabetes is a complex syndrome of polygenic nature; the genetic susceptibility of the pancreas β cells determines the risk of developing the disease. Increased plasma glucose and free fatty acids may exert, in the long term, toxic influences on β-cell function. When glucose

is in excess, instead of flowing uniquely and normally through oxidative phosphorylation, metabolites overflow into alternative pathways causing oxidative stress and leading to β-cell dysfunction.[15]

Comments on the Obesity Epidemic

Adipocyte number is settled early in life during childhood and adolescence. An increasing number of nations face childhood obesity problems. Obese children are at a high risk of becoming irreversibly obese adults. Most obese adults have been obese since childhood, with less than 10 percent of children with normal weight going on to develop adult obesity. By contrast, more than three-fourths of obese children go on to become obese adults. Obesity has its genesis in childhood. Interventional focus should be placed in early life.[16] Risk factors and causes of obesity in children include a number of parameters (ie, genetic, antenatal life, auxologic parameters at birth, early postnatal development, socioeconomic conditions of the parents, physical activity, dieting, etc).

Increased lipid storage in already developed fat cells (adipocytes) is thought to be the most important event of fat mass expansion. Adipocyte number is a major determinant for the fat mass in adults. As previously suspected in the 1970s, a recent study has confirmed that the number of adipocytes existing in adulthood is set during childhood and adolescence. The number of fat cells stays constant in adulthood in lean and obese individuals, even after marked weight loss. Approximately 10 percent of fat cells are renewed annually at all adult ages and levels of body mass index. A tight regulation of fat cell numbers occurs during adulthood.[17] Thus, it is clear that an excess number of fat cells represent an important element of the future of fat mass status. The number of adipocytes for lean and obese individuals is set before the age of 20 years. Adipocyte number is subject to little variation during adulthood; changes are limited to variations in cell size. Even after significant weight loss in adulthood and reduced adipocyte volume, the adipocyte number remains the same.

Glucose uptake is essential for triacylglycerol synthesis in human fat cells. Glucose uptake by fat cells operates under the control of the Glut 4 glucose transporter. Insulin stimulates fatty acids and glucose uptake and activates lipoprotein lipase activity and triglyceride synthesis.[18] It is easily understandable that whenever insulin release is potently stimulated by high GI food or SSB intake, a potent signal for fat storage will be provided to the fat cell by insulin. Erratic and/or frequent intake of SSBs could represent a risk of fat storage in patients at risk of developing obesity, depending on their activity level. Cumulative daily imbalances in energy intake affect body fat mass.[19] If intake exceeds expenditure by 2 percent daily (ie, <1 can of SSBs) for a year, the result would be an increase of 75 312 kJ, or approximately 2.3 kg. A major program to control childhood obesity must be established at all the levels of health care delivery. The necessary measures include education of the public regarding the risk factors for childhood obesity: (1) limit consumption of sucrose- and fructose-containing drinks and foods with high carbohydrate and fat contents, (2) assume correct hydration by water drinking, and (3) promote exercise programs at home and at school.

What Do Epidemiological Studies Tell Us: Interest and Limits of Cross-sectional, Longitudinal, and Intervention Studies?

Overweight among children has increased dramatically during the past 2 decades and is reaching epidemic proportions. The obesity epidemic is a crisis that requires action before all the scientific evidence is settled. A number of questions have been raised concerning the putative impact of SSBs on health and obesity epidemics. Energy intake is positively associated with consumption of soft drinks.[20] For example, mean adjusted energy intake was 7656 kJ/d for school-aged children who were not consumers of SSBs, compared with 8443 kJ/d for children who consumed an average of 250 mL of soda per day.[21]

Influential global reports have asserted that SSBs play a key role in the etiology of overweight and obesity.[22,23] Cross-sectional studies are the most common. A number of comprehensive scientific reviews of the evidence have tended to be cautious, less straightforward, and with a number of controversies that cannot be detailed here. A recent systematic review and meta-analysis have concluded that the strength of the relationship was near zero and contested some previous positive results.[24] However, this meta-analysis was open to criticisms. Concerning longitudinal studies, half of a group of 18 showed a significant positive result between SSB intake and body mass index; the effect appears to be rather small. The effects of potential confounding factors from other components of the diet, physical activity, and other lifestyle factors are not sufficiently assessed in the majority of such studies, as recently discussed.[25]

Intervention trials represent the best level of evidence to test a hypothesis. Avoidance of SSBs may help to prevent further weight gain in overweight children or obese subjects.[26, 27] The relative effects of dietary sugars (glucose vs fructose) were compared during a 10-week consumption period. Overweight and obese subjects consumed glucose- or fructose-sweetened beverages providing 25 percent of energy requirements for 10 weeks. It was demonstrated that dietary fructose specifically increases hepatic de novo lipogenesis, promotes dyslipidemia, decreases insulin sensitivity, and increases visceral adiposity in overweight/obese adults.[28] Results of intervention trials are promising, although they remain quite rare, difficult to settle, and expensive.

Conclusions and Future Trends

Despite the large number of studies on the role of sugar intake in beverages on overweight and health, definitive conclusions are not easily drawn from studies. Publication biases have been highlighted recently.[25] Industry-funded studies tend to reveal smaller effects than other studies. Cross-sectional studies are the most abundant types of studies but they cannot establish cause-effect relationships and are rarely conclusive. The effects observed in longitudinal studies are often seen in the studies of smaller size, but could be affected by modification of other aspects of diet and lifestyle. It is necessary to be careful with industry-funded studies, which have a tendency to reveal smaller effects.

The recent results of an intervention study provide the best arguments to infer causality. It is expected that this kind of intervention approach will be expanded in the future in the different populations of the planet because nutritional habits and sugar composition of SSBs could differ noticeably. Intervention trials must be developed to delineate the doses of SSBs promoting adverse changes of plasma lipids and a decrease in insulin sensitivity in different populations at risk for health problems. More studies of adequate duration must also be performed among children and in overweight consumers of SSBs. When considering weight changes and obesity-related questions related to SSB consumption, it is important to take into account population differences and genetic parameters. Lifestyle influences (eg, other components of the diet and physical activity) must also be considered in the studies.

References

1. Bray GA, Nielsen SJ, Popkin BM. Consumption of high-fructose corn syrup in beverages may play a role in the epidemic of obesity. *Am J Clin Nutr.* 2004;79:537–543.
2. Havel PJ. Dietary fructose: implications for dysregulation of energy homeostasis and lipid/carbohydrate metabolism. *Nutr Rev.* 2005;63:133–157.
3. Johnson RJ, Segal MS, Sautin Y, et al. Potential role of sugar (fructose) in the epidemic of hypertension, obesity and the metabolic syndrome, diabetes, kidney disease, and cardiovascular disease. *Am J Clin Nutr.* 2007;86:899–906.
4. Foster-Powell K, Holt SH, Brand-Miller JC. International table of glycemic index and glycemic load values: 2002. *Am J Clin Nutr.* 2002;76:5–56.
5. Cummings DE, Overduin J. Gastrointestinal regulation of food intake. *J Clin Invest.* 2007;117:13–23.
6. Rozengurt E. Taste receptors in the gastrointestinal tract. I. Bitter taste receptors and alpha-gustducin in the mammalian gut. *Am J Physiol Gastrointest Liver Physiol.* 2006;291:G171–G177.
7. Li X, Staszewski L, Xu H, et al. Human receptors for sweet and umami taste. *Proc Natl Acad Sci USA.* 2002;99:4692–4696.
8. Postic C, Dentin R, Denechaud PD, et al. ChREBP, a transcriptional regulator of glucose and lipid metabolism. *Annu Rev Nutr.* 2007;27:179–192.
9. Johnson RJ, Perez-Pozo SE, Sautin YY, et al. Hypothesis: could excessive fructose intake and uric acid cause type 2 diabetes? *Endocr Rev.* 2009;30:96–116.
10. Gonzalez JA, Reimann F, Burdakov D. Dissociation between sensing and metabolism of glucose in sugar sensing neurones. *J Physiol.* 2009;587:41–48.
11. Lane MD, Cha SH. Effect of glucose and fructose on food intake via malonyl-CoA signaling in the brain. *Biochem Biophys Res Commun.* 2009;382:1–5.
12. Beauchamp GK, Mennella JA. Early flavor learning and its impact on later feeding behavior. *J Pediatr Gastroenterol Nutr.* 2009;48(1 suppl):S25–S30.

13. Small DM, Gregory MD, Mak YE, et al. Dissociation of neural representation of intensity and affective valuation in human gustation. *Neuron.* 2003;39:701–711.

14. Willett W, Manson J, Liu S. Glycemic index, glycemic load, and risk of type 2 diabetes. *Am J Clin Nutr.* 2002;76:274S–280S.

15. Poitout V, Robertson RP. Glucolipotoxicity: fuel excess and beta-cell dysfunction. *Endocr Rev.* 2008;29:351–366.

16. August GP, Caprio S, Fennoy I, et al. Prevention and treatment of pediatric obesity: an endocrine society clinical practice guideline based on expert opinion. *J Clin Endocrinol Metab.* 2008;93:4576–4599.

17. Spalding KL, Arner E, Westermark PO, et al. Dynamics of fat cell turnover in humans. *Nature.* 2008;453:783–787.

18. Lafontan M. Advances in adipose tissue metabolism. *Int J Obes (Lond).* 2008;32(suppl 7):S39–S51.

19. Rosenbaum M, Leibel RL, Hirsch J. Obesity. *N Engl J Med.* 1997;337:396–407.

20. Ludwig DS, Peterson KE, Gortmaker SL. Relation between consumption of sugar-sweetened drinks and childhood obesity: a prospective, observational analysis. *Lancet.* 2001;357:505–508.

21. Harnack L, Stang J, Story M. Soft drink consumption among US children and adolescents: nutritional consequences. *J Am Diet Assoc.* 1999;99:436–441.

22. World Health Organization and Food and Agriculture Organization. *Diet, Nutrition and the Prevention of Chronic Diseases.* Geneva, Switzerland: WHO; 2003.

23. World Cancer Fund Food. *Nutrition, Physical activity and the Prevention of Cancer.* Washington, DC: American Institute for Cancer Research; 2007.

24. Forshee RA, Anderson PA, Storey ML. Sugar-sweetened beverages and body mass index in children and adolescents: a meta-analysis. *Am J Clin Nutr.* 2008;87:1662–1671.

25. Gibson S. Sugar-sweetened soft drinks and obesity: a systematic review of the evidence from observational studies and interventions. *Nutr Res Rev.* 2008;21:134–147.

26. Ebbeling CB, Feldman HA, Osganian SK, et al. Effects of decreasing sugar-sweetened beverage consumption on body weight in adolescents: a randomized, controlled pilot study. *Pediatrics.* 2006;117:673–680.

27. Sichieri R, Paula Trotte A, de Souza RA, et al. School randomised trial on prevention of excessive weight gain by discouraging students from drinking sodas. *Public Health Nutr.* 2009;12:197–202.

28. Stanhope KL, Schwarz JM, Keim NL, et al. Consuming fructose-sweetened, not glucose-sweetened, beverages increases visceral adiposity and lipids and decreases insulin sensitivity in overweight/obese humans. *J Clin Invest.* 2009;119:1322–1334.

Critical Thinking

1. Compare and contrast the physiological actions of glucose vs fructose in the body.

2. List the diseases caused by excess intake of fructose, particularly from high-fructose sweeteners.

3. Explain why fructose is implicated in the increased prevalence of type 2 diabetes and obesity.

4. Evaluate why the results from the majority of research on fructose, diabetes, and obesity are rarely conclusive. What type of research needs to be conducted to provide more conclusive evidence?

MAX LAFONTAN, PHD, is director of research, Unité Inserm 858, Institut de Médecine Moléculaire de Rangueil, and Université Paul Sabatier, Toulouse, France. The author is not receiving any funding for research investigations from Danone Waters but has received consulting fees from a paid advisory board for the review. Dr Lafontan has received speaker and consultancy honorarium from Danone Waters R&D.

When the Liver Gets Fatty

Havard Health Letter

A s Americans have gotten fatter, so have their livers, and some hearts may suffer as a result.

There's a fair amount of guesswork to the estimates, but perhaps as many as 20 percent of American adults have some degree of fatty liver disease, a condition that used to occur almost exclusively in people who drink excessively. The epidemics of obesity and diabetes are to blame. Fatty liver affects between 70 percent and 90 percent of people with those conditions, so as obesity and diabetes have become more common, so has fatty liver disease.

Fatty liver disease isn't confined to any one group, and there don't seem to be pronounced gender differences, but studies suggest that Latinos are disproportionately affected. It's primarily a condition of middle age, although children may get it, too. Fatty liver disease is rapidly becoming more common in Asia, and some research suggests that men in India may be especially susceptible.

Plumped-up Liver Cells

The prevailing theory is that the condition gets started because of insulin resistance, which is, in turn, frequently a consequence of obesity and excess fat tissue in the abdomen. When people are insulin resistant, their muscle, fat, and liver cells don't respond normally to insulin, so levels of the hormone—and the blood sugar it ushers into cells—build up in the blood. As a result, the risk of developing diabetes and heart disease increases. But insulin resistance is a complicated metabolic state that also includes an increase in the amount of free fatty acids circulating in the blood.

Fatty liver disease occurs when some of those fat molecules accumulate inside liver cells. The presence of those fattened cells can then lead to inflammation in the liver and damage to surrounding liver tissue. Once that happens, if excess alcohol is not involved, the condition is called nonalcoholic steatohepatitis (*steato-* for fat and *–hepatitis* because the liver is inflamed). Fortunately, that unwieldy name boils down to a handier acronym, NASH. Estimates vary quite a bit, but it seems that 5 percent to 10 percent of people with fatty liver disease go on to develop NASH.

NASH is often a relatively stable, low-grade condition that people live with for years, with few if any symptoms. But it can also start a cascade of serious damage to the liver and attempts by the organ to regenerate itself that culminate in an abundance of scar tissue and impaired liver function—a condition called cirrhosis. Cirrhosis is irreversible and can lead to total failure of the liver. It also is associated with an increased risk for developing liver cancer.

Some studies have shown as few as 3 percent of people with NASH developing cirrhosis, while others have shown as many as 26 percent doing so. There's no test or risk factor that predicts who will develop cirrhosis and who won't, although one study did find that people who are older or whose initial liver biopsies showed more inflammation were at greater risk. It's clear, though, that the prognosis for NASH is far better than it is for steatohepatitis that's the result of heavy alcohol consumption. Perhaps as many as half of all those with alcoholic steatohepatitis (which lacks a handy acronym) go on to develop cirrhosis.

It's just a theory at this point, but people with fatty liver disease and NASH may need to be more worried about heart disease and stroke than about serious liver problems. An article published in *The New England Journal of Medicine* in late 2009 argued that the inflammatory and other factors pumped out by a fat-afflicted liver promote the atherosclerotic process that damages the insides of arteries and makes blood more likely to clot, a combination that can lead to heart attack or stroke. The evidence the authors cited is intriguing, if circumstantial. They pointed to a study showing that people with NASH are twice as likely to die from heart attack or stroke as people without it. And NASH seems to add to the risks that come with excess weight. Overweight men with NASH have higher levels of C-reactive protein, an inflammatory factor, and fibrinogen, a clotting factor, than overweight men without NASH. Moreover, the levels of those and other factors go up as NASH gets more severe.

Diagnosis Requires a Biopsy

Most people with fatty liver disease don't have symptoms, and that's true even if it has developed into NASH. Only occasionally do people feel run-down, or they have an achy feeling in the upper right side of the abdomen, where the liver is located. So, more often than not, fatty liver disease and NASH are discovered incidentally, starting with higher than normal levels of

The Fatty Liver

How it Starts and What it can Lead To
Abdominal obesity and metabolic syndrome* cause insulin resistance Insulin resistance increases fatty acid levels in the blood

Fat accumulates in liver cells

- Up to 20 percent of Americans have fatty livers
- Usually there are no symptoms
- Weight loss can make the liver less fatty
- Excessive alcohol also make the liver fatty

Fat in liver cells causes inflammation and damage to liver tissue

- The medical term is *steatohepatitis* (*steato-* for fat and *-hepatitis* for liver inflammation)
- Steatohepatitis that's not related to alcohol is called nonalcoholic steatohepatitis, or NASH
- A liver biopsy is the only way to definitely diagnose NASH
- Weight loss is the main treatment; vitamin E has shown some promise

Further liver damage results in liver fibrosis and cirrhosis

- Fibrosis is a buildup of fibrous tissue; cirrhosis is a buildup of scar tissue
- Between 3 percent and 26 percent of NASH patients develop cirrhosis
- A small number of people with cirrhosis develop liver cancer

NASH has been linked to an increased risk of heart attack and stroke

- A liver affected by NASH may produce inflammatory factors that promote the atherosclerotic process that narrows blood vessels
- NASH may be just another aspect of metabolic syndrome
- The cause of NASH, not NASH itself, may increase heart attack and stroke risk

* Metabolic syndrome is abdominal obesity along with high triglycerides, high blood pressure, high blood sugar, and low HDL cholesterol.

liver enzymes on a routine blood test. Ultrasound imaging, the same technology used to get pictures of developing fetuses, can be informative: the liver looks bright because the fat shows up as white on the image. But neither an ultrasound nor a CT or MRI scan is completely reliable for making a diagnosis. The fat in the liver is visible, but not the NASH-related inflammation. Some researchers have developed formulas that use a simple blood test and measurements of various hormones, inflammatory factors, and liver enzymes to arrive at a diagnosis, but this work is at a preliminary stage.

Currently, a liver biopsy is the only way to make a definitive diagnosis of fatty liver or NASH. Liver biopsies involve inserting a long needle into the right side of the abdomen and extracting a small piece of liver tissue that can be examined under a microscope. Liver biopsies are an invasive procedure, so they aren't entirely free of risk and complications, but they're also fairly routine these days and can be done on an outpatient basis.

Whether a doctor will order a biopsy to nail down a diagnosis depends on many factors, including whether the person is obese or has diabetes or shows other signs of liver trouble.

Weight Loss is the Treatment

There's been a fair amount of research into using diabetes drugs to treat NASH, even in people who don't have diabetes. Rosiglitazone (sold as Avandia) and pioglitazone (sold as Actos) have been the leading candidates because they reduce insulin resistance, the root cause of fatty livers. They're not looking so promising these days. The FDA has moved to sharply curtail the use of Avandia because it seems to cause heart problems. The results of an important trial published in 2010 in *The New England Journal of Medicine* showed Actos to be no better than a placebo in improving NASH in people without diabetes.

Another diabetes drug, metformin (Glucophage), might prove to be an effective treatment, but there isn't enough evidence yet. Vitamin E is a possibility: the same trial that showed Actos wasn't effective showed some improvement in the livers of people who took large doses (800 IU daily) of the vitamin. But many doctors are wary about prescribing large doses of vitamin E because they've been associated with an increased risk of bleeding. Besides, the improvements in the liver were limited. Fish oil has produced some favorable results, and clinical trials are under way, but it can't be endorsed yet.

These setbacks and uncertainties have left weight loss (ideally from changes in diet and an increase in physical activity) as the only recommended treatment for most cases of fatty liver disease and NASH. In many cases, weight loss seems to have a very direct effect: as people lose weight, the fatty liver becomes less fatty. Crash dieting is a bad idea, though, because rapid weight loss (losing 4 pounds a week or more) can wind up damaging the liver. Of course, if sustained weight loss were easy, a lot of today's health problems would be solved, not just fatty liver disease and NASH.

In addition to encouraging people to lose weight, doctors will often advise people with diabetes who have fatty liver disease or NASH to be vigilant about controlling their blood sugar.

The Bottom Line

Many parts of the body come to grief once people become obese or develop diabetes. It's not surprising that our livers do too, given how central they are to a whole suite of metabolic processes. There's some evidence that a fatty liver may add to the already high risk of heart disease among people who are obese or have diabetes. Fatty livers can also develop into cirrhotic ones if the inflammatory processes take off.

But there are two bright spots in the take-home message about fatty livers. First, most cases stay relatively stable and don't result in serious liver disease. Second, the treatment is not an expensive drug with side effects, but losing weight—and that will benefit many other parts of the body besides the liver.

Critical Thinking

1. Define non-alcoholic steatohepatitis.
2. Explain the relationship of type 2 diabetes and obesity, insulin resistance, and fatty liver disease.
3. How does the prognosis of liver disease caused by excessive alcohol differ from NASH?
4. What is the most effective treatment currently available for NASH?

Nutrition and Immunity

Balancing Diet and Immune Function

SUSAN S. PERCIVAL, PhD

This article briefly reviews the components of the immune system with emphasis on a particular leukocyte, the gamma delta (γδ) T cell. The importance of nutrition in this large and complex system cannot be underestimated. All nutrients, macro and micro, are required in an optimum balance for the proper function of immunity. The issue is that an optimum balance specifically for the role of immunity in humans is not well understood. This article describes some of the consequences of nutrient deficiencies, but more importantly discusses foods that help maintain or balance the immune response by the γδ T cell. The consequences of an immune system that is out of balance are also discussed.

Functional Immunity

Parts and Location

Immune cells originate in the bone marrow. Some cells differentiate there, in the marrow (neutrophils, other granulocytes, and B cells), whereas others travel to the thymus (T cells) to differentiate. Some cells, for example, monocytes, travel through the blood and differentiate into macrophages in the tissues. Whereas the blood cells are the best studied because of their accessibility, many of our immune cells reside in the skin and the epithelial linings of the gut, lung, and reproductive system. The gut, because of its large surface area, is the largest immune organ in the body.

Three Modes of Operation

The first mode of operation is known as surveillance (Figure). To survey their environment, the immune cells migrate in and out of the lymph, blood, and tissues. Some maintain residence in tissues or lymph, whereas others never stop moving. Both static cells and migrating cells can be "samplers," testing their immediate surroundings for evidence of foreign invaders. Surveillance destroys foreign invaders without any symptoms of illness. One particular cell involved in surveillance is the γδ T cell, whose importance is a central focus of this report.

The second mode of operation is the activation or response. If surveillance is not enough to combat the foreign invader, the immune system goes into action, which is known as the response mode. First, signaling molecules such as cytokines (peptides), leukotrienes, and prostaglandins (lipids) are synthesized and secreted, resulting in a complex network of communication signals to other cells of the immune system. Cell numbers expand greatly, and eventually, the foreigner is destroyed by cytotoxic activity of the immune cells. Symptoms of illness, including inflammation and fever, accompany the response.

To understand the response capacity of immunity, the general organization will be covered first. In most of the literature, immunity is organized into 2 systems, the innate immune system and the adaptive (or acquired) immune system (Table). The cells of our innate immune system react within minutes to a foreign invasion. They kill pathogen using free radicals and other toxic chemicals, and they recognize foreign invaders by their nonspecific patterns. The innate cells express receptors on their cell surfaces that recognize nonspecific patterns known as pathogen-associated molecular patterns (PAMPs). Bacteria, for example, contain unique molecules such as lipopolysaccharide, not found in any other plant or animal. Other PAMPs are derived from viruses, protozoa, and fungi and include molecules such as peptidoglycans, lipoproteins, flagellin, double-stranded and single-stranded RNA from viruses, imidazoquinolines, CpG DNA motifs, and teichoic acids. Our innate immune system uses pattern recognition receptors to detect PAMP, and this recognition results in an immune response. Interaction of the PAMP with the pattern recognition receptors sets off a chain reaction of signaling molecules such as cytokines,

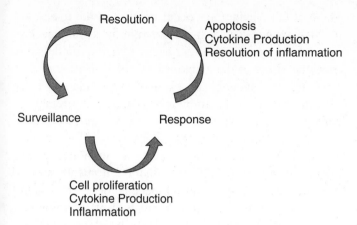

Figure. The cyclic nature of immunity. Surveillance is the nonsymptomatic mode of handling foreign invaders. When surveillance is not enough, activation of the immune response occurs, driven by cytokines and lipid mediators. Once the foreign invader has been disposed of, then an active process operates to resolve inflammation so that it returns to surveillance.

prostaglandins, and leukotrienes. These mediators, in turn, cause activation of the adaptive (or acquired) immune cells, the alpha beta ($\alpha\beta$) T cells and the B cells. The adaptive cells may take up to days to fully respond. They get their signals not only from the innate cells' signaling molecules but also from antigen-presenting cells. Each T or B cell of the adaptive immune system produces a unique receptor, and each cell responds to very specific antigens, not just a generalized pattern. Cells of the adaptive immune system have the ability to distinguish between self and nonself. Their mode of killing is by initiating apoptosis or programmed cell death. These cells are influenced by previous exposures to pathogens and thus are said to have memory.

Finally, the third mode is the return to normal surveillance. When the pathogen has been destroyed, the immune system returns to surveillance mode. This return to normal surveillance is an active process utilizing specific cells such as $\gamma\delta$ T cells, macrophages, natural killer cells, and CD8$^+$ T cells to destroy activated immune cells to end the response. The consequence of not ending the response is chronic inflammation and is discussed in the following section.

Nutritional Aspects
Nutrient Deficiencies
Many examples exist in the literature of specific nutrient deficiencies that result in impaired immunity and an impaired immune response. Protein-calorie malnutrition, essential lipid deficiency, and vitamin and mineral deficits all result in some aspect of impaired immunity. Nutrients are important for synthesis and secretion of signaling molecules, cell proliferation, free radical generation, and the active process of immune suppression at the end of the response. Lacking any nutrient would impair the response.

Nutrition for Surveillance and for the Response
A healthy, balanced diet provides all nutrients necessary for adequate operation of the surveillance mode because that is the normal condition under which nutrient requirements were determined. However, it is much more difficult to study the increased nutrient requirements during the immune response, but considering that cell proliferation is a major part of the response, all nutrients are required in greater quantity. To determine how much of an increased need occurs during the response, nutrient requirements would have to be studied at the onset of illness. Some of the nutrients for which information is available and that show a greater need in the context of the immune response include conditionally essential amino acids,[1,2] zinc,[3] and magnesium.[4] An exception to the generalized statement that all nutrients are needed in greater

Table. Origin and Function of Immune Cells

Branch	Cell	Differentiation Location	Specialized Function
Acquired	B cell	Bone marrow	Secret antibodies
	Tcell	Thymus	Cytotoxic, helper, regulatory
Innate	Monocyte	Bone marrow	Further differentiates to macrophages
	Macrophage	Tissues (see monocyte)	Phagocytosis, respiratory burst
	Neutrophils	Bone marrow	Phagocytosis, respiratory burst
	Other granulocytes:	Bone marrow	Various: basophils, eosinophils, mast cells
Characteristics of both	$\gamma\delta$ T cell	Thymus	Cytotoxic, regulatory
	Natural killer cell	Bone marrow	Cytotoxic

amounts is iron, because it appears to be sequestered during an immune response.

Other indirect evidence that suggests initiating an immune response requires more nutrients is due to the nature of the response itself: in addition to the demands for cellular proliferation, the immune response must synthesize and secrete signaling molecules and antibodies. Although it is difficult to pinpoint exactly how much more of a specific nutrient is needed, some research suggests that greater doses of nutrients may reduce the severity of a cold or flu. A meta-analysis[5] suggests that gram quantities of vitamin C taken regularly had no effect on the incidence of common cold symptoms but were beneficial in that they reduced the duration of the cold. However, a subgroup exposed to extreme conditions (exercise and/or cold weather) did have a reduced incidence when supplemented with gram quantities of vitamin C. The mechanism by which vitamin C works to reduce severity of an illness is not clear.

Folic acid and other B vitamins that are involved in 1-carbon metabolism are also considered critical nutrients for the response mode. Because of the rapid proliferation of many immune cell types, the need to synthesize DNA, transcribe message, and translate proteins may require more of these vitamins.

Vitamins A and D, because of their role in cellular differentiation and transcription, are theoretically required in greater amount when mounting an immune response. The stores of nutrients may be enough to handle the increased need without requiring an increased intake, but nonetheless are used by the body to a greater extent for an immune response.

During the response, assessing nutrient requirements is more challenging. Nutrients are required in greater quantity when the immune system is responding, but what ones, and how much, is not known. Studying simple illness in humans is not easy, unless perhaps it is under controlled conditions, such as a viral challenge. Humans are genetically or environmentally dissimilar, but even more challenging is that humans have differences in vaccination histories as well as immunological memories. In other words, different people will respond in different ways to the same challenge.

Consequences of Not Ending an Immune Response

Inflammation is a necessary component of the immune response. What is inflammation, exactly? It is a collection of symptoms described more than 2000 years ago as swelling, due to increased permeability of the capillaries resulting in edema, redness, and heat due to increased blood flow, and pain due to stimulation of nerve endings.

Some of these symptoms occur because of the release of reactive oxygen species that are part of the killing mechanism of the innate immune system. Other symptoms are from the effect of the cytokines and lipid mediators that drive the inflammatory process and set the stage for both the eradication of the foreign invader and the repair of damaged tissues. Normally, mechanisms are in place to restore the immune response to its surveillance mode. However, in some circumstances, the immune system inappropriately stays "on" because it is chronically stimulated by some foreign invasion that cannot be eradicated, or the mechanism to turn inflammation off is impaired. Chronic inflammation is thought to be responsible for many diseases.

Conversely, the disease itself might be a cause of chronic inflammation. Heart disease, cancer, rheumatoid arthritis, inflammatory bowel disease, and some neurological disorders have symptoms that suggest chronic inflammation may be involved in the disease process. Reactive oxygen species that are generated during chronic inflammation may cause damage to host macromolecules if not contained or neutralized. For example, oxidized low-density lipoprotein molecules may be viewed as foreign by the immune system and are taken up by macrophages in the arterial vessel walls. Reactive oxygen species may damage cellular DNA, and this damage may have some relationship to cancer, although cancer is much more complex than simple DNA damage. Oxidation of proteins affects the elasticity of cell membranes and may impair function of enzymes. Some neurological disorders are associated with oxidized proteins in the brain. Damage to carbohydrate moieties, specifically those in the joint fluids such as hyaluronic acid, is thought to be associated with some forms of arthritis. To summarize, inflammation is important for an immune response, but there are circumstances where it may be dysregulated. Can diet help alleviate some of the repercussions of chronic inflammation? And, importantly, can dietary factors be helpful in helping to resolve the inflammation after it is no longer needed for the immune response?

Good evidence has been published that omega-3 fatty acids play a role in resolving inflammation when the response is no longer needed. The omega-3 fatty acids of importance are eicosapentaenoic acid and docosahexaenoic acid, 20:5n-3 and 20:6n-3, respectively. The synthesis of lipid mediators from these fatty acids produces inflammatory products of lower bioactivity compared with those derived from arachidonic acid, 20:4n-6. Moreover, eicosapentaenoic acid and docosahexaenoic acid can produce lipid mediators with anti-inflammatory activity. The potent anti-inflammatory mediators are known as the resolvins and protectins.[6]

Priming as a Means to Optimize Immune Response

The ability to prime our immune cells is poorly defined, mechanistically. B cells are primed as a result of vaccinations. In this sense, B cells are trained to recognize an attenuated foreign invader and forms memory cells that can respond faster and more effectively in the event that foreign invader is encountered again.

Certain molecules prime the immune cell without overtly activating the cell because they interact only weakly. Known as nonmicrobial priming, it is a fairly new concept in relation to dietary compounds and results in upregulation of mRNA transcripts but no translation of protein.[7] The immune cell is primed by certain food ingredients and is now able to respond quicker and more effectively to eradicate the real foreign invader because the building blocks are already present. Some of the molecules that can weakly interact with immune cells and prime them are found in foods of plant origin. The complex molecular structure of some phytochemicals may look similar to a PAMP, but not similar enough to result in activation.

Evidence That Some Food Ingredients Prime Immune Cells

This portion of the article discusses recent research showing evidence of priming of the γδ T cell by food and food components. First, the γδ T cell is briefly described, and then, the food components that prime this cell are briefly reviewed.

The γδ T cell resides mainly in the skin and in the epithelial linings of the gut, lungs, and reproductive tract. There they act as a first line of defense against pathogens that are eaten or inhaled. About 5 percent to 8 percent of human T cells in the blood are the γδ T cells, with the remainder circulating T cells the more common αβ T cell. Although they are a T cell, carrying the T-cell receptor (TCR), they behave more like innate cells in that they recognize PAMPs and do not require recognition of the major histocompatibility complex as does the αβ T cell.

Generally, the γδ T cells are studied with those isolated from the blood because acquiring them from tissue, in humans, at least, is not feasible. Some of the γδ T cells may be naive, meaning they have not interacted with pathogen. But some may have already surveyed their environment, have interacted with foreign objects, and are now migrating through the blood to other locations.[8] Thus, some of the γδ T cells isolated from the blood have been exposed to food components in the gut, and the functional changes due to diet can be measured in γδ T cells obtained from blood samples, regardless of whether the food components have been absorbed.

In addition to the ability of γδ T cells to kill pathogen-infected cells and malignant cells, they are also necessary to turn off the immune response. In animal models where the γδ TCR is knocked out, the animals are inflamed.[9,10] Adding another inflammatory stress to γδ-TCR knock-out mouse model is fatal. The researchers showed that γδ cells physically interacted with activated macrophages, resulting in macrophage cell death, and were required to end the response. If dietary compounds can enhance the function of γδ T cells, then diet may be instrumental in providing anti-inflammatory activity as well.

The relationship between diet and the γδ T cell was first published in 1999.[11,12] These studies showed that drinking tea beverage compared with coffee resulted in an increased γδ T-cell proliferation and interferon γ synthesis. The mechanism by which tea was thought to work was through a unique amino acid, L-theanine. After L-theanine is consumed, it is hydrolyzed to glutamic acid and ethylamine by the kidney.[13,14] Ethylamine is thought to be the nonmicrobial antigen that interacts with the γδ T cell.

If a compound from tea interacts with the γδ T cell, we asked if other fruits and/or vegetables also interact with this cell. In 2 studies, γδ T-cell numbers were increased in the blood when subjects were fed a fruit and vegetable concentrate[15] or grape juice from Concord grapes (publication in review). The cellular proliferative capacity was not changed, but in 1 study,[15] a reduction in circulating interferon γ was observed, which suggests lower inflammatory activity.

A capsule containing a standardized mixture of tea components, L-theanine and catechins, showed an ability to functionally change γδ T cells after consumption.[16,17] In these studies, people consumed a defined amount of L-theanine with tea catechins for 10 weeks. White blood cells from the subjects were then incubated ex vivo, with the compound responsible for priming them, ethylamine, and the results showed a greater activation and proliferation of γδ T cells from subjects consuming L-theanine compared with those obtained from people consuming the placebo. A greater concentration of interferon γ was also produced by the cells from the L-theanine consumers. One of the inflammatory biomarkers that were measured was reduced, whereas a second one went unchanged.[16] The subjects taking the tea components experienced fewer cold and flu symptoms during the study.

Results of these studies led to the hypothesis that the phytochemicals found in plants can prime the γδ T cell. Other in vitro research showed that γδ T cells interact with proanthocyanidins and result in increased proliferation and activation.[18] Despite limitations to in vitro cell culture studies, we hypothesize that in vivo the γδ T cells obtained from blood may have interacted with phytochemicals while residing in the gut. $\gamma\delta$ T cells migrate out of the gut into the bloodstream where they are isolated and shown to have functional changes. The hypothesis of nonmicrobial priming suggests that the weak interaction of food phytochemicals with the cells does not activate the cell, but only primes it to respond better and faster to a secondary stimulus.[7] Although phytochemicals are not essential for life, as is a classic nutrient, they are beneficial to health.

Summary

All nutrients are important for maintaining immunity and providing appropriate amounts of protein, fat, carbohydrate, vitamins, and minerals for the surveillance mode of keeping us from getting sick. More nutrients are required during pathogen invasion, but it proves more difficult to study exactly what is the "right" balance of nutrients that are required to provide an optimal response when invaded by pathogen.

The food ingredients mentioned in relation to priming of the $\gamma\delta$ T cells are plant-derived compounds. Thus, the best advice for a healthy immune system is to consume fruits and vegetables and includes tea. Vitamin C, folic acid and other B vitamins, vitamins A and D, phytochemicals, and food fiber all work to keep the immune system functioning without overresponsiveness (inflammation) or underresponsiveness (illness). These compounds do not appear to be stored in the body; therefore, to maintain a primed state requires daily consumption, to maximize exposure and thus benefits. Priming immune cells promotes a faster and stronger response. $\gamma\delta$ T cells are unique cells that are important in surveillance, response, and ending the response. They appear to be supported by dietary compounds in a manner consistent with health benefits.

References

1. Furst P. Conditionally indispensable amino acids (glutamine, cyst(e)ine, tyrosine, arginine, ornithine, taurine) in enteral feeding and the dipeptide concept. *Nestle Nutr Workshop Ser Clin Perform Prog.* 2000;3:199–217; discussion 217–219, 199–217.
2. Manhart N, Stehle P. Nutritive amino acids—effective modulators of the immune response. *Forum Nutr.* 2003;56:151–154.
3. Raqib R, Roy SK, Rahman MJ, et al. Effect of zinc supplementation on immune and inflammatory responses in pediatric patients with shigellosis. *Am J Clin Nutr.* 2004;79:444–450.
4. Tam M, Gomez S, Gonzalez-Gross M, Marcos A. Possible roles of magnesium on the immune system. *Eur J Clin Nutr.* 2003;57:1193–1197.
5. Douglas RM, Hemila H, Chalker E, Treacy B. Vitamin C for preventing and treating the common cold. *Cochrane Database Syst Rev.* 2007:CD000980.c.
6. Galli C, Calder PC. Effects of fat and fatty acid intake on inflammatory and immune responses: a critical review. *Ann Nutr Metab.* 2009;55:123–139.
7. Jutila MA, Holderness J, Graff JC, Hedges JF. Antigen-independent priming: a transitional response of bovine gamma delta T-cells to infection. *Anim Health Res Rev.* 2008;17:1–11.
8. Brandes M, Willimann K, Lang AB, et al. Flexible migration program regulates gamma delta T-cell involvement in humoral immunity. *Blood.* 2003;102:3693–3701.
9. Carding SR, Egan PJ. Gamma delta T cells: functional plasticity and heterogeneity. *Nat Rev Immunol.* 2002;2:336–345.
10. Egan PJ, Carding SR. Downmodulation of the inflammatory response to bacterial infection by gamma delta T cells cytotoxic for activated macrophages. *J Exp Med.* 2000;191:2145–2158.
11. Bukowski JF, Morita CT, Brenner MB. Human $\gamma\delta$ T cells recognize alkylamines derived from microbes, edible plants, and tea: implications for innate immunity. *Immunity.* 1999;11:57–65.
12. Kamath AB, Wang L, Das H, Li L, Reinhold VN, Bukowski JF. Antigens in tea-beverage prime human Vgamma 2Vdelta 2 T cells in vitro and in vivo for memory and nonmemory antibacterial cytokine responses. *Proc Natl Acad Sci U S A.* 2003;100:6009–6014.
13. Mitchell SC, Zhang AQ, Smith RL. Ethylamine in human urine. *Clin Chim Acta.* 2000;302:69–78.
14. Unno T, Suzuki Y, Kakuda T, Hayakawa T, Tsuge H. Metabolism of theanine, gamma-glutamylethylamide, in rats. *J Agric Food Chem.* 1999;47:1593–1596.
15. Nantz MP, Rowe CA, Nieves C Jr, Percival SS. Immunity and antioxidant capacity in humans is enhanced by consumption of a dried, encapsulated fruit and vegetable juice concentrate. *J Nutr.* 2006;136:2606–2610.
16. Nantz MP, Rowe CA, Bukowski JF, Percival SS. Standardized capsule of *Camellia sinensis* lowers cardiovascular risk factors in a randomized, double-blind, placebo-controlled study. *Nutrition.* 2009;25:147–154.
17. Rowe CA, Nantz MP, Bukowski JF, Percival SS. Specific formulation of *Camellia sinensis* prevents cold and flu symptoms and enhances $\gamma\delta$ T cell function: a randomized, double-blind, placebo-controlled study. *J Am Coll Nutr.* 2007;26:445–452.
18. Holderness J, Jackiw L, Kimmel E, et al. Select plant tannins induce IL-2Ralpha up-regulation and augment cell division in gamma delta T cells. *J Immunol.* 2007;179:6468–6478.

Critical Thinking

1. List the nutrients that support the proper function of T cells.

2. Summarize the immune response to a pathogen and the type of nutrients involved in each phase.

3. Discuss the challenges of conducting research on the nutrient requirements of the immune response.

SUSAN S. PERCIVAL, PHD, is a professor of nutritional sciences in the Department of Food Science and Human Nutrition at the University of Florida, Gainesville. Her educational background includes a master's of science degree from the University of California, Davis, and a PhD from the University of Texas, Austin. She did her postdoctoral research in the Department of Biochemistry and Biophysics at Texas A&M University. From 1978 to 1981, she was tenure track faculty at the University of Rhode Island prior to an educational leave to pursue her doctorate. In 2004, she took an 8-month sabbatical leave at the National Institutes of Health with the Nutritional Sciences Research Group at the National Cancer Institute. She currently teaches courses on current issues in dietary supplements, research planning, and nutrition and immunity. Her current research deals with how dietary components influence immunity. Experimental models in cell culture, mice, and in humans reveal that certain dietary components including bioactive compounds from fruits and vegetables, herbs and spices, red wine, and green tea affect specific branches of immunity. These plant bioactive food components have benefits not only with their protective antioxidant capacity, but also through their ability to affect intracellular signaling pathways and prime immune cells to activate faster and to a greater extent when stimulated to do so. Funding acknowledgements: University of Florida Agriculture Experiment Station, IFAS.

From *Nutrition Today*, vol. 46, no. 1, January/February 2011, pp. 12–17. Copyright © 2011 by Lippincott, Williams & Wilkins/Wolters Kluwer Health. Reprinted by permission via Rightslink.

UNIT 5

Obesity and Weight Control

Unit Selections

Learning Outcomes

After reading this Unit, you will be able to:

- Identify the primary factors that have contributed to the obesity epidemic in the world.

- Describe the behavioral approach to weight loss and why it is so effective.

- Compare the actions of the hormones that influence food intake.

- Define food deserts. Where are they more likely to occur?

- Summarize the "food environment" in the United States. Explain why many health professionals refer to our food environment as toxic.

- Develop recommendations of how families can effectively impact the nutrition and health of their children.

- Discuss how excessive maternal weight gain during pregnancy can impact the health of the fetus.

- Describe how the Federal Trade Commission, the Centers for Disease Control and Prevention, the Food and Drug Administration, and the Department of Agriculture together are tackling the way food is marketed to children.

- Discuss the health consequences associated with children being overweight or obese.

- Explain how negative stigmas and prevalence of negative messages regarding obesity can potentiate the development of eating disorders.

Student Website

www.mhhe.com/cls

Internet References

American Society of Exercise Physiologists (ASEP)
www.asep.org
Calorie Control Council
www.caloriecontrol.org
Centers for Disease Control and Prevention: Overweight & Obesity
www.cdc.gov/obesity
Shape Up America!
www.shapeup.org

Overweight and obesity have become epidemic in the United States during the last century and are rising at a dangerous rate worldwide. Approximately 5 million adults are overweight or obese according to the standards set by the U.S. government using a body mass index (BMI) range of 30 to 39.9. Reports suggest that by the year 2050, half of the U.S. population will be considered obese if current trends continue; however, recent analysis indicates that the rate of increase in overweight and obesity in the United States is nearing a plateau rather than the upward slope. Overweight and obesity is prevalent in males and females of all ages, races, and ethnic groups.

Prevention efforts are geared toward curtailing obese children from maturing into obese adults who burden our current healthcare system and government supported healthcare reimbursement programs with exorbitant costs of obesity-related chronic diseases. The major health consequences of obesity are heart disease, diabetes, gallbladder disease, osteoarthritis, and some cancers. The cost for treating the degenerative diseases secondary to obesity is approximately $100 billion per year in the United States.

Even though health and nutrition professionals have tried to prevent and combat obesity with behavior modification, a healthy diet, and exercise, it seems that these traditional ways have not proven effective. Fast-food restaurants are the mainstay for many Americans because they offer quick, inexpensive food. Supersizing has become the norm because, in many instances, it's cheaper to order a biggie combo than smaller items individually. Americans are so accustomed to our fast food nation that many people become infuriated when asked to pull up and wait an extra minute for a 2,400-calorie meal. The problem is exacerbated by the food industry's historical plight to earn profit and market share by providing U.S. consumers with the fatty, sugary, and salty foods that we demand.

Food companies spend millions of dollars in advertising foods loaded with simple sugars, fat, and salt. Their aggressive advertising, coupled with food accessibility and large portion sizes, has impacted the current obesity pandemic. Other obstacles to maintaining a healthy diet are low accessibility and the high cost of eating a healthy diet.

More recently, scientists have reported that fat is a dynamically active endocrine organ that releases hormones and inflammatory proteins that may predispose a person to chronic diseases such as heart disease. In addition, research has discovered the role of the "hunger hormone" and how individual differences affect our ability to lose weight. A positive association was recently found between obesity, especially central obesity, and different types of cancer. Thus, there is a great need for a multifaceted public health approach that would involve mobilization of private and public sectors and focus on building better coping skills and increasing activity.

Globalization is causing the rest of the world and especially developing third world countries to mimic the unhealthy Western diet that contributes to obesity. Obesity and its health consequences are now becoming a global epidemic. Sweetened beverages and the sedentary Western way of life that has been adopted by many developing countries are some of the major contributors of this epidemic.

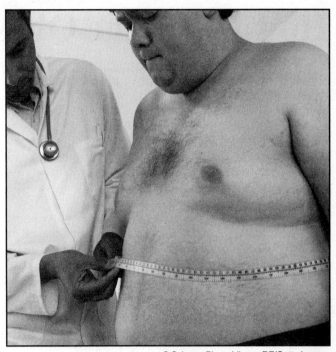

© Science Photo Library RF/Getty Images

Intervention and prevention should be the top priorities of policymakers. At the public sector, inclusion of health officials, researchers, educators, legislators, transportation experts, urban planners, and businesses to cooperate in formulating ways to combat obesity is crucial. A sound public health policy would require that weight-loss therapies have long-term maintenance and relapse-prevention measures built into them. Healthy People 2010 is the U.S. government's prevention agenda designed to ensure high quality of life and reduce health risks. One of the 28 areas it focuses on is overweight and obesity. Its main objectives are to reduce the proportion of overweight and obese children, teens, and adults by half and to increase the proportion of adults who are at a healthy weight.

Another perspective to consider about the obesogenic environment in the United States is the affect it is having on people who have or may develop disordered eating. An obesogenic environment is an environment that has norms of inadequate physical activity, consumes too many calories, promotes energy-dense foods, has a large number of obese people with biological predispositions to weight challenges and food addictions, and societal discrimination and media manipulation of ideal body image. This environment may contribute to disordered eating behavior in people prone to the disease. Conflicting messages such as very thin is beautiful and eating energy-dense foods is attractive and desirable can lead to feelings of helplessness, psychological distress, and self-dislike.

The articles in this chapter may be used to supplement information presented in the energy balance section of general nutrition courses.

How to Fix the Obesity Crisis

Although science has revealed a lot about metabolic processes that influence our weight, the key to success may lie elsewhere.

DAVID H. FREEDMAN

Obesity is a national health crisis—that much we know. If current trends continue, it will soon surpass smoking in the U.S. as the biggest single factor in early death, reduced quality of life and added health care costs. A third of adults in the U.S. are obese, according to the Centers for Disease Control and Prevention, and another third are overweight, with Americans getting fatter every year. Obesity is responsible for more than 160,000 "excess" deaths a year, according to a study in the Journal of the American Medical Association. The average obese person costs society more than $7,000 a year in lost productivity and added medical treatment, say researchers at George Washington University. Lifetime added medical costs alone for a person 70 pounds or more overweight amount to as much as $30,000, depending on race and gender.

All this lends urgency to the question: Why are extra pounds so difficult to shed and keep off? It doesn't seem as though it should be so hard. The basic formula for weight loss is simple and widely known: consume fewer calories than you expend. And yet if it really were easy, obesity would not be the nation's number-one lifestyle-related health concern. For a species that evolved to consume energy-dense foods in an environment where famine was a constant threat, losing weight and staying trimmer in a modern world of plenty fueled by marketing messages and cheap empty calories is, in fact, terrifically difficult. Almost everybody who tries to diet seems to fail in the long run—a review in 2007 by the American Psychological Association of 31 diet studies found that as many as two thirds of dieters end up two years later weighing more than they did before their diet.

Science has trained its big guns on the problem. The National Institutes of Health has been spending nearly $800 million a year on studies to understand the metabolic, genetic and neurological foundations of obesity. In its proposed plan for obesity research funding in 2011, the NIH lists promising research avenues in this order: animal models highlighting protein functions in specific tissues; complex signaling pathways in the brain and between the brain and other organs; identification of obesity-related gene variants; and epigenetic mechanisms regulating metabolism.

This research has provided important insights into the ways proteins interact in our body to extract and distribute energy from food and produce and store fat; how our brains tell us we are hungry; why some of us seem to have been born more likely to be obese than others; and whether exposure to certain foods and toxic substances might modify and mitigate some of these factors. The work has also given pharmaceutical companies numerous potential targets for drug development. What the research has not done, unfortunately, is make a dent in solving the national epidemic.

Maybe someday biology will provide us with a pill that readjusts our metabolism so we burn more calories or resets our built-in cravings so we prefer broccoli to burgers. But until then, the best approach may simply be to build on reliable behavioral-psychology methods developed over 50 years and proved to work in hundreds of studies. These tried-and-true techniques, which are being refined with new research that should make them more effective with a wider range of individuals, are gaining new attention. As the NIH puts it in its proposed strategic plan for obesity research: "Research findings are yielding new and important insights about social and behavioral factors that influence diet, physical activity, and sedentary behavior."

How We Got Here

The desperation of the obese and overweight is reflected in the steady stream of advice pouring daily from sources as disparate as peer-reviewed scientific journals, best-selling books, newspapers and blogs. Our appetite for any diet twist or gimmick that will take the pounds off quickly and for good seems to be as insatiable as our appetite for the rich food that puts the pounds on. We, the public, love to believe in neat fixes, and the media oblige by playing up new scientific findings in headline after headline as if they are solutions.

It doesn't help that the scientific findings on which these headlines are based sometimes appear to conflict. For example, a study in September's *American Journal of Clinical Nutrition* found a link between increased dairy intake and weight loss, although a meta-analysis in the May 2008 *Nutrition Reviews* discovered no such link. A paper in the *Journal of Occupational and Environmental Medicine* in January 2010 postulated a connection between job stress and obesity, but in October a report in the journal *Obesity* concluded there was no such correlation. Part of the problem, too, is that obesity researchers are in some ways akin to the metaphorical blind men groping at different parts of the elephant, their individual study findings addressing only narrow pieces of a complex puzzle.

When the research is taken together, it is clear that the obesity fix cannot be boiled down to eating this or that food type or to taking any other simple action. Many factors contribute to the problem. It is partly environment—the eating habits of your friends, what food is most available in your home and your local stores, how much opportunity you have to move around at work. It is partly biology—there are genetic predispositions for storing fat, for having higher satiety thresholds, even for having more sensitive taste buds. It is partly economics—junk food has become much cheaper than fresh produce. And it is marketing, too—food companies have become masterful at playing on human social nature and our evolutionary "programming" to steer us toward unhealthy but profitable fare. That is why the narrow "eat this" kinds of solutions, like all simple solutions, fail.

When we go on diets and exercise regimens, we rely on willpower to overcome all these pushes to overeat relative to our activity level. And we count on the reward of getting trimmer and fitter to keep us on the wagon. It *is* rewarding to lose the weight, of course. Unfortunately, time works against us. As the weight comes off, we get hungrier and develop stronger cravings and become more annoyed by the exercise. Meanwhile the weight loss inevitably slows as our metabolism tries to compensate for this deprivation by becoming more parsimonious with calories. Thus, the punishment for sticking to our regimen becomes increasingly severe and constant, and the expected reward recedes into the future. "That gap between the reinforcement of eating and the reinforcement of maybe losing weight months later is a huge challenge," says Sung-Woo Kahng, a neurobehaviorist who studies obesity at the Johns Hopkins University School of Medicine and the Kennedy Krieger Institute.

We would be more likely to stick with the regimen if it remained less punishing and more reliably rewarding. Is there a way to make that happen?

From Biology to Brain

The most successful way to date to lose at least modest amounts of weight and keep it off with diet and exercise employs programs that focus on changing behavior. The behavioral approach, tested over decades, involves making many small, sustainable adjustments in eating and exercise habits that are prompted and encouraged by the people and the rest of the environment around us.

The research in support of behavioral weight-loss approaches extends back more than half a century to Harvard University psychologist B. F. Skinner's development of the science of behavioral analysis. The field is founded on the notion

Advances in the Lab

The Biology of Obesity

The National Institutes of Health has spent nearly $800 million a year on studies to understand the neurological, metabolic and genetic foundations of obesity. In the process, scientists have uncovered complex biochemical pathways and feedback loops that connect the brain and digestive system; a new appreciation for the regulatory functions of fat tissues; subtle hereditary changes that make some groups more prone to obesity than others; and the strong possibility that exposure to certain foods and toxic substances might modify and mitigate some of these factors. Given that it will likely take decades to understand the various causes of obesity, more surprises are no doubt in store.

- **Brain:** Scientists have long known that the hypothalamus and brain stem help to regulate feelings of hunger and fullness. Over the past several years researchers have found that the pleasure-reward centers of the limbic system and the evaluating functions of the prefrontal cortex are also heavily involved. Indeed, chronic overeating bears biochemical similarities to drug addiction.

- **Metabolism:** The ability to burn and store energy varies greatly from cell to cell. In 2009 three studies in the *New England Journal of Medicine* demonstrated that at least some women and men continue to benefit well into adulthood from small stores of brown fat, which, unlike white fat, is associated with being lean. Brown fat helps to generate heat and is apparently more closely related to muscle than to white fat, whose primary purpose is to store excess energy.

- **Genes:** Researchers have confirmed variations in 20-odd genes that predispose people to gaining weight easily. But further investigation shows that the effects are modest at best and cannot account for the current obesity epidemic. Genes may still play a role, however, through the environment's influence on which ones get turned on or off. So far most such genetic switches for obesity have been identified in mice, although a few likely human candidates are known.

that scientists cannot really know what is going on inside a person's brain—after all, even functional MRIs, the state of the art for peering into the mind, are crude, highly interpretable proxies for cognition and emotion that reduce the detailed firing of billions of neurons in complex circuits to a few blobs of color. But researchers can objectively and reproducibly observe and measure physical behavior and the immediate environment in which the behavior occurs, allowing them to identify links between environment and behavior. That typically includes trying to spot events or situations that may be prompting or triggering certain behaviors and noting what may be rewarding and thus reinforcing of some behaviors or punishing and thus inhibiting of others.

The effectiveness of behavioral interventions has been extensively documented for a wide variety of disorders and problem behaviors. A 2009 meta-analysis in the *Journal of Clinical Child & Adolescent Psychology* concluded that "early intensive behavioral intervention should be an intervention of choice for children with autism." A systematic review sponsored by the U.S. Preventive Services Task Force found that even brief behavioral counseling interventions reduced the number of drinks taken by problem drinkers by 13 to 34 percent for as long as four years. Review studies have found similar behavioral-intervention successes in challenges as diverse as reducing stuttering, increasing athletic performance and improving employee productivity.

To combat obesity, behavioral analysts examine related environmental influences: Which external factors prompt people to overeat or to eat junk food, and which tend to encourage healthful eating? In what situations are the behaviors and comments of others affecting unhealthful eating? What seems to effectively reward eating healthfully over the long term? What reinforces being active? Behavior-focused studies of obesity and diets as early as the 1960s recognized some basic conditions that seemed correlated with a greater chance of losing weight and keeping it off: rigorously measuring and recording calories, exercise and weight; making modest, gradual changes rather than severe ones; eating balanced diets that go easy on fats and sugar rather than dropping major food groups; setting clear, modest goals; focusing on lifelong habits rather than short-term diets; and especially attending groups where dieters could receive encouragement to stick with their efforts and praise for having done so.

If these strategies today sound like well-worn, commonsense advice, it is because they have been popularized for nearly half a century by Weight Watchers. Founded in 1963 to provide support groups for dieters, Weight Watchers added other approaches and advice in keeping with the findings of behavioral studies and used to bill itself as a "behavior-modification" program. "Whatever the details are of how you lose weight, the magic in the sauce is always going to be changing behavior," says nutrition researcher and Weight Watchers chief science officer Karen Miller-Kovach. "Doing that is a learnable skill."

Studies back the behavioral approach to weight loss. A 2003 review commissioned by the U.S. Department of Health and Human Services found that "counseling and behavioral interventions showed small to moderate degrees of weight loss sustained over at least one year"—a year being an eon in the world of weight loss. An analysis of eight popular weight-loss programs published in 2005 in the *Annals of Internal Medicine* found Weight Watchers (at that time in its pre-2010 points-overhaul incarnation) to be the only effective program, enabling a 3 percent maintained body-weight loss for the two years of the study. Meanwhile a 2005 *JAMA* study found that Weight Watchers, along with the Zone diet (which, like Weight Watchers, recommends a balanced diet of protein, carbohydrates and fat), achieved the highest percentage (65 percent) of one-year diet adherence of several popular diets, noting that

"adherence level rather than diet type was the key determinant of clinical benefits." A 2010 study in the *Journal of Pediatrics* found that after one year children receiving behavioral therapy maintained a body mass index that was 1.9 to 3.3 lower than children who did not. (BMI is a numerical height-weight relation in which 18.5 is held to be borderline underweight and 25 borderline overweight.) The *Pediatrics* report noted that "more limited evidence suggests that these improvements can be maintained over the 12 months after the end of treatments." A 2010 study in *Obesity* found that continuing members of Take Off Pounds Sensibly (TOPS), a national, nonprofit behaviorally focused weight-loss organization, maintained a weight loss of 5 to 7 percent of their body weight for the three years of the investigation. The UK's Medical Research Council last year declared that its own long-term study had shown that programs based on behavioral principles are more likely to help people take and keep the weight off than other approaches. (The study was funded by Weight Watchers, but without its participation.)

Mass-market programs tend to fall short when it comes to enlisting a full range of behavioral techniques and customizing them to meet the varied needs of individuals.

But Weight Watchers and other mass-market programs tend to fall short when it comes to enlisting a full range of behavioral techniques and customizing them to meet the varied needs of individuals. They cannot routinely provide individual counseling, adapt their advice to specific challenges, assess environmental factors in a member's home, workplace or community, provide much outreach to members who do not come to meetings, or prevent their members from shooting for fast, dramatic, short-term weight loss or from restricting food groups. As a for-profit company, Weight Watchers sometimes even mildly panders to these self-defeating notions in its marketing. "Some people join us to drop 10 pounds for a high school reunion," says Weight Watchers's Miller-Kovach. "They achieve that goal, then stop coming."

To close that gap, a number of researchers have turned their attention in recent years to improving, expanding and tailoring behavioral techniques, with encouraging results. For example, Michael Cameron, head of the graduate behavioral analysis department at Simmons College and a faculty member at Harvard Medical School, is now focusing his research on behavioral weight-loss techniques. He is one year into a four-person study—behavioral analysts generally do very small group or even single-subject studies to more closely tailor the intervention and observe individual effects—in which the subjects meet together with him via online videoconferencing for reinforcement, weigh themselves on scales that transmit results via wireless networks, and have their diets optimized to both reduce caloric density and address individual food preferences.

Favorite foods are used as a reward for exercise. So far the subjects have lost between 8 and 20 percent of their body weight.

Matt Normand, a behavioral analyst at the University of the Pacific, has focused on finding ways to more precisely track subjects' calorie intake and expenditure by, for example, collecting receipts for food purchases, providing food checklists to record what is eaten, and enlisting various types of pedometers and other devices for measuring physical activity. He then provides participants with daily detailed accounts of their calorie flow and in one published study showed three of four subjects reduced calorie intake to recommended levels. Richard Fleming, a researcher at the University of Massachusetts Medical School's Shriver Center, has in *Obesity* looked at ways to encourage parents to steer their children to healthier choices. He has found, among other techniques, that showing parents in person what appropriate serving sizes of foods look like on plates is helpful. Another successful Fleming trick: letting children pick out a small treat at a food store—as long as they walk there. "Kids can really respond to that reward for being active," he says.

Our environment is one in which ubiquitous, sophisticated marketing efforts prey on our need for sensory gratification as well as our vulnerability to misinformation.

Why are behavioral interventions effective? Laurette Dubé, a lifestyle psychology and marketing researcher at McGill University's Faculty of Management, notes that our environment is currently one in which ubiquitous, sophisticated marketing efforts prey on our need for sensory gratification as well as our vulnerability to misinformation. In addition, the poor eating and exercise habits we observe in our friends, family and colleagues encourage us to follow suit. In essence, behavioral interventions seek to reconfigure this environment into one in which our needs for information, gratification and social encouragement are tapped to pull us toward healthy food and exercise choices rather than away from them. "When we are getting the right messages in enough ways, we have a better chance of resisting the urge to eat more than we need," Dubé says.

Changing Policy

There is no one-size-fits-all solution, behavioral or otherwise, to the problem of obesity. But although behavioral interventions work best when they are customized to individuals, mass-market behavioral approaches such as Weight Watchers and TOPS are at least fairly effective. Why don't more people lose weight with them? The main reason is that people simply do not sign up for them, often because would-be weight losers are chasing fad diets or supplements or have read that obesity is locked into our genes. Weight Watchers, by far the most popular behavioral weight-loss program, counts only 600,000 meeting-attending members in its ranks in North America. That means that fewer than one out of 100 obese people in the U.S.

What Works?

Four Steps to Losing Weight

Behavior-focused studies of obesity and diets have identified some basic conditions that seem correlated with a greater chance of losing weight and keeping it off: setting clear, modest goals and focusing on lifelong habits, among others. Most of these behavior changes fall into four main categories.

Initial Assessment

Research underscores the need to determine baseline measurements. How much does an individual weigh? What rituals and routines contribute to overeating (eating under stress) or underexercising (unrealistic expectations)? A physician, a nurse practitioner or a nutrition counselor can help with the assessment.

Behavior Shifts

Many people find it is easier to make small changes at first—such as taking the stairs instead of an elevator. Studies show that surveying the entire buffet before serving themselves will help people put less food on their plate.

Self-Monitoring

Recording body weight, counting the calories eaten and logging steps taken provide objective feedback on how well individuals are changing their habits. Behavior studies have found both low-tech paper logs and wireless monitoring systems to be of benefit.

Support Groups

Studies document the benefits of encouragement by others. Being part of a group—whether an exercise group, a formal support group or even a virtual group—lets participants share triumphs, bemoan setbacks and strategize solutions.

and about one out of 200 overweight people are part of a formal behavioral-modification program.

Public policy may be changing, however. The U.S. Surgeon General's office and the CDC have both publicly lined up behind behavioral approaches as the main weapon in what is becoming a war on obesity. First Lady Michelle Obama's high-profile Let's Move campaign against childhood obesity consists almost entirely of behavioral weight-loss wisdom—that is, find ways to encourage children to eat less-calorie-dense foods, to become more active, and to enjoy doing it. The recent proposed ban of toys in Happy Meals in San Francisco suggests that more officials may be getting ready to pressure the food industry into easing up on contaminating the environment with what are essentially obesity-supportive marketing tactics. To make it easier and more tempting to buy healthier food in poorer, disproportionately overweight communities, the White House has proposed subsidizing the costs of fruits and vegetables. Approaching the problem from the other direction, New York City Mayor Michael Bloomberg is among those who have advocated modifying food-assistance programs to restrict the purchase of high-sugar beverages, and last year Washington, D.C., enacted a 6 percent tax on sugary drinks. New York City has also offered vouchers for buying produce at farmers' markets to low-income families and incentives to stores to offer healthier fare.

Some experts are trying to push the government to rewrite zoning and building codes to ensure that neighborhoods and buildings become friendlier to walkers, bikers and stair climbers. A 2009 study by researchers at Louisiana State University Medical School found that a mere 2.8 percent increase in a person's stair usage alone would keep off almost a pound a year. "The correlation between activity levels and healthy weight is one of the best-established ones in all of obesity research," says William M. Hartman, a psychologist and director of the behavioral program of the highly regarded Weight Management Program of the California Pacific Medical Center in San Francisco.

Increasing access to behavior therapy would help, too. Many overweight people might only need online behavioral monitoring, support and progress-sharing tools, which have proved moderately effective in studies. Others may need much more intensive, more personal interventions of the kind Cameron is developing. Given that obesity especially plagues the economically disadvantaged, fees for these programs may have to be heavily subsidized by the government and health care insurers. A weekly session with a behavioral therapist costing $50 would amount to $2,500 a year, or a bit more than a third of the $7,000 per year societal and medical costs of obesity—and the sessions might only be needed for a year or two to establish new, permanent eating and exercise habits, whereas the savings would continue on for a lifetime.

It is too soon to say whether the public will accept government efforts to push it toward healthier choices. In San Francisco, a community known to be especially friendly to public health initiatives, the plan to ban Happy Meals has provoked angry reactions, and Mayor Gavin Newsom vetoed it. Efforts by Let's Move to bring healthier food to school cafeterias have been intensely criticized by some as overly intrusive. Even if these efforts are eventually fully implemented nationwide, there is no way of being sure they will significantly reduce obesity. The current rate of obesity is far beyond any ever seen before on the planet, and thus a large-scale solution will necessarily be an experiment in mass behavior change. But the research suggests that such a grand experiment would be our best shot at fixing obesity and that there is reason to be hopeful it will succeed. Given that more and more scientists, public policy experts and government officials seem eager to get it off the ground, we may well have early findings within this decade.

More to Explore

About Behaviorism. B. F. Skinner. Vintage, 1974. A classic in behavior modification. You on a Diet: The Owner's Manual for Waist Management. Michael F. Roizen and Mehmet C. Oz. Free Press, 2006. Good layperson's guide to various aspects of weight management.

Determining the Effectiveness of Take Off Pounds Sensibly (TOPS), a Nationally Available Nonprofit Weight Loss Program. Nia S. Mitchell et al., in *Obesity.* Published online September 23, 2010. www.nature.com/oby/journal/vaop/ncurrent/full/oby2010202a .html

The entry portal to the range of NIH research on obesity: obesityresearch.nih.gov.

Critical Thinking

1. Describe the neurological, metabolic, and genetic causes of obesity.

2. Describe the behavioral approach to weight loss and why it is so effective.

3. How do the rewards/punishments for positive lifestyle modification change over time?

DAVID H. FREEDMAN has been covering science, business and technology for 30 years. His most recent book, *Wrong,* explores the forces that lead scientists and other top experts to mislead us.

The Fat Plateau

Americans are no longer getting fatter, it appears.

THE ECONOMIST

A few years ago, Burger King, a fast-food chain, conducted a study of the eating habits of some of its most frequent customers. A few dozen "SuperFans", as the firm calls them, recorded and photographed everything they ate for two weeks. The results were collected in a book called "Food for Thought". Unsurprisingly, this book is not publicly available: amateur photos of heaps of junk food are hardly an enticing advertisement for a firm that supplies the stuff. Nonetheless, "Food for Thought" gives an insight into why some Americans have such poor diets.

The fast-food fans in the book typically lead chaotic lives. They often toil long, irregular hours for not much money. They grab food when they can, skipping many meals and gorging at unorthodox times. They favour whatever is quick, convenient and comforting. ("I selected the pie because it was easy to grab out of the fridge," says one.) They often have an imperfect grasp of nutritional science. ("I am eating chocolate muffins at work because they are not too heavy," says another.) Oddly for a piece of corporate research, the book contains passages that are quite moving. One single dad's diary shows him eating nothing but junk for days on end. Then, one evening, he visits his aunt's house and she cooks him a feast of real food: pork, okra stew, collard greens and corn bread.

At 33.8%, America's obesity rate is ten times higher than Japan's. In all, 68% of Americans are either obese or overweight. (Some studies yield lower numbers, but since they typically ask people how much they weigh, rather than weighing them, scepticism is in order.) Few problems, besides death, afflict more people. Americans are more likely to be overweight than to pay federal income tax.

But the good news is that the nation may have stopped getting fatter. A study published this month in the *Journal of the American Medical Association (JAMA)* found that American women were no more likely to be obese in 2008 than they were nearly a decade before. For men, there was a small rise in obesity over the same period, but no change in the past three years. Among children, too, there was no change in obesity rates except among the very heaviest boys, whose numbers increased slightly. Could it be that the American obesity epidemic has reached a plateau?

If the national girth really has stopped expanding, that would be a blessing, though of course it is a big fall in obesity that is really required. Although a little extra heft is no big deal, many Americans are so ample that it ruins their health. That places a burden on the health-care system: each obese American racks up medical bills 42% higher than an American of normal weight, according to Eric Finkelstein and Justin Trogdon, writing in *Health Affairs*. Add to that the indirect costs of obesity, such as lost productivity due to sickness or premature death.

The startling Republican victory in Massachusetts this week throws Barack Obama's health reforms up in the air. But the issue will not go away. And a plateau in the obesity rate would make some kind of reform a bit less expensive. It will not lead to a sudden dip in health-care costs, predicts Mr Trogdon. But it could substantially slow the rate at which they are rising. Previous projections typically assumed that Americans would keep on ballooning. As a thought experiment in 2008, Youfa Wang of the Johns Hopkins Centre for Global Health drew a line from recent trends and projected that 100% of Americans would be over-weight by 2048. By 2030, his model showed health-care costs attributable to excess weight approaching a trillion dollars a year.

The latest numbers remind us how little is known about public health. Of course, people put on weight when they consume more calories than they burn off. But no one knows for sure why America's obesity has trebled since 1960. Plausible theories abound. As people grow richer food becomes relatively cheaper. Time grows more precious: hence the lure of fast food. Desk work burns fewer calories than spadework. And labour-saving devices do just that if we still washed dishes and clothes by hand, we would burn off five pounds of flesh each year, reckons Barry Popkin, the author of a book called "The World is Fat". All this is no doubt true, but it does not explain why Americans are fatter than people in other rich countries, nor why they appear to have stopped getting fatter.

No to Nannies

Kathleen Sebelius, the health secretary, says that "fighting obesity is at the heart" of health reform. But telling people to eat more healthily is like telling them not to have risky sex. Americans are suspicious of the nanny state at the best of times, let alone when it nags them to curb their most basic instincts. Some regulations help: forcing restaurants to post calorie counts on dishes, for example, prompts diners to pick less calorific treats. But politicians are reluctant to attack voters' favourite vices too vigorously. A recent proposal to tax sugary drinks, for example, went nowhere. Opponents argued that it would disproportionately affect the poor. True enough, but the poor are disproportionately likely to be overweight.

The constant barrage of pro-vegetable propaganda in schools may have raised awareness of the need for a balanced diet, reckons Mr Trogdon. And popular pressure has prompted many fast-food outlets to offer salads and other wholesome fare. But even if good food were freely available, losing weight is hard. Every year, 25% of American men and 43% of American women attempt it. "[F]ailure rates are exceedingly high," notes a *JAMA* editorial. But there is hope. Eating is social. Studies suggest that people guzzle more if they have overweight friends and relatives, and less if they don't. So if Americans have stopped getting fatter, their children have a better shot at staying trim.

Critical Thinking

1. What are the primary factors that have contributed to the obesity epidemic in the United States?

2. What is the latest percentage of obese or overweight Americans? How does this percentage differ from the obesity rate percentage?

3. Describe the typical fast food fan depicted in the book, *Food for Thought.*

The Hungry Brain

The urge to eat too much is wired into our heads. **Tackling obesity may require bypassing the stomach** and short-circuiting our brains.

DAN HURLEY

At 10:19 P.M. on a Monday evening in October, I sat in a booth at Chevys Fresh Mex in Clifton, New Jersey, reviewing the latest research into the neurobiology of hunger and obesity. While I read I ate a shrimp and crab enchilada, consuming two-thirds of it, maybe less. With all this information in front of me, I thought, I had an edge over my brain's wily efforts to thwart my months-long campaign to get under 190 pounds. But even as I was taking in a study about the powerful lure of guacamole and other salty, fatty foods, I experienced something extraordinary. That bowl of chips and salsa at the edge of the table? It was whispering to me: *Just one more. You know you want us. Aren't we delicious?* In 10 minutes, all that was left of the chips, and my willpower, were crumbs.

I am not alone. An overabundance of chips, Baconator Double burgers, and Venti White Chocolate Mochas have aided a widespread epidemic of obesity in this country. Our waists are laying waste to our health and to our health-care economy: According to a study published by the Centers for Disease Control and Prevention in 2010, nine states had an obesity rate of at least 30 percent—compared with zero states some 10 years earlier—and the cost of treatment for obesity-related conditions had reached nearly 10 percent of total U.S. medical expenditure. So-called normal weight is no longer normal, with two-thirds of adults and one third of children and adolescents now classified as overweight or obese. Dubbed the "Age of Obesity and Inactivity" by the *Journal of the American Medical Association,* this runaway weight gain threatens to decrease average U.S. life span, reversing gains made over the past century by lowering risk factors from smoking, hypertension, and cholesterol. We all know what we should do—eat less, exercise more—but to no avail. An estimated 25 percent of American men and 43 percent of women attempt to lose weight each year; of those who succeed in their diets, between 5 and 20 percent (and it is closer to 5 percent) manage to keep it off for the long haul.

The urgent question is, why do our bodies seem to be fighting against our own good health? According to a growing number of neurobiologists, the fault lies not in our stomachs but in our heads. No matter how convincing our conscious plans and resolutions, they pale beside the brain's power to goad us into noshing and hanging on to as much fat as we can. With that in mind, some scientists were hopeful that careful studies of the brain might uncover an all-powerful hormone that regulates food consumption or a single spot where the cortical equivalent of a neon sign blinks "Eat Heavy," all the better to shut it off.

After extensive research, the idea of a single, simple cure has been replaced by a much more nuanced view. The latest studies show that a multitude of systems in the brain act in concert to encourage eating. Targeting a single neuronal system is probably doomed to the same ill fate as the failed diets themselves. Because the brain has so many backup systems all geared toward the same thing—maximizing the body's intake of calories—no single silver bullet will ever work.

The brain's prime directive to eat and defend against the loss of fat emerged early in evolution.

"I call it the 'hungry brain syndrome'," says Hans-Rudolf Berthoud, an expert in the neurobiology of nutrition at the Pennington Biomedical Research Center in Baton Rouge, Louisiana. The brain's prime directive to eat and defend against the loss of fat emerged early in evolution, because just about every creature that ever trotted, crawled, swam, or floated was beset by the uncertainty of that next meal. "The system has evolved to defend against the slightest threat of weight loss, so you have to attack it from different directions at once."

With the obesity epidemic raging, the race for countermeasures has kicked into high gear. Neuroscientists are still seeking hormones that inhibit hunger, but they have other tactics as well. One fruitful new avenue comes from the revelation that hunger, blood sugar, and weight gained per calorie consumed all ratchet up when our sleep is disrupted and our circadian rhythms—the 24-hour cycle responding to light and dark—[are] thrown into disarray. All this is compounded by stress, which decreases metabolism while increasing the yen for high-calorie food. We might feel in sync with our high-tech world, but the obesity epidemic is a somber sign that our biology and lifestyles have diverged.

Seeking Silver Bullets, Shooting Blanks

The path forward seemed so simple back in 1995, when three papers in *Science* suggested a panacea for the overweight: A hormone that made animals shed pounds, rapidly losing body fat until they were slim. Based on the research, it seemed that doctors might soon be able to treat obesity the way they treat diabetes, with a simple metabolic drug.

Fat cells release that "diet" hormone—today named leptin, from the Greek *leptos,* meaning thin—to begin a journey across the blood-brain barrier to the hypothalamus, the pea-size structure above the pituitary gland. The hypothalamus serves as a kind of thermostat, setting not only body temperature but playing a key role in hunger, thirst, fatigue, and sleep cycles. Leptin signals the hypothalamus to reduce the sense of hunger so that we stop eating.

In early lab experiments, obese mice given extra leptin by injection seemed sated. They ate less, their body temperature increased, and their weight plummeted. Even normal-weight mice became skinnier when given injections of the hormone.

Once the pharmaceutical industry created a synthetic version of human leptin, clinical trials were begun. But when injected into hundreds of obese human volunteers, leptin's effect was clinically insignificant. It soon became clear why. In humans, as in mice, fat cells of the obese already produced plenty of leptin—more in fact than those of their thin counterparts, since the level of leptin was directly proportional to the amount of fat. The early studies had worked largely because the test mice were, by experimental design, leptin-deficient. Subsequent experiments showed that in normal mice—as in humans—increases in leptin made little difference to the brain, which looked to *low* leptin levels as a signal to eat more, essentially disregarding the kind of high levels that had caused deficient mice to eat less. This made leptin a good drug for maintaining weight loss but not a great candidate for getting the pounds off up front.

Despite that disappointment, the discovery of leptin unleashed a scientific gold rush to find other molecules that could talk the brain into turning hunger off. By 1999 researchers from Japan's National Cardiovascular Center Research Institute in Osaka had announced the discovery of ghrelin, a kind of antileptin that is released primarily by the gut rather than by fat cells. Ghrelin signals hunger rather than satiety to the hypothalamus. Then, in 2002, a team from the University of Washington found that ghrelin levels rise before a meal and fall immediately after. Ghrelin (from the Indo-European root for the word "grow") increased hunger while jamming on the metabolic brakes to promote the body's storage of fat.

So began another line of attack on obesity. Rather than turning leptin on, researchers began exploring ways to turn ghrelin

off. Some of them began looking at animal models, but progress has been slow; the concept of a ghrelin "vaccine" has been floated, but clinical trials are still years off.

Seeking a better understanding of the hormone, University of Washington endocrinologist David Cummings compared ghrelin levels in people who had lost considerable amounts of weight through diet with those who shed pounds by means of gastric bypass surgery—a technique that reduces the capacity of the stomach and seems to damage its ghrelin-producing capacity as well. The results were remarkable. For dieters, the more weight lost, the greater the rise in ghrelin, as if the body were telling the brain to get hungry and regain that weight. By contrast, the big losers in the surgical group saw ghrelin levels fall to the floor. Surgical patients never felt increases in appetite and had an easier time maintaining their weight loss as a result. (A newer weight-loss surgery removes most of the ghrelin-producing cells outright.)

Based on such findings, a ghrelin-blocking drug called rimonabant was approved and sold in 32 countries, though not in the United States. It remained available as recently as 2008, even though it also increased the risk of depression and suicidal thinking; it has since been withdrawn everywhere. The verdict is still out on a newer generation of combination pharmaceuticals, including one that contains synthetic versions of leptin and the neurohormone amylin, known to help regulate appetite. In a six-month clinical trial, the combination therapy resulted in an average weight loss of 25 pounds, or 12.7 percent of body weight, with greater weight loss when continued for a full 52 weeks; those who stopped taking the drug midway regained most of their weight.

The Circadian Connection

The limited results from tackling the hypothalamus sent many scientists looking at the other gyres and gears driving obesity in the brain, especially in regions associated with sleep. The first big breakthrough came in 2005, when *Science* published a landmark paper on mice with a mutated version of the Clock gene, which plays a key role in the regulation of the body's circadian rhythms. The mutant mice not only failed to follow the strict eat-by-night, sleep-by-day schedule of normally nocturnal mice, they also became overweight and developed diabetes. "There was a difference in weight gain based on when the food was eaten, whether during day or night," says the study's senior author, endocrinologist Joe Bass of Northwestern University. "That means the metabolic rate must differ under those two conditions."

Could *my* late-night hours be the undoing of my weight-loss plans? Four days after my humiliating defeat by a bowl of tortilla chips, I met with Alex Keene, a postdoctoral researcher at New York University with a Matisse nude tattooed on his right forearm and a penchant for studying flies. His latest study asked whether a starved fly would take normal naps or sacrifice sleep to keep searching for food. He found that like humans (and most other creatures), flies have a neurological toggle between two fundamental yet incompatible drives: to eat or to sleep. "Flies only live a day or two when they're starved,"

Keene told me as we walked past graduate students peering at flies under microscopes. "If they decide to sleep through the night when they're starved, it's a bad decision on their part. So their brains are finely tuned to suppress their sleep when they don't have food and to sleep well after a meal."

For a major study published last year, Keene bred flies with dysfunctional mutations of the Clock gene and also of Cycle, another gene involved in circadian rhythms. He found that the genes together regulate the interaction between the two mutually exclusive behaviors, sleep and feeding, kicking in to suppress sleep when a fly is hungry.

Even when fed, flies without working versions of the Clock and Cycle genes tended to sleep poorly—about 30 percent as much as normal flies. "It was as if they were starving right away," Keene explains. Keene went even further, pinpointing where, amid the 100,000 or so neurons in the fly brain, the Clock gene acts to regulate the sleeping-feeding interaction: a region of just four to eight cells at the top of the fly brain.

"My father is an anthropologist," Keene told me as we stood in the fly room, its air pungent with the corn meal and molasses the flies feed on. "It's ironic, right? He looks at how culture determines behavior, while I look at how genes determine behavior. I used to get him so mad he'd storm out of the house."

Perhaps it takes an anthropologist's son to see that the excess availability of cheap, high-calorie chow cannot fully explain the magnitude and persistence of the problem in our culture. The rebellion against our inborn circadian rhythms wrought by a 24-hour lifestyle, lit by neon and fueled by caffeine, also bears part of the blame. The powerful effect of disordered sleep on metabolism has been seen not just in flies but also in humans. A 2009 study by Harvard University researchers showed that in just 10 days, three of eight healthy volunteers developed prediabetic blood-sugar levels when their sleep-wake schedule was gradually shifted out of alignment.

"It's clear from these types of studies that the way we're keeping the lights on until late at night, the way in which society demands that we stay active for so much longer, could well be contributing to aspects of the metabolic disease we're seeing now," says Steve Kay, a molecular geneticist at the University of California, San Diego.

These insights have fostered collaboration between once-diverse groups. "Physicians who specialized in obesity and diabetes for years are now discovering the importance of circadian effects," Kay says. At the same time, "basic research scientists like me, who have been studying the circadian system for so many years, are now looking at its metabolic effects. When so many people's research from so many areas starts to converge, you know we're in the midst of a paradigm shift. This is the slow rumbling before the volcano blows."

This past April, the National Institute of Diabetes and Digestive and Kidney Diseases (NIDDK) of the National Institutes of Health organized a first-ever national conference focused solely on how circadian rhythms affect metabolism. "What has become obvious over the past few years is that metabolism, all those pathways regulating how fats and carbohydrates are used, is affected by the circadian clock," says biochemist Corinne Silva, a program director at the NIDDK. Her goal is to find drugs

that treat diabetes and obesity by targeting circadian pathways. "The mechanisms by which circadian rhythms are maintained and the cross talk with metabolic signaling are just beginning to be elucidated," she says, but they should lead to novel therapeutic approaches in the years ahead.

In Keene's view, the newfound link between sleep and obesity could be put to use right now. "People who are susceptible to diabetes or have weight issues might just get more sleep. I get only about six hours of sleep myself. I usually run in the middle of the night. I'm not a morning person," the enviably thin, 29-year-old Keene states.

My visit to his fly room convinced me to try a new angle in my quest to get under 190 pounds: Rather than focus on *how much* food I put in my mouth, I would focus on *when* I eat. I decided I would no longer eat after 10 P.M.

The Pleasure Factor

Timing may be everything for some folks, but it wasn't for me. No wonder: The brain has no shortage of techniques to goad us into eating. Another line of evidence suggests that the brains of overweight people are wired to feel more pleasure in response to food. Sleep deprived or not, they just enjoy eating more. To study such differences, clinical psychologist Eric Stice of the Oregon Research Institute mastered the delicate task of conducting fMRI brain scans while people were eating. The food he chose to give the volunteers inside the tunnel-like scanners was a milk shake. And let the record show, it was a *chocolate* milk shake.

Brains of the overweight are wired to feel more pleasure in response to food.

Obese adolescent girls, Stice found, showed greater activation compared with their lean peers in regions of the brain that encode the sensory experience of eating food—the so-called gustatory cortex and the somatosensory regions, archipelagoes of neurons that reach across different structures in the brain. At the same time, the obese girls sipping milk shakes showed decreased activation in the striatum, a region near the center of the brain that is studded with dopamine receptors and known to respond to stimuli associated with rewards. Stice wondered whether, even among normal-weight girls, such a pattern might predict an increased risk of overeating and weight gain.

To test his hypothesis, he followed a group of subjects over time, finding that those with reduced activation in the dorsal (rear) region of the striatum while sipping a milk shake were ultimately more likely to gain weight than those with normal activation. The most vulnerable of these girls were also more likely to have a DNA polymorphism—not a mutation, per se, but a rather routine genetic variation—in a dopamine receptor gene, causing reduced dopamine signaling in the striatum and placing them at higher risk. "Individuals may overeat," Stice and his colleagues concluded, "to compensate for a hypofunctioning dorsal striatum, particularly those with genetic polymorphisms thought to attenuate dopamine signaling in this region."

Stice was initially surprised by the results. "It's totally weird," he admits. "Those who experienced less pleasure were at increased risk for weight gain." But his more recent studies have convinced him that the reduced pleasure is a result of years of overeating among the obese girls—the same phenomenon seen in drug addicts who require ever-greater amounts of their drug to feel the same reward. "Imagine a classroom of third graders, and everyone is skinny," he says. "The people who initially find that milk shake most orgasmic will want more of it, but in so doing they cause neuroplastic changes that downregulate the reward circuitry, driving them to eat more and more to regain that same feeling they crave."

Even among people of normal weight, individual differences in brain functioning can directly affect eating behaviors, according to a 2009 study by Michael Lowe, a research psychologist at Drexel University. He took fMRI brain scans of 19 people, all of them of normal weight. Nine of the volunteers reported following strict diets; the other 10 typically ate whenever and whatever they wanted. Lowe had all of them sip a milk shake immediately before getting scanned. The brains of the nondieters, he found, lit up just as one would expect, showing activations in areas associated with satiation and memory, as if saying, "Mmmm, that was good." The chronic dieters showed activations in areas of the brain associated with desire and expectation of reward, however. If anything, the milk shake had made them hungrier.

"What we have shown is that these chronic dieters may actually have a reason to restrain themselves, because they are more susceptible than average to overeating," Lowe says.

Yet inborn differences in hunger and desire, too, turn out to be only part of the weighting game. Eating behaviors are also linked to areas of the brain associated with self-control (such as the left superior frontal region) and visual attention (such as the right middle temporal region). A recent fMRI study led by Jeanne McCaffery, a psychologist at Brown Medical School, showed that successful weight losers had greater activation in those regions, compared with normal-weight people and obese people, when viewing images of food.

The effects of stress on eating behaviors also has a neurobiological basis, according to University of Pennsylvania neurobiologist Tracy Bale. She showed that neural pathways associated with stress link directly to areas of the brain associated with seeking rewards. "Few things are more rewarding evolutionarily than calorie-dense food," Bale told me a few days after presenting a seminar on the subject at last fall's Society for Neuroscience meeting in San Diego. "Under stress people don't crave a salad; they crave something high-calorie. It's because those stress pathways in the limbic system feed into the reward centers, and they drive reward-seeking behaviors. What that tells us is that in addition to drug companies' trying to target appetite, they need to look at the reward centers. We're not necessarily fat because we're hungry but because we're looking for something to deal with stress."

Aha! Perhaps it was stress that was messing with my latest, clock-based diet. Back in March 2010, a tree had fallen on my family's home during a major storm, crushing the roof, destroying half the house, and forcing us to flee to a nearby apartment. By November, as I researched this story, we had finally moved back into our rebuilt house. With nerves fully frayed, I found myself drawn as never before to the Tick Tock Diner, where the motto literally is "Eat Heavy," and where the french fries never tasted better. Instead of losing a few pounds to get under 190, by Thanksgiving I had hit 196.

How to Fix a Hungry Brain

Neuroscience has yet to deliver a weight-loss elixir for paunchy 53-year-old journalists like me, much less for those suffering from serious obesity. But that day will come, Steve Kay asserts, once researchers figure out the correct combination of drugs that work simultaneously on multiple triggers of eating and metabolism, just as hypertension is now routinely treated with two- or three-drug combinations.

Some scientists think a more radical approach is called for. Since the triggers of obesity lie in the brain, neurosurgeons at West Virginia University Health Sciences Center are attempting to rewire those triggers directly using deep brain stimulation (DBS). Since 2009 they have performed surgery on three obese patients to implant electrodes that emit rhythmic electric shocks into the hypothalamus. Having failed other medical therapies for obesity, the three agreed to volunteer for DBS, a treatment already approved for treating the tremors and dystonia of Parkinson's disease. "These patients weren't eating all that much; it was mainly a problem of having very slow metabolisms," says Donald M. Whiting, one of the neurosurgeons leading the study. "Our goal was to speed it up." On the basis of successful animal studies, he adds, "we thought we'd switch on the energy and collect our Nobel Prize."

All three patients experienced significantly less hunger when the electrodes were switched on, and all regained their normal hunger when the electrodes were switched off. Unfortunately, none lost a significant amount of weight in the study's first year. The problem, Whiting concludes, is that there are many ways to adjust DBS. With four contact points on the electrodes, each placed half a millimeter apart and each adjustable for voltage, frequency, and pulse width, the research team has been seeking the combination of settings that most effectively rev up metabolism. So far they have found settings that work only temporarily.

"The brain is really pretty smart," Whiting says. "It tends to want to reboot to factory settings whenever it can. We find that we can reset things for a week or two, but then the brain gets back to where it wants." Despite the challenges, Whiting remains convinced that finding a safe and effective medical treatment for weight control will be essential to turn the obesity epidemic around—and that no amount of preaching from Oprah, no behavior program from Weight Watchers nor food from Jenny Craig, will ever suffice.

"This mystification that obesity is caused by a lack of willpower or just eating the wrong foods is simply a misconception," Joe Bass of Northwestern told me. "There is so much social stigma attached to weight that we make a lot of value judgments. The effort in science is to peel back those layers of belief and try to understand things in an experimental, rational mode. Just as we have made progress against heart disease with statins and blood pressure drugs, we will find medications that can safely and substantially lower weight."

Months after my investigation of the brain-gut connection began, I faced the acid test. In early March I stepped back onto my bathroom scale for a final weigh-in. Rather than slip below 190, for the first time in my life I had tipped, by a single pound, over 200. You might blame it on insufficient exercise or on the cheese and crackers I failed to remove from my late-night work ritual. I'm blaming it on my brain.

Critical Thinking

1. Describe the hormones that impact food intake and explain their actions in the body.

2. Explain how sleep and circadian rhythms influence feeding behavior and metabolism.

3. How does the limbic system dictate the types of foods that we crave during stress?

In Your Face
How the Food Industry Drives Us to Eat

Bonnie Liebman, and Kelly Brownell

Excess pounds raise the risk of diabetes, heart disease, stroke, cancer (of the breast, colon, esophagus, kidney, and uterus), gallbladder disease, arthritis, and more. And once people gain weight, the odds of losing it and keeping it off are slim.

"Estimates are that this generation of children may be the first to live fewer years than their parents," says Kelly Brownell. "Health care costs for obesity are now $147 billion annually."

What are we doing about it? Not enough.

"The conditions that are driving the obesity epidemic need to change," says Brownell. Here's why and how.

Q: Why do you call our food environment toxic?
A: Because people who are exposed to it get sick. They develop chronic diseases like diabetes and obesity in record numbers.

Q: How does the environment influence what we eat?
A: When I was a boy, there weren't aisles of food in the drugstore, and gas stations weren't places where you could eat lunch. Vending machines in workplaces were few and far between, and schools didn't have junk food. Fast food restaurants didn't serve breakfast or stay open 24 hours. Today, access to unhealthy choices is nearly ubiquitous.

Burgers, fries, pizza, soda, candy, and chips are everywhere. Apples and bananas aren't. And we have large portion sizes—bigger bagels, burgers, steaks, muffins, cookies, popcorn, and sodas. We have the relentless marketing of unhealthy food, and too little access to healthy foods.

Q: Does the price structure of food push us to buy more?
A: Yes. People buy a Value Meal partly because that large burger, fries, and soft drink cost less than a salad and bottle of water. A large popcorn doesn't cost much more than a small. A Cinnabon doesn't cost much more than a Minibon.

Q: And most stores are pushing junk food, not fresh fruit?
A: Yes. There's a Dunkin' Donuts at our Stop 'n Shop supermarket and at the Wal-Mart near us. And if you look at retail stores, they're set up in ways that maximize the likelihood of impulse purchases.

For example, the candy is on display at the checkout line at the supermarket. And when you go to a modern drugstore, the things you usually go to a drugstore to buy—like bandages, cough medicine, pain reliever, your prescriptions—are all at the back. People typically have to walk by the soda, chips, and other junk food to navigate their way there and back.

Old Genes, New World

Q: You've said that our biology is mismatched with the modern world, How?
A: Thousands of years ago, our ancestors faced unpredictable food supplies and looming starvation. Those who adapted ate voraciously when food was available and stored body fat so they could survive times of scarcity.

Our bodies were programmed to seek calorie-dense foods. They were exquisitely efficient calorie-conservation machines, which matched nicely with a scarce food supply.

But now we have abundance. And there's no need for the extreme physical exertion that our ancestors needed to hunt and gather food. It's a mismatch.

Q: How do ads encourage overeating?
A: Overeating is written into the language that companies use—names like Big Gulp, Super Gulp, Extreme Gulp. At one point, Frito-Lay sold dollar bags of snack foods called the Big Grab. The burger companies describe their biggest burgers with words like the Monster Burger, the Whopper, the Big Mac. The industry capitalizes on our belief that bigger is better and promotes large amounts of their least healthy foods.

Q: Why do we want a good deal on a bad food?
A: Everybody likes value. Getting more of something for your money isn't a bad idea. You like to do that when you buy an automobile or clothing or laundry detergent or anything.

But when the incentives are set up in a way that offers value for unhealthy food, it's a problem. If you buy the big bag of Cheetos, you get a better deal than if you buy the little bag. A big Coke is a better deal than a little Coke. But if you buy six apples, you don't always get a better deal than if you buy three.

Q: Is indulgence a code word for overeating?
A: Right. You deserve a reward and we're here to offer it to you. And ads describe foods as sinful. Or we make light of eating too much, like the ad that said "I can't believe I ate the whole thing."

Are We Irresponsible?

Q: *How does the food industry blame people for the obesity epidemic?*

A: The two words it uses most frequently are personal responsibility. It plays well in America because of this idea that people should take charge of their own lives and because some people have the biological fortune to be able to resist our risky environment.

But it also serves to shift blame from the industry and government to the individuals with a weight problem. It's right out of the tobacco-industry playbook.

Q: *What else is in the food industry's playbook?*

A: Industry spokespeople raise fears that government action usurps personal freedom. Or they vilify critics with totalitarian language, characterizing them as the food police, leaders of a nanny state, and even food fascists, and accuse them of trying to strip people of their civil liberties.

They also criticize studies that hurt the food industry as "junk science." And they argue that there are no good or bad foods—only good or bad diets. That way, soft drinks, fast foods, and other foods can't be targeted for change.

Q: *So people think it's their fault?*

A: Many people who struggle with weight problems believe it's their own fault anyway. So exacerbating that is not helpful. But removing the mandate for business and government to take action has been very harmful.

For example, if you look at funding to reduce obesity, it has lagged far behind the extent of the problem. It's because of this idea that people are responsible for the way they are, so why should government do anything about it?

Q: *Are people irresponsible?*

A: There's been increasing obesity for years in the United States. It's hard to believe that people in 2010 are less responsible than they were 10 or 20 years ago. You have increasing obesity in literally every country in the world. Are people in every country becoming less responsible?

We looked into the literature to find data on other health behaviors like mammograms, seat belt use, heavy drinking, and smoking. All those other behaviors have remained constant or have improved in the U.S. population.

If irresponsibility is the cause of obesity, one might expect evidence that people are becoming less responsible overall. But studies suggest the opposite.

So if people are having trouble acting responsibly in the food arena, the question is why? There must be enormous pressure bearing down on them to override their otherwise responsible behavior.

Q: *It's not as though society rewards obesity.*

A: No. Obesity is stigmatized. Overweight people, especially children, are teased and victimized by discrimination. Obese children have lower self-esteem and a higher risk of depression. They're less likely to be admitted to college. And obese adults are less likely to be hired, have lower salaries, and are often viewed as lazy and less competent. So the pressure to overeat must be overwhelming.

Q: *Are the pressures worse for children?*

A: Yes. Kids don't have the natural cognitive defenses against marketing. And they're developing brand loyalty and food preferences that can last a lifetime.

To allow the food industry to have free range with our children has come at a tremendous cost. A third of kids are now overweight or obese. And when you project ahead to the adult diseases that will cause, it's incredible. Someday, our children may wonder why we didn't protect them from the food companies.

Q: *Do we do anything to protect kids?*

A: We do some nutrition education in schools, but it's a drop against the tidal wave of what the food industry is doing to educate those children.

The Robert Wood Johnson Foundation is by far the biggest funder of work on childhood obesity, and it's now spending $100 million a year on the problem. The food industry spends that much every year by January 4th to market unhealthy food to children. There's no way the government can compete with that just through education.

If parents ate every meal with their children, that would amount to 1,000 teaching opportunities per year. Yet the average child sees 10,000 food ads each year. And parents don't have Beyoncé, LeBron, and Kobe on their side.

Q: *So if irresponsibility isn't to blame, what is?*

A: When you give lab animals access to the diets that are marketed so aggressively in the United States, they become obese. We have abundant science that the environment is the causative agent here. So the environment needs to be changed.

That's what public policy is all about. We require that children get vaccinated and ride in child safety seats. We have high taxes on cigarettes. Your car has an air bag. The government could educate us to be safe drivers and hope for the best. Or it could just put an air bag in every car. Those are examples of government taking action to create better defaults.

Keeping It off

Q: *Why is it so important to prevent obesity?*

A: Because it's so difficult to fix. The results of studies on treating obesity are very discouraging, especially if one looks at long-term results. The exception is surgery, but that's expensive and can't be used on a broad scale. So this is a problem that screams out to be prevented.

Q: *Why is it so hard to keep weight off?*

A: There's good research, much of it done by Rudolph Leibel and colleagues at Columbia University, that shows that when people are overweight and lose weight, their biology changes in a way that makes it hard to keep the weight off.

Take two women who weigh 150 pounds. One has always weighed 150 and the other was at 170 and reduced down to 150. Metabolically, they look very different. To maintain her 150-pound weight, the woman who has dropped from 170 is going to have to exist on about 15 percent fewer calories than the woman who was always at 150.

Q: *Why?*

A: It's as if the body senses that it's in starvation mode so it becomes more metabolically efficient. People who have lost weight burn fewer calories than those who haven't, so they have to keep taking in fewer calories to keep the weight off. That's tough to do day after day, especially when the environment is pushing us to eat more, not less.

And Leibel and others have shown that there are changes in hormones, including leptin, that explain why people who lose weight are hungry much of the time.

Q: *Are you saying that our bodies think we're starving when we lose just 10 percent of our body weight?*

A: Right. It's not hopeless, but the data can be discouraging. The results of weight-loss studies are clear. Not many people lose a significant amount of weight and keep it off. All these environmental cues force people to eat, and then this biology makes it hard to lose weight and keep it off.

Q: *Does genetics play a role in obesity?*

A: Yes. Genetics can help explain why some people are prone to gain weight and some are not. But genetics can't explain why there are so many overweight people. The reason we have more obesity than Somalia, let's say, is not because we're genetically different. The fact that so many people are overweight is all environment.

Addictive Foods

Q: *Are some foods addictive?*

A: My prediction is that the issue of food and addiction will explode onto the scene relatively soon, because the science is building almost by the day and it's very compelling. I think it's important to put the focus on the food, rather than the person. There are people who consider themselves food addicts, and they might be, but the more important question is whether there's enough addictive properties in some foods to keep people coming back for more and more. That's where the public health problem resides.

Q: *What are those properties?*

A: What's been studied most so far is sugar. There are brain-imaging studies in humans and a variety of animal studies showing that sugar acts on the brain very much like morphine, alcohol, and nicotine. It doesn't have as strong an effect, but it has a similar effect on reward pathways in the brain. So when kids get out of school and they feel like having a sugared beverage, how much of that is their brain calling out for this addictive substance? Are we consuming so many foods of poor nutrient quality partly because of the addictive properties of the food itself?

Q: *What do you mean by reward pathways?*

A: There are pathways in the brain that get activated when we experience pleasure, and drugs of abuse like heroin hijack that system. The drugs take over the system to make those substances extremely reinforcing and to make us want those things when we don't have them.

The drugs do that by setting up withdrawal symptoms when we don't have them. The drugs set up the addiction by creating tolerance, so you need more over time to produce the same effect. The drugs set us up to have cravings. The same reward system is activated by foods, especially foods high in sugar.

Q: *Do we need more research in people?*

A: Yes, but we already have animal and human studies, some done by highly distinguished researchers. I think this is a top priority because if we get to the point where we say that food can be addictive, the whole landscape can change.

Think of the morality or legality of marketing these foods to children. Could the industry ever be held accountable for the intentional manipulation of ingredients that activate the brain in that way? The stakes are very high.

Q: *How much does exercise matter to losing weight?*

A: Exercise has so many health benefits that it's hard to count them. It lowers the risk for cancer, heart disease, and cognitive impairment as people age. There's a very long list of reasons to be physically active, but weight control may not be one of them. Recent studies have suggested that the food part of the equation is much more important than the activity part.

Q: *Because you can undo an hour of exercise with one muffin?*

A: Yes. The food industry has been front and center in promoting exercise as the way to address the nation's obesity problem. The industry talks about the importance of physical activity continuously, and they've been quite involved in funding programs that emphasize physical activity. The skeptics claim that that's the way to divert attention away from food.

Answers

Q: *So what's the answer to the obesity epidemic?*

A: The broad answer is to change the environmental conditions that are driving obesity. Some of the most powerful drivers are food marketing and the economics of food, so I would start there. I don't think we have much chance of succeeding with the obesity problem unless the marketing of unhealthy foods is curtailed.

Q: *Not just to kids?*

A: No, but children would be a great place to start. Second would be to change the economics so that healthy food costs less and unhealthy food costs more. So a small tax on sugar-sweetened beverages—say, one penny per ounce—would be part of that effort.

Ideally, the tax revenues would be used to subsidize the cost of fruits and vegetables. That creates a better set of economic defaults. Now, especially if you're poor, all the incentives are pushing you toward unhealthy foods.

Q: *Like zip codes where there are no grocery stores?*

A: That's a great example of a bad default. Another, which applies not just to the poor, would be what children have available in schools. You can sell a lot of junk in schools and then try to educate your way out of it. Or you can just get rid of the junk food and kids will have healthier defaults. They'll eat healthier food if that's what's available. You can inspire that just by changing the default.

Imagine the optimal environment to combat obesity. We would have affordable and healthful food, especially fresh fruits and vegetables, easily accessible to people in low-income neighborhoods. TV commercials for children would encourage them to eat fresh fruits and vegetables rather than pushing processed snacks that are associated with TV and movie characters. And every community would have safe sidewalks and walking trails to encourage physical activity.

Q: *So people wouldn't have to struggle to avoid eating junk?*

A: Right. We have a terrible set of defaults with food: big portions, bad marketing, bad food in schools. These conditions produce incentives for the wrong behaviors. So the question is: can we create an environment that supports healthy eating, rather than undermines it?

If you count the number of places where you can buy sugared beverages and salty snack foods and candy, it's enormous. If you count the number of places where you can buy baby carrots and oranges, it's a fraction of that.

So if you were creating an environment from scratch, you would do the opposite of what we have. The population deserves a better set of defaults.

Critical Thinking

1. What is meant by the quote, "our biology is mismatched with the modern world"?

2. What types of foods are considered addictive?

3. The author talks about the U.S. food defaults. What are the U.S. food defaults that are causative factors in our toxic food environment?

KELLY BROWNELL is a professor in the Department of Psychology at Yale University. He is also a professor of epidemiology and public health. Brownell co-founded and directs Yale's Rudd Center for Food Policy and Obesity, which works to improve the world's diet, prevent obesity, and reduce weight stigma. Brownell, who is a member of *Nutrition Action*'s scientific advisory board, has published more than 300 scientific articles and chapters and 14 books including *Food Fight: The Inside Story of the Food Industry, America's Obesity Crisis, and What We Can Do About It* (McGraw-Hill). He spoke to *Nutrition Action*'s Bonnie Liebman from New Haven.

Birth Weight Strongly Linked to Obesity

New evidence suggests gain during pregnancy is key.

NANCI HELLMICH

Women who gain a lot of weight during pregnancy are more likely to have high-birth-weight babies, which may increase the children's risk of becoming obese later in life, a new study suggests.

The findings add to growing evidence of the importance of appropriate weight gain during pregnancy.

For several decades, researchers have observed that a high birth weight increases the risk that a child will gain too much weight later in life. Some studies of animals suggest excess calories affect the fetus, including the fat tissue and the organs that regulate body weight.

Now researchers at Children's Hospital in Boston and Columbia University in New York have studied the medical records of more than 500,000 women who had two or more pregnancies, a total of more than 1 million babies. A newborn who weighed more than 8½ pounds at birth was considered at a high birth weight.

By comparing siblings, researchers for the first time were able to control for mothers' genetic influences on birth weight.

The findings, reported online in The Lancet: The women gained an average of 30 pounds during pregnancy; those who gained 50 pounds were twice as likely to have a high-birth-weight baby than those who gained 20.

"Although birth weight is not the only determinant of adult weight, these findings suggest that an optimal time to begin obesity prevention efforts is before birth," says pediatric endocrinologist David Ludwig of Children's Hospital, lead author of the study.

Matthew Gillman of Harvard Medical School, who is also researching pregnancy and weight gain, says follow-up studies are needed to establish the link between gestational weight gain and childhood obesity.

In the meantime, there are other reasons to be concerned, Ludwig says. Pregnant women who are overweight or obese are at greater risk of problems such as complications during labor and delivery (including C-sections), gestational diabetes and high blood pressure.

How much should you gain?

Recommendations for total weight gain during pregnancy based on pre-pregnancy weight:

Pre-pregnancy weight (Body mass index)	Recommended weight gain
Underweight (Less than 18.5)	28–40 lbs
Normal weight (18.5–24.9)	25–35 lbs
Overweight (25–29.9)	15–25 lbs
Obese (30 or greater)	11–20 lbs

Source: Institute of Medicine   By Frank Pompa, USA TODAY

A word of caution: "Being severely underweight during pregnancy, as well as severely limiting food intake, can also be problematic to fetal growth and development," says Alan Fleischman, medical director for the March of Dimes, which works to improve babies' health. Too little weight gain increases the risk of having a low-birth-weight baby of less than 5½ pounds.

Critical Thinking

1. Pregnant women who are overweight or obese are at greater risk for developing certain medical conditions. What are three of these medical conditions?

2. How does excessive maternal weight gain during pregnancy impact the health of the fetus?

3. What is the recommended weight gain for a normal weight pregnant woman? How does this recommendation differ from the recommended weight gain for an obese pregnant woman?

Eating Disorders in an Obesogenic Environment

Joyce A. Corsica, PhD, and Megan M. Hood, PhD

A n obesogenic environment is an environment that produces and supports overweight and obesity through several intersecting mechanisms. Obesogenic environments and behavior, particularly in the context of genetic susceptibility to obesity, are believed to account for the increased prevalence of overweight and obesity in the world today. Such an environment includes decreased physical activity, increased energy intake, heavy promotion of energy-dense foods, greater number of overweight people, biological predisposition to weight difficulties, food addiction and changes in neurochemistry, and impact of both social discrimination and media manipulation of the ideal body image. Together these factors pose substantial problems for individuals with disordered eating behaviors, as will be discussed in this article. Although the development of eating disorders is complex and multifactorial, the combination of these factors in the obesogenic environment has the potential to contribute to the disordered eating behavior and cognitions to which some young people are vulnerable.

The Obesogenic Environment

Contributors to the obesogenic environment include the current physical environment, behavior (including energy intake and decreased physical activity), and the social environment, as well as a biological predisposition to positive energy balance (1). In the past 3 decades, environmental changes have reduced physical activity via labor-saving devices such as cars, elevators, escalators, motorized walkways, and remote controls, which have had a cumulative impact in decreasing daily energy expenditure (2,3). At the same time, energy expended in leisure-time physical activities has decreased as people spend more time sitting passively in front of computers, televisions, DVD players, and video games rather than participating in physical activities that require movement and greater amounts of energy expenditure. National statistics confirm that fewer than one third of Americans engage in the recommended amounts of physical activity of at least 30 minutes most days (4). There is no federal standard or education mandate for physical education in schools (5), and physical activity programs are among the first areas to succumb to budget cuts (6).

Obesogenic behavior includes the consumption of larger portions of food, particularly high-fat, high-sugar foods, often combined with greater time spent in passive or sedentary activity. The current environment promotes the overconsumption of energy-dense, nutrient-poor food (7,8), which is typically considered obesogenic. Processed foods in particular pose difficulties for weight management. Comprised of primarily refined grains, sugars, and preservatives, processed foods (most packaged foods) are generally inexpensive, highly palatable, energy-dense, and convenient. When the diet includes higher amounts of processed foods, higher levels of hunger are reported (9). Excess consumption of processed food can also displace the consumption of healthier, whole foods and promote repeated cycles of eating (and craving) more processed, highly palatable foods. Moreover, these high-calorie and low-cost items are readily available at convenience stores, drug stores, and 24-hour service stations, in addition to fast-food restaurants, grocery stores, and food courts (7). In addition, more sugar-sweetened beverages are being consumed than ever before (10), which has been shown to be an independent risk factor for obesity in children (11). Lastly, many of these problematic foods are being served and consumed in increasingly large portion sizes, particularly in restaurants. Eating away from home, especially at fast-food restaurants, is associated with higher energy and higher fat intake (12) and is a significant contributor to weight gain and the increasing prevalence of overweight (13–15).

The obesogenic social environment includes constant advertising as well as opportunities and pressure to eat. Unhealthy foods, including many breakfast cereals and pastries, are often marketed selectively to children and vulnerable populations. The average child watches 10,000 advertisements for food each year, an astonishing 95 percent of which are for sugared cereals, candy, fast foods, and soft drinks (16). Television-watching is often accompanied by snacking on energy-dense foods (which are often being advertised) and is associated with higher body weight (17).

Finally, it is recognized that all of these environmental factors occur on a foundation of biology. Biological factors include a genetic predisposition to positive calorie balance, which was formerly an adaptive and protective response to environmental changes in energy availability. Several convergent lines of evidence support that there are individual differences in the predisposition to weight gain and suggests that genetic variation has much to do with the risk of becoming obese (18). In summary, the obesogenic environment is characterized as a confluence of highly palatable, readily available, heavily advertised foods; larger portion sizes; increased pressure to eat; and significantly decreased work and leisure activity, all in the context of biology that predisposes many to weight gain.

The Impact of the Media

The media's portrayal (and some would say, idealization) of a very thin female body type has long been viewed as an important sociocultural risk factor for eating disorders (19,20). The media's impact on potential body dissatisfaction, disordered eating, and obesity is actually twofold. Media sources, including television shows, commercials, movies, and fashion magazines, encourage a generally unattainable, very thin ideal body image. For example, the average fashion model weighs 24 percent less than the average female today (21). Viewing of such images in fashion magazines seems to be associated with increased eating disorder symptomatology in adolescent girls (22,23). Yet, at the same time that a thin body is idealized, media-based advertising reinforces the availability and even the sex appeal of high-energy-dense foods. Taken together, the average woman faces conflicting messages: very thin equals beautiful, but eating energy-dense foods is attractive and desirable. The combination of what many perceive as an unhealthy, unattainable, but highly valued body image perpetuated in the media, with the realities of the obesogenic environment, sets up a virtually no-win situation that can lead to feelings of learned helplessness, psychological distress, and potential self-dislike/hatred and increased rates of both disordered eating and obesity. Although the media's influence has been longstanding, it has a far greater presence now than ever before (24).

Psychosocial Consequences of Obesity: Impact on Disordered Eating and Dieting

The obesogenic environment, by definition, promotes obesity, and obesity can and does result in considerable social discrimination and psychological distress. Social consequences associated with obesity (which result from the widespread but mistaken belief that overweight people lack self-control) include bias, stigmatization, and discrimination, consequences that can be highly detrimental to psychological well-being (25). Negative attitudes toward obese people have been reported by children as well as adults, by health care professionals as well as the general public, and by overweight individuals themselves (26,27). Discrimination due to obesity may well be the last socially acceptable form of widespread prejudice. The impact of this prejudice on young people, in terms of their body image, food choices, and behaviors, cannot be understated. Discrimination or bias may compel more restriction in the current environment, and the high rates of obesity make this more likely. Exposure to critical comments by family about shape, weight, or eating behaviors, as well as weight-related teasing, have been identified as risk factors for a range of eating disordered behaviors (28,29).

Up to one in four 11-year-olds has already tried to diet once (30). This is concerning because children who diet may actually end up gaining more weight in the long term compared with children who do not diet due to the fact that dieting may cause a cycle of restrictive eating followed by overeating or binge-eating (31). The risk for obesity may be more than 300 percent higher for adolescent girls who describe themselves as dieters compared with those who do not diet (32). Adolescent girls who are obese or at risk for becoming obese are also more likely to use unhealthy weight practices, such as vomiting and using diet pills or laxatives (33).

Notably, an obesogenic environment confers more potential for parents to be overweight. Rates of overweight in this county

have now reached 68 percent (34), which means it is likely that a child will have at least one parent who is overweight. In some children and adolescents, a combination of genetics and environmental factors related to having an overweight parent may increase perception/risk for eating disorders (22). This is especially true if overweight parents allow energy-dense foods in the diet (and in the house), promote the use of food to modulate mood states, promulgate weight and shape biases, make critical comments about shape or weight, and do not tend to encourage leisure-time physical activity.

Newer Research: Food Addiction and External Food Sensitivity as Contributors to Intake Regulation Difficulties and Disordered Eating

Many people report addiction-like symptoms, including cravings and loss of control over eating, related to eating the very foods previously discussed as contributing to the obesogenic environment (high-sugar, high-fat, processed foods) (35,36). Recent research suggests that addiction-like processes may underlie some intake regulation difficulties in some people and may contribute to disordered eating and weight-control difficulties (37). For example, sugar is thought to have addiction potential as a highly palatable food that releases opioids and dopamine (38), but researchers have demonstrated in animals that it is a pattern of restriction alternated with brief availability that seems to produce an addictive pattern of eating. Recent evidence suggests that behavioral and neural pathway changes may be induced by the restriction/exposure pattern, including tendency to self-medicate, restricting/bingeing pattern, or tendency to eat certain foods while hungry. It has been suggested that some disordered eating behaviors, including the frequently seen pattern of daytime restriction and nighttime overeating/loss of control, binge eating, or even diet cycling, may replicate the restriction/exposure pattern found in animal studies, resulting in food addiction symptoms (36).

Another recently identified factor that may encourage increased energy intake is susceptibility to environmental cues (known as external food sensitivity), which has been demonstrated via functional resonance imagery to serve as a predisposing factor to food cravings and food intake (39). This means that the sight, smell, or suggestion of food can serve as a potent eating trigger in susceptible people. Given the obesogenic environment, replete with easily available, heavily advertised, and palatable foods, this increased exposure may induce cravings, loss of control, and binge cycling as early as childhood and adolescence in those who are susceptible to these environmental cues, which, as previously discussed, are pervasive in our current environment.

Eating Disorders in the Obesogenic Environment

Rates of eating disorders in women are increasing (40), and eating disorders are being diagnosed at younger ages and with greater frequency (41). Although most teens do not suffer from a diagnosable eating disorder or from obesity, many engage in disordered eating behaviors such as binge-eating, purging, and dieting that are sustained across the next decade of life (42). These behaviors can be associated with serious physical and emotional difficulties, as well as ongoing and unremitting symptomatology across many years.

In an obesogenic environment, it is a far greater challenge to maintain healthy eating habits in light of the environmental and biological factors discussed thus far. Exposure to this environment, with its energy-dense food choices that are constantly available, low levels of physical activity, greater likelihood of overweight parents, bias/discrimination either received or observed, and very early dieting, combined with conflicting messages in the media can together, or even in isolation, lead to feelings of loss of control, food restriction, bingeing, and weight gain. Considering that those with binge-eating behaviors are more susceptible than non–binge-eaters to the variety of processed, sweetened, high-fat foods that are available (as they report receiving greater enjoyment out of the taste, smell, and texture of food [43] and tend to have lower dietary restraint than those with restricting eating disorders), this environmental onslaught of food availability poses considerable and constant challenges to those who engage in binge-eating behavior (44).

Even in very young children, there is a substantial impact of the environment on the development of obesity and disordered eating. Binge-eating episodes have been reported in 2 percent of children age 5 to 6 years and presence of these episodes is associated with obesity (45). Moreover, the presence of binge-eating in these children is strongly associated with eating disturbances in their mothers. Warning signs of possible disordered eating behavior in children include eating in the absence of hunger, eating to modulate strong or negative affect, eating in secret, or hiding food (46).

Prevention: Changing the Obesogenic Environment

Efforts toward prevention of weight- and eating-related problems must occur on multiple levels, including, perhaps most importantly, changes in the obesogenic environment (47). Current efforts at prevention, such as taxes on soda and processed foods, and reduced availability of sugar-sweetened soft drinks and vending machines in schools, have the potential to reduce exposure to some especially obesogenic foods. Interventions targeting the school environment are particularly important given the potential to dramatically impact awareness and eating habits for children and adolescents during key developmental periods (see references [48–51] for reviews of obesity-prevention programs). To improve the obesogenic environment, we offer the following suggestions (adapted from reference [52]), which lend themselves to reducing the potential for disordered eating in this environment.

Continue to Intervene in Schools

Schools are in a unique position to support the promotion of healthy lifestyles. Interventions in the school environment can result in beneficial changes in both diet and physical activity. School-based physical activity programs that provide for enjoyable and regular exercise participation for all students are a necessity. In addition, schools should promote healthy eating patterns by ensuring that cafeterias and vending machines offer a variety of low-cost, nutritious foods and snacks. Continuing to address processed food availability, including fast-food operations on school premises, is necessary. It is imperative that we decrease access to high-calorie, nutritionally poor foods and provide greater opportunities for students to select healthy foods. In addition, an effective school-based intervention may require multiple components, including a behavioral curriculum, parent involvement, changes in the school food program, and support from the food industry.

Regulate Advertising of Junk Foods

Restaurant, soft drink, and candy companies spend more than $400 billion per year to advertise their products, often targeting their messages to young people, whereas very little is spent on advertising to promote healthy dietary practices (7). This dramatic inequity requires attention, and more stringent regulation is needed to decrease the advertising of unhealthy foods, particularly during children's shows. It may be helpful to require TV commercials to disclose prominently the nutrient values (eg, calories, calories from fats, serving size) of advertised products, particularly snack foods. The concept of food addiction makes a strong case for reducing, limiting, or controlling foods with addiction potential in the environment (36).

Impose a "Sugared Beverage Tax"

For many years, Brownell and his colleagues (53,54) have recommended adopting a tax on unhealthy foods, with the revenues from such a tax used to fund public health initiatives to promote healthy eating and exercise habits. A modest tax per 12-oz soft drink or per pound of snack foods would go toward subsidizing healthier food choices, underwriting the cost of a national campaign to improve the nation's eating habits, or reducing health care costs. A recent national survey showed that 60 percent to 70 percent of adults would support such a tax if the revenues were used to reduce health care costs (55).

Prevention in the Home: Helping Adolescents Develop Healthy Eating Attitudes and Behaviors in an Obesogenic Environment

Adults can serve as positive role models for their children. Because children of overweight parents are more likely to be overweight, and daughters of mothers who diet are more likely to diet than other girls, it is critical that adults, particularly women, model healthy eating attitudes and behaviors. The following guidelines are adapted from BodyWise and Bodyworks, which are initiatives of the US Department of Health and Human Services Office on Women's Health (56).

- Assist children in attaining a positive relationship with food. Serve and eat a variety of foods and balanced meals, plan meals in advance, and keep healthy snacks available. Skipping meals should be discouraged, and food should not be used as a reward.
- Help children learn control of their own eating behaviors. Avoid forcing food on children and adolescents (including cleaning the plate) and avoid forbidding or restricting certain foods. Studies show that when mothers restrict their children's food, the children tend to eat more when unsupervised (57). Encourage eating until satisfied, and discourage eating outside of hunger.
- Encourage family meals and eating breakfast. Eating meals as a family has emerged as a possible buffer against the development of eating disorders in adolescent girls (33). Likewise, breakfast-eating may also play a role in preventing the development of eating problems (58) and improving dietary quality and physical activity among adolescents (59).
- Be aware of children's emotional health. Depression, anxiety, and the use of food to cope with emotional states may signal both the need for intervention and increased risk for disordered eating patterns.

- Provide opportunities for children to participate in a variety of physical activities, including sporting activities, dancing, hiking, swimming, and anything that is enjoyable and gets them moving. Encourage both a wide range of activities and mindful physical activity choices (eg, stairs vs elevator). Parents and other adults and older siblings should model increased activity so that it is a natural part of the environment. At the same time, exposure and opportunity for sedentary activities, such as computer use and television-viewing, should be limited.

- Discuss unrealistic media messages about females' bodies as well as the mixed messages conveyed in the media. It is important to discuss how media images are manipulated by computers and airbrushing and how they are not real images of real females. Create a positive focus on health and health-promoting behaviors and activities to build and foster self-esteem. It may be particularly important to address the internalized aesthetic standards that produce faulty weight-related expectations, to resist the social pressure to achieve an "ideal" body, to adopt non-derogatory self-statements about large body size, and to uncouple the association between body weight and self-esteem (60).

References

1. Bouchard C, Rankinen T. Exciting advances and new opportunities. In: Clement K, Sorensen T (eds). *Obesity: Genomics and Postgenomics.* New York, NY: Informa Healthcare; 2008. 549–562.

2. Hill JO, Wyatt HR, Melanson EL. Genetic and environmental contributions to obesity. *Med Clin North Am.* 2000;84:333–346.

3. James WP. A public health approach to the problem of obesity. Int J Obes. 1995;19(suppl 3):S37–S45.

4. US Department of Health and Human Services, Centers for Disease Control and Prevention. Vital and Health Statistics Summary. Health Statistics for US Adults: National Health Interview Survey, 2009. US Department of Health and Human Services, Centers for Disease Control and Prevention. 2010. www.cdc.gov/nchs/data/series/sr_10/sr1_249.pdf. Accessed March 31, 2011.

5. Plaza C. School nutrition & physical education legislation: An overview of 2005 state activity. Robert Wood Johnson Foundation Web site. www.rwjf.org/files/research/ NCSL%20-%20April%202005%20Quarterly%20Report.pdf. Accessed March 31, 2011.

6. Lee SM, Burgeson CR, Fulton JE, Spain CG. Physical education and physical activity: Results from the School Health Policies and Programs Study 2006. *J Sch Health.* 2007;77:435–463.

7. Battle EK, Brownell KD. Confronting a rising tide of eating disorders and obesity: Treatment vs prevention and policy. *Addict Behav.* 1996;21:755–765.

8. Kant AK. Consumption of energy-dense, nutrient-poor foods by adult Americans: Nutritional and health implications. The Third National Health and Nutrition Examination Survey, 1988–1994. *Am J Clin Nutr.* 2000;72:929–936.

9. Fuhrman J, Sarter B, Glaser D, Acocella S. Changing perceptions of hunger on a high nutrient density diet. *Nutr J.* 2010;9:51.

10. Nielsen SJ, Popkin BM. Changes in beverage intake between 1977 and 2001. *Am J Prev Med.* 2004;27:205–210.

11. Ludwig DS, Peterson KE, Gortmaker SL. Relations between consumption of sugar-sweetened drinks and childhood obesity. *Lancet.* 2001;357:505–508.

12. French SA, Harnack L, Jeffery RW. Fast food restaurant use among women in the Pound of Prevention study: Dietary, behavioral and demographic correlates. *Int J Obes.* 2000;24:1353–1359.

13. Binkley JK, Eales J, Jekanowski M. The relation between dietary change and rising U.S. obesity. *Int J Obes.* 2000;24:1032–1039.

14. McCrory MA, Fuss PJ, Hays NP, Vinken AG, Greenberg AS, Roberts SB. Overeating in America: Association between restaurant food consumption and body fatness in healthy adult men and women ages 19 to 80. *Obes Res.* 1999;7:564–571.

15. Pereira M, Kartashov AI, Ebbeling CB, Van Horn L, Slattery ML, Jacobs Jr. M, Ludwig DS. Fast-food habits, weight gain, and insulin resistance (The CARDIA Study): 15-year prospective analysis. *Lancet.* 2005;365:36–42.

16. Brownell K. The environment and obesity. In: Fairburn CG, Brownell KD, eds. *Eating Disorders and Obesity,* 2nd ed. New York, NY: Guilford Press; 2002:433–438.

17. Harris JL, Bargh JA, Brownell KD. Priming effects of television food advertising on eating behavior. *Health Psychol.* 2009;28:404–413.

18. Bouchard C. The biological predisposition to obesity: Beyond the thrifty gene scenario [commentary]. *Int J Obes.* 2007;31:1337–1339.

19. Levine M, Harrison K. Media's role in the perpetuation and prevention of negative body image and disordered eating. In: Thompson JK, ed. *Handbook of Eating Disorders and Obesity.* Hoboken, NJ: John Wiley & Sons, Inc; 2004:695–717.

20. Stice E, Schupak-Neuberg E, Shaw H, Stein RI. Relation of media exposure to eating disorder symptomatology: An examination of mediating mechanisms. *J Abnorm Psychol.* 1994;103:836–840.

21. Kilbourne J. *Deadly Persuasion: Why Women Must Fight the Addictive Power of Advertising.* New York, NY: Free Press, 1999.

22. Bulik CM. Genetic and biological risk factors. In: Thompson JK, ed. *Handbook of Eating Disorders and Obesity.* Hoboken, NJ: John Wiley & Sons, Inc; 2004:3–16.

23. Vaughan K, Fouts G. Changes in television and magazine exposure and eating disorder symptomatology. *Sex Roles.* 2003;49:313–320.

24. Derenne, JL, Eugene V. Beresin, EV. Body Image, Media, and Eating Disorders. *Acad Psychiatry.* 2006;30:257–261.

25. Stunkard AJ, Sobal J. Psychosocial consequences of obesity. In: Brownell KD, Fairburn CG, eds. *Eating Disorders and Obesity: A Comprehensive Handbook.* New York, NY: Guilford Press; 1995:417–421.

26. Crandall CS, Biernat M. The ideology of antifat attitudes. *J Appl Soc Psychol.* 1990;20:227–243.

27. Rand CS, Macgregor AM. Morbidly obese patients' perceptions of social discrimination before and after surgery for obesity. *South Med J.* 1990;83:1390–1395.

28. Wade T, Gillespie N, Martin NG. A comparison of early family life events amongst monozygotic twin women with lifetime anorexia nervosa, bulimia nervosa, or major depression. *Int J Eat Disord.* 2007;40:679–686.

29. Fairburn C, Doll HA, Welch SL, Hay PJ, Davies BA, O'Connor ME. Risk factors for binge-eatingdisorder: A community-based, case-control study. *Arch Gen Psychiatry.* 1998;55:425–432.

30. Hill AJ. Prevalence and demographics of dieting. In: Fairburn CG, Brownell KD eds. *Eating Disorders and Obesity,* 2nd ed. New York, NY: Guilford Press; 2002:80–83.

31. Field AE, Austin SB, Taylor CB, Malspeis S, Rosner B, Rockett HR, Gillman MW, Colditz GA. Relation between dieting and weight change among preadolescents and adolescents. *Pediatrics.* 2003;112:900–906.

32. Stice E, Cameron RP, Killen JD, Hayward C, Taylor CB. Naturalistic weight-reduction efforts prospectively predict growth in relative weight and onset of obesity among female adolescents. *Consult Clin Psychol.* 1999;67:967–974.

33. Neumark-Sztainer D, Eisenberg ME, Fulkerson JA, Story M, Larson NI. Family meals and disordered eating in adolescents: Longitudinal findings from project EAT. *Arch Pediatr Adolesc Med.* 2008;162:17–22.

34. Flegal KM, Carroll MD, Ogden CL, Curtin LR. Prevalence and trends in obesity among US adults, 1999–2008. *JAMA.* 2010;303:235–241.

35. Bjorvell H, Ronnberg S, Rosner S. Eating patterns described by a group of treatment seeking overweight women and normal weight women. *Scand J Behav Trier.* 1985;14:147–156.

36. Gearhardt AN, Corbin WR, Brownell KB. Preliminary validation of the Yale Food Addiction Questionnaire. *Appetite.* 2008;52:430–436.

37. Corsica JA, Pelchat ML. Food addiction: True or false? *Curr Opin Gastroenterol.* 2010;26:165–169.

38. Avena NM, Rada P, Hoebel BG. Evidence for sugar addiction: Behavioral and neurochemical effects of intermittent, excessive sugar intake. *Neurosci Biobehav Rev.* 2008;32:20–29.

39. Passamonti L, Rowe JB, Schwarzbauer C, Ewbank MP, von dem Hagen E, Calder AJ. Personality predicts the brains response to viewing appetizing foods: The neural basis of a risk factor for overeating. *J Neurosci.* 2009;29:43–51.

40. Borzekowski DL, Bayer AM. Body image and media use among adolescents. *Adolesc Med.* 2005;16:289–313.

41. Field AE, Carmargo, CA, Taylor, CB. Peer, parent, and media influences on the development and frequent dieting among preadolescent and adolescent girls and boys. *Pediatrics.* 2001;107:54–60.

42. Neumark-Sztainer D, Wall, M, Larson, NI, Eisenberg, ME, Loth, K. Dieting and disordered eating behaviors from adolescence to young adulthood: Findings from a 10-year longitudinal study. *J Am Diet Assoc.* 2011;111:1004–1011.

43. Mitchell JE, Mussell MP, Peterson CB, Crow S, Wonderlich SA, Crosby RD, Davis T, Weller C. Hedonics of binge eating in women with bulimia nervosa and binge eating disorder. *Int J Eat Disord.* 1999;26:165–170.

44. Wilfley DE, Schwartz MB, Spurrell EB, Fairburn CG. Using the eating disorder examination to identify the specific psychopathology of binge eating disorder. *Int J Eat Disord.* 2000;27:259–269.

45. Lamerz A, Kuepper-Nybelen J, Bruning N, Wehle C, Trost-Brinkhues G, Brenner H, Hebebrand J, Herpertz-Dahlmann B. Prevalence of obesity, binge eating, and night eating in a cross-sectional field survey of 6-year-old children and their parents in a German urban population. *J Child Psychol Psychiatry.* 2005;46:385–393.

46. Marcus MD, Kalarchian MA. Binge eating in children and adolescents. *Int J Eat Disord.* 2003;34(suppl 1):S47–S57.

47. Brownell K. The humbling experience of treating obesity: Should we persist or desist? *Behav Res Ther.* 2010;48:717–719.

48. Baranowski T, Cullen KW, Nicklas T, Thompson D, Baranowski J. School-based obesity prevention: A blueprint for taming the epidemic. *Am J Health Behav.* 2002;26:486–493.

49. Doak CM, Visscher TM, Renders CL, Seidell J. The prevention of overweight and obesity in children and adolescents: A review of interventions and programmes. *Obes Rev.* 2006;7:111–136.

50. Kropski JA, Keckley PH, Jensen GL. School-based obesity prevention programs: An evidence-based review. *Obesity.* 2008;16:1009–1018.

51. Stice E, Shaw H, Marti CN. A meta-analytic review of obesity prevention programs for children and adolescents: The skinny on interventions that work. *Psychol Bull.* 2006;132:667–691.

52. Corsica JA, Perri MG. Obesity. In: Nezu A. ed. *Handbook of Psychology.* Vol 9. 2nd ed. Hoboken, NJ: John Wiley & Sons, Inc. In press.

53. Brownell KD. Get slim with higher taxes. *The New York Times.* Dec 15, 1994;A29.

54. Jacobson MF, Brownell KD. Small taxes on soft drinks and snack foods to promote health. *Am J Public Health.* 2000;90:854–857.

55. Center for Science in the Public Interest. Taxing sugared beverages would help trim state budget deficits, consumers' bulging waistlines, and health care costs. Center for Science in the Public Interest Web site. www.cspinet.org/new/pdf/state_budget_report_-_sugar_tax.pdf. 2010. Accessed March 31, 2011.

56. US Department of Health and Human Services Office on Women's Health. US Department of Health and Human Services Web site. www.4woman.gov. Accessed March 15, 2011.

57. Birch L. Acquisition of food preferences and eating patterns in children. In: Fairburn CG, Brownell, KD eds. *Eating Disorders and Obesity,* 2nd ed. New York, NY: Guilford Press; 2002:75–79.

58. Fernández-Aranda F, Krug I, Granero R, Ramon JM, Badia A, Giménez L, Solano R, Collier D, Karwautz A, Treasure J. Individual and family eating patterns during childhood and early adolescence: An analysis of associated eating disorder factors. *Appetite.* 2007;49:476–485.

59. Timlin M, Pereira MA, Story M, Neumark-Sztainer D. Breakfast eating and weight change in a 5-year prospective analysis of adolescents: Project EAT (Eating Among Teens). *Pediatrics.* 2008;121:e638–e645.

60. Foster GD, Kendall PC. The realistic treatment of obesity: Changing the scales of success. *Clin Psychol Rev.* 1994;14:701–736.

Critical Thinking

1. Describe the obesogenic environment in the United States.

2. Explain how negative stigmas and prevalence of negative messages regarding obesity can potentiate the development of eating disorders.

2. List five ways adults can address the impact of the obesogenic environment on the development of eating disorders.

J. A. CORSICA AND M. M. HOOD are assistant professors, Rush University Medical Center, Chicago, IL.

UNIT 6

Health Claims

Unit Selections

Learning Outcomes

After reading this Unit, you will be able to:

- Defend the claim that chocolate is good for the heart and cardiovascular system.

- Identify the three flavanols (phytochemicals) found in chocolate.

- Compare the effects of the dietary substances that are touted to increase brain function.

- Discuss the challenges of evaluating the "brain-boosting power" of dietary substances.

- List the nutrients that are required to be included on the Nutrition Facts panel.

- Contrast the types of health claims that can be published on product labels: nutrient content claims and structure/function claims.

- Identify the form of omega-3 fatty acid found in flax.

- Explain why fish oil is considered the more potent source omega-3 fatty acids compared to flax oil.

- List the beneficial characteristics of flax, other than containing omega-3 fatty acids.

Student Website
www.mhhe.com/cls

Internet References

Federal Trade Commission (FTC): Diet, Health & Fitness
www.ftc.gov/bcp/menus/consumer/health.shtm
Food and Drug Administration (FDA)
www.fda.gov/default.htm
National Council against Health Fraud (NCAHF)
www.ncahf.org
Office of Dietary Supplements: Health Information
http://ods.od.nih.gov/Health_Information/Health_Information.aspx
QuackWatch
www.quackwatch.com

Technological advances in the 21st century have resulted in high-speed communication of scientific results and the possibility for miscommunication. Even if the scientific protocol, study, design, data collection, and analysis are impeccable, it is still possible to report the findings in a confusing and biased manner. According to an American Dietetic Association (ADA) survey, 90 percent of consumers polled get their nutrition information from television, magazines, and newspapers.

Some Americans are so confused and overwhelmed by the controversies surrounding food and health that they have stopped paying attention to the contradictory claims reported by news media. The media very frequently misinterpret results, simplify the message, and do not provide the proper context to accurately interpret the information. In addition, the media are eager to publish sensational information and not wait for evidence to be evaluated for validity and reliability.

One of the most popular health messages that has not been missed by many is that chocolate is good for your heart. The research refers to dark chocolate with high cocoa content and lower saturated fat than the milk chocolate that is so plentiful. The article by Hara Estroff Marano summarizes the research that supports chocolate as a heart healthy brain food and also provides a brief, interesting history of chocolate as a health food.

A topic of current interest with many touted health claims is omega-3 fatty acids and the best source for these beneficial fats. Demand for supplements and fortified foods containing omega-3s has culminated in a vast number of products on the market. Since the metabolic pathways of these PUFAs are complex, there is a great deal of confusion when it comes to information presented on the label and in the media. "Brain Boosters," by Janet Raloff, provides advice on how to intelligently interpret the claims about nutritional supplements touted to enhance brain function. Flax meal, flax seeds, and flax oil are all products derived from flax, which has been reported to lower heart disease risk, reduce inflammation, diabetes, depression, and anxiety among other health benefits. Consumers are increasingly interested in purchasing and using flax for its health-promoting properties. "The Benefits of Flax" from *Consumer Reports on Health* discusses the difference between omega-3s from flax seed oil versus fish oil.

Interest in nutrition's impact on brain function and energy level is growing. Because of this, there are many dietary

© ULTRA.F/Getty Images

supplements on the market that supposedly improve cognitive function and provide energy. One of the articles in this unit provides information on foods, food components, and other products that are thought to improve mental performance and energy level. Caffeine, caffeine derivatives, glucose, ginkgo biloba, Chinese ginseng, and cocoa flavanols are on the "mental menu" as improving brain function in the article by Janet Raloff.

Articles in this unit were selected based on the common interests in the topics. Our society is inundated with health claims of foods and dietary supplements. People want an easy fix and the next greatest product that will make them healthy without all the troublesome work of diet and physical activity. The articles in Unit 6 provide a few items of good news as well as practical information about product labeling.

The Scoop on Chocolate

Is chocolate really healthy?

HARA ESTROFF MARANO

The cocoa bean formally belongs to the genus *Theobroma,* or food of the gods. Not many mortals would disagree. And science now rewards their taste. Researchers are finding that consumption of cocoa-rich chocolate, loaded with classy antioxidants, offers a growing array of benefits to brain and body. Most surprising is that, when processed to preserve its fullest complement of natural antioxidants, cocoa may have therapeutic benefits against cardiovascular ills that take a special toll on the aging brain.

Native to South America, the bean of *Theobroma cacao* was ground and consumed as a warm beverage 2,000 years ago by Mayans and, later, by the Aztecs, who called it "bitter water." Columbus was the first European to sample the beverage, often spiced with pepper, but it was only after Cortes conquered the Aztecs that it became a prized drink in Spain, despite the fact that the hot and spicy drink was considered morally dangerous. Mixing it with milk and sugar made it more palatable to Europeans.

Long before chocolate was transformed into a dessert, it was valued for promoting health. Cortes wrote to King Carlos I of Spain that he had found a "drink that builds up resistance and fights fatigue" and brought tons of beans back with him. When Thomas Jefferson got his first sip in France, he wrote John Adams: "The superiority of chocolate, both for health and nourishment, will soon give it the same preference over tea and coffee in America which it has in Spain." European doctors recommended cacao for angina, respiratory problems, dysentery, indigestion, weakness, gout, liver and kidney disease, and general revitalization.

Long before chocolate was transformed into a dessert, it was valued for promoting health.

Cacao begins its transcendence into chocolate with fermentation after harvesting. The large, rugby-ball-shaped fruit of *Theobroma* contain about 40 cocoa beans embedded in a sticky, white pulp. The beans are scooped out and placed in trays for open-air fermentation, during which the pulp sugars alter the chemical composition of the bitter beans. Then the beans are dried, typically outdoors. An average tree produces 30 viable pods a year—yielding two pounds of chocolate.

Shipped off to factories, the dried beans undergo roasting for flavor development—at high temperatures for a short time, which boosts chocolate flavor, or lower temperatures for a longer time, believed to preserve more subtle flavors and more of the antioxidants. Then they are ground.

The resulting chocolate liquor may—with the variable addition of sugar, vanilla, and powdered milk—head straight for molding into chocolate bars or undergo pressing to separate the fatty cocoa butter from the cocoa solids, which are pulverized into cocoa powder. The cocoa butter—about a third of which is oleic acid, the same fat found in olive oil—is typically mixed back into chocolate as it later undergoes kneading and hot-and-cold tempering to further develop flavor and impart gloss. Cocoa butter also contains saturated fats, primarily stearic acid, which does not raise cholesterol levels.

During processing, cocoa beans may be washed to neutralize acids and decrease bitterness. Such so-called Dutch processing darkens the cocoa but halves its naturally high antioxidant level.

Cocoa and cocoa-laden dark chocolate have been identified as rich sources of antioxidants known as flavanols. Cocoa has more cardioprotective proanthocyanidins than blueberries, more brain-saving catechins than green tea, more heart-healthy phenols than red wine. Two tablespoons of cocoa have more antioxidants than four cups of green tea.

For over two decades, chocolate has been linked to protecting the cardiovascular system, and especially to lowering blood pressure, shielding the brain from stroke and the heart from overwork.

Researchers at Johns Hopkins have shown that a few squares of chocolate—the equivalent of two tablespoons of dark cocoa—can halve the risk of heart attack by decreasing the tendency of blood platelets to clot. The effect is similar to that of aspirin. Italian investigators have found that a small square of chocolate two or three times a week reduces levels of C-reactive protein, an inflammatory substance that is a risk factor for heart attack and stroke.

How to Choose [and Eat] Your Treat

What makes chocolate so appealing to you and me is what excites scientists about the health value of chocolate: People don't have to retrain habits to partake of the merits. They just have to make sure to buy a cocoa-rich version, but not too much. A square of dark chocolate a day will do it. More promotes weight gain, which offsets cardiovascular benefits. And the milk in milk chocolate interferes with antioxidant absorption.

The finest cocoa beans come from the tropics of Madagascar and the Americas, but Africa is the bulk producer; the single largest supplier of cocoa is the Ivory Coast.

Look for a product with the highest cocoa content (above 70 percent) and the fewest other ingredients. The best chocolate, says Jacques Torres, renowned New York chocolatier, contains only cocoa, sugar, cocoa butter, and lecithin, an emulsifier.

In a German study, a mere 30 calories worth of dark chocolate significantly lowered both systolic and diastolic blood pressure in middle-age and older men and women—without adding weight. Prevalence of hypertension dropped from 86 to 68 percent over 18 weeks of chocolate-eating, which, by boosting flavanols in blood, stimulated production of arterial nitric oxide, a compound known to relax blood vessels and increase blood flow through them (it's the source of Viagra's power). Swedish researchers have found that dark chocolate also biochemically mimics the first-choice drugs for hypertension by inhibiting the ACE enzyme known to raise blood pressure.

A German study that followed nearly 20,000 men and women age 35 to 65 for 10 years observed a 39 percent decrease in risk of stroke and heart attack among those who ate a small square of chocolate daily. Canadian researchers determined that eating 50 grams of dark chocolate a week markedly reduces the risk of death in those who have already suffered a stroke. What's more, chocolate seems to protect against heart failure and to lower the risk of death among those already diagnosed with the condition.

By increasing blood flow to the brain, chocolate also significantly protects against cognitive decline among those over 60, a separate study found. And Oxford University researchers who tested older chocolate eaters confirmed that they perform significantly better on a range of cognitive tests than those who do not partake.

But chocolate's benefits are not limited to any age group. "If you're going to have a treat," says Murray Mittelman, who directs a cardiovascular research unit at Harvard, "dark chocolate is probably a good choice, as long as it's in moderation."

Critical Thinking

1. Describe the processing of cocoa beans.

2. Why does "Dutch chocolate" have half of the antioxidant content?

3. Name the three flavanols (phytochemicals) found in chocolate.

4. Discuss how chocolate is good for the heart and cardiovascular system.

From *Psychology Today*, March/April 2011, pp. 44–45. Copyright © 2011 by Sussex Publishers, LLC. Reprinted by permission.

The Benefits of Flax

Flax products have been popping up all over grocery-store shelves lately, with claims such as "special protection for women's health" and "fights the blues." Here's our take on the seed's potential benefits, as well as some advice on how to incorporate it into your diet.

As Good as Fish Oil?

Flax products come in three forms: supplements, oil, and the seed itself. All of those, like fish oil, contain omega-3 fatty acids. In fish oil, those substances protect the heart in several ways, notably thinning the blood and lowering levels of LDL (bad) cholesterol and triglycerides. Moreover, those fatty acids might offer other health benefits, including protection against mild depression, Alzheimer's disease, and macular degeneration.

But it's unclear if the fatty acids in flax, which come in the form of alpha-linolenic acid (ALA), provide the same benefits. That's because the body has to convert ALA into the two fatty acids, eicosapentaenoic acid (EPA) and docosahexaenoic acid (DHA), found in fish oil. And to get meaningful amounts of those compounds you may have to consume lots of flax, according to a September 2008 study in the American Journal of Clinical Nutrition. It found that even large doses of flax oil—four to six 600-milligram capsules—boosted blood levels of EPA by only about 35 percent and had no effect on DHA.

Benefits Beyond the Heart

Still, flax oil might provide at least some coronary protection. And flaxseeds, especially crushed or ground, may offer certain benefits that fish oil does not. For example, they are rich sources of lignans, compounds that alter the way the body handles estrogen. That may explain why preliminary research hints that flaxseed can lower the risk of breast cancer. And one small study of women with mild menopausal symptoms found that about 3 tablespoons of flaxseed a day eased their hot flashes and night sweats as effectively as supplemental estrogen. Finally, the seeds contain lots of fiber, protein, magnesium, and thiamin.

How to Get more into Your Diet

- Add a tablespoon of crushed or ground flaxseed to your hot or cold breakfast cereal or yogurt.
- Add a teaspoon of crushed or ground flaxseed to mayonnaise or mustard when making a sandwich.
- Use crushed or ground flaxseed in place of eggs in baking. Mix 1 tablespoon with 3 tablespoons of water as a substitute for 1 large egg, and let it sit for a few minutes. Note that this will change the texture of the food.
- Look for products that contain flax, including cereals, granola bars, and breads.

Recommendation

Flax-oil supplements might be worth a try for people who want some of the benefits of fish oil but don't like the taste of fish or fish-oil pills, or avoid fish because they're vegetarians. But the supplements aren't good for people who can't take fish oil for safety reasons, because they may interact with the same blood-thinning drugs. And women with a history of breast, ovarian, or uterine cancers, as well as endometriosis or fibroids, should talk with their doctor before consuming flaxseeds because of their possible effect on estrogen. But most other people can safely add flaxseed to their diet.

Critical Thinking

1. Define alpha-linolenic acid (ALA), eicospentaenoic acid (EPA), and docosahexaenoic acid (DHA).

2. Explain why fish oil is considered the more potent source of omega-3 fatty acids compared to flax oil.

3. Describe the beneficial characteristics of flax, other than containing omega-3 fatty acids.

Brain Boosters

Some Nutritional Supplements Provide Real Food for Thought

JANET RALOFF

On his third consecutive evening of air combat, a military pilot closes in on the night's quarry, a suspected Taliban fuel depot in Afghanistan. Fatigued, his alertness flagging, the pilot throws some chewing gum into his mouth. Laced with caffeine, it's the cockpit alternative to a cup of coffee.

This pilot would probably suspect that the gum is just a perk-me-up. But several caffeinated military rations—including this relatively new one—do more than stave off sleepiness. Emerging data indicate that these rations boost not only attention but also cognitive performance, features that do not necessarily climb in lockstep.

The U.S. Department of Defense has been investigating such supplements to improve the ability of U.S. armed forces to maintain sustained periods of intense vigilance and focus, explains Harris Lieberman, a psychologist at the Army Research Institute of Environmental Medicine in Natick, Mass. Another hope, he notes: These dietary aids might minimize the risk of "friendly fire."

Army researchers at the institute, including Lieberman, are at the forefront of a small but growing cadre of investigators exploring how to boost what they call mental energy. This rather fuzzy phrase embraces wakefulness, but also includes mood, motivation and the capacity to perform key mental tasks.

Increasing mental energy is important for those enervated because of a lack of sleep or for those whose jobs, like those of fighter pilots, require vigilance even in the face of sleep deprivation. Compounds that keep you awake, it turns out, can also boost other aspects of mental performance. Improved cognition is emerging as a quantifiable side benefit of many of these substances—in some cases, even for those folks who aren't sleepy to begin with.

But the data can be hard to interpret, primarily because no test exists to directly measure mental energy, explains Patrick O'Connor of the University of Georgia in Athens. It must be inferred from other indicators. Still, it is fair to view fatigue and mental energy as anchoring opposite poles of a common spectrum, he says.

Similarly, caffeine anchors the stimulatory end of a spectrum of natural products exhibiting promise in hiking or sustaining cognitive aspects of mental energy. Others include L-theanine in tea, guarana, cocoa constituents and ginseng.

Learning how these compounds work, at what doses and under what circumstances, is important, argues O'Connor, because "mental energy underlies everything in our lives." It's key, he says, to achieving goals at home and work—and even to the success of the economy.

Perky Brews

More data has emerged on caffeine's role in promoting mental energy than on any other dietary constituent. The stimulant blocks the activity of adenosine, a molecule that slows heart rate and induces drowsiness. Caffeine perks people up, Lieberman says, "by blocking something that normally slows you down."

At the Experimental Biology 2010 meeting in April in Anaheim, Calif., he described how, some 25 years ago, his team found that as little as 32 milligrams of caffeine—equivalent to what's in a 12-ounce can of cola or less than a cup of regular coffee—improved attentiveness for auditory and visual cues.

People had thought that any improved performance from caffeine might be limited to people who were tired. Here, though, the young men in the study were well rested, suggesting broader benefits.

Lieberman's more recent work has tested caffeine's effects on tasks especially relevant to the military. For instance, a study conducted during the training of 68 Navy SEALs assayed the effects of caffeine after 72 hours of sleep deprivation and round-the-clock exposure to cold and other stressors. The men were taking part in a weeklong test of endurance known as Hell Week.

Not surprisingly, the exhausted trainees didn't do nearly as well on tests of vigilance and other measures of cognitive performance three days into Hell Week as they had before the training marathon began. But those who got between 100 and

300 milligrams of caffeine an hour before a battery of mental tests made fewer mistakes and responded more quickly.

One task asked SEALs to scan for faint images that appeared for a couple of seconds on a computer monitor. Trainees who got no caffeine scored an average of 7.9 correct hits out of 20, while those given caffeine averaged between 10.6 and 12.2 correct responses. Caffeine recipients also had nearly 30 percent shorter response times. Scores on several other tasks, including a test of marksmanship, were unaffected.

Other scientists have been exploring caffeine's impacts on the brain. Andrew Smith of Cardiff University in Wales, for instance, asked 118 students to watch a computer screen where three-digit numbers appeared at a rate of 100 per minute. When two consecutive numbers matched, participants were to note it with a keystroke. Before the tests, 84 students were given chewing gum; roughly half (41) got gum laced with 40 milligrams of caffeine.

Students reported feeling substantially more alert after chewing the caffeinated gum. They also performed better on some tests, including the one in which they had to identify repeated numbers. Those given caffeine were 4.4 percent faster than those who worked gum-free and 4 percent faster than non-caffeinated-gum chewers. The stimulant also appeared to speed up people's ability to learn new information, Smith reported in the April 2009 *Human Psychopharmacology*.

Tea's Bonus

Tea, which people worldwide drink more of than any other beverage except water, is a major dietary source of caffeine. Unlike coffee, it contains another potentially powerful ingredient for brain activity: L-theanine, an amino acid that can alter alpha brain wave rhythms, inducing wakeful relaxation.

In 2008 in *Nutrition Reviews,* Janet Bryan of the University of South Australia in Adelaide observed that alpha wave activity has been linked to "increased performance under stress and improved learning and concentration" and reduced anxiety. L-theanine seems to enhance caffeine's mental benefits, she noted.

Unilever, which owns Lipton, is actively investigating L-theanine's effects. Neither caffeine nor tea's caffeine-theanine combo augment performance on all types of mental tests, says Eveline De Bruin, a cognitive neuroscientist with Unilever's R&D facility in Vlaardingen, the Netherlands. The biggest impacts, she says, are in enhancing what's known as executive function—the ability to perform complex tasks that rely on planning or decision making.

For instance, in an upcoming issue of *Appetite,* De Bruin's team reports that tea brings boosts in executive function that increase with dose. On each day of a two-day study, 26 volunteers drank either strong tea or a tealike placebo before testing. One test asked participants to listen to rules on how to respond to sounds or images on a computer screen—and the rules changed every few seconds during each five-minute session. The men and women responded correctly in the auditory test almost twice as often (around 15 to 20 percent of the time versus 8 or 9 percent) after drinking tea rather than the placebo.

Participants were also marginally—but reliably—more accurate after tea on a test that looked at the ability to plan and execute decisions.

While Unilever has demonstrated that tea enriched with triple the normal amount of L-theanine improves attention, De Bruin says Lipton has no plans to market such a product. "It is an interesting idea," she concedes, "but at present Lipton is proud of producing an all-natural leaf-tea product that is unmodified yet capable of noticeably improving attention and alertness."

Sweet Paradox

Thinking, calculating, planning, learning, remembering—such mental tasks consume plenty of energy. Because glucose, better known as blood sugar, fuels body and brain, it might seem that a good dose of something sweet would be just what Mother Nature ordered to kick-start your neural hardware. Yet people with diabetes and high blood sugar levels can suffer from cognitive impairments.

Studies have begun probing this seeming contradiction. Two papers in August in *Psychopharmacology,* for instance, report a boost in mental performance when healthy people down a drink fortified with at least 50 grams of glucose (about 10 teaspoons worth) following a 12-hour overnight fast.

Christine Gagnon of the University of Quebec at Montreal and colleagues showed that in 44 people age 60 and up, drinking the glucose 15 minutes before the start of testing led to better scores on some tests than did the sugar-free alternative. Those on a sugar rush performed faster and accrued fewer errors when asked to quickly read a color name or name the color of words (even if a color word, such as *green,* appeared in a different color, say red). Glucose appeared especially beneficial in tasks that required switching and dividing attention, the researchers observed.

Among 90 undergrads, a sugary drink improved immediate recall of words, not faces, compared with a sugar-free one, reported a team led by Lauren Owen of the Brain Sciences Institute at the Swinburne University of Technology in Melbourne, Australia. Recall of large numbers that had appeared in earlier math calculations also improved.

Doses given in each study were high and would be ill-advised for people with trouble controlling their blood sugar, such as those with diabetes or metabolic syndrome. But David Benton of Swansea University in Wales has shown there may be a way to get the benefits of a glucose burst without overdoing sugary drinks. At the experimental biology meeting, he presented data indicating that for mental performance, it's actually better to deliver glucose parsimoniously. He does it by giving subjects foods containing carbohydrates that digest slowly.

In an early study, Benton's team gave cereals, breakfast bars or biscuits with roughly equal calories to 106 undergraduate women. The main difference between the meals was their glycemic index—how quickly the carbs break down into glucose.

Thirty minutes later and at regular intervals thereafter, the women took memory tests. Those who got the low-glycemic breakfast performed progressively better than those eating the rapidly digested meals. The difference was most dramatic for a later testing, 3.5 hours after breakfast, Benton says.

His group ran a similar test in rats, feeding them either quickly or slowly digested carbs. The rodents exhibited a similar improvement in learning when they got the slowly digested chow.

In a follow-up test, Benton's group administered breakfast to kids in an elementary school class for four weeks. Kids got a meal with high-glycemic carbs on one-third of the days, low-glycemic foods on another third, and carbs that broke down at an intermediate rate on the remaining days.

On various days throughout the trial, hidden cameras recorded the 19 children while they were supposed to be working independently on a reading or math assignment. The behavior of each child was recorded over a 30-minute period and scientists later logged what the youngster had been doing: working, looking around the room, talking to others, fidgeting, acting out or moving around the room. On days when the kids had eaten the low-glycemic breakfast, they were much more likely to remain on task—26 percent of the time versus 18 percent or less on the other days.

The kids also took simple memory tests and played with a video game that was rigged to be frustratingly difficult to master. On days they had eaten the slow-to-digest breakfast, kids exhibited more initial patience with the game. Their recall was also better—"about 10 percent better," Benton says. It's a small difference, he acknowledges. "But if your child came home with 10 percent better scores on a test, would it matter to you? Most parents would say yes."

Herbal Therapies

Tea and coffee aren't the only natural stimulant-laced plant extracts to show energizing as well as brain-boosting attributes. There's also guarana. Seeds of this Amazonian plant are an especially potent source of caffeine, which can constitute 5 percent of dried extracts. But guarana may have more than caffeine going for it.

At the experimental biology meeting, David Kennedy of Northumbria University in Newcastle upon Tyne, England, described cognitive benefits in young adults given small amounts of guarana—more benefits than when those volunteers received high doses. Indeed, Kennedy noted, guarana amounts needed to boost test scores and mood contained just 4 to 9 milligrams of caffeine. "That's only about a tenth as much as you'd find in a cup of coffee," Kennedy points out. "So guarana was doing something that wasn't attributable to its caffeine"—although his team doesn't yet know what.

He and colleagues have also been investigating other natural products that might elevate energy, attention and mental performance. Among these: Chinese ginseng (*Panax ginseng*). Young adults scored better on a battery of mental tests—including serial subtraction of numbers in their heads—and exhibited less mental fatigue after getting this herbal supplement rather than a placebo.

How Chinese ginseng may improve performance is unknown, but Kennedy suspects the effect might have to do with ginseng's ability to moderate blood sugar levels. At least at the 200-milligram dose used by his group, this supplement caused a drop in blood-glucose levels one hour after consumption.

On the Mental Menu

Recent work suggests dietary substances such as caffeine and glucose may boost mental skills. Evidence for others ("Emerging substances") is preliminary.

Caffeine

Increases visual and auditory vigilance; speeds reaction times, improves accuracy and limits false positives on vigilance tasks; and increases learning and short-term memory on computer tests that require keystroke responses.

L-theanine

Increases speed and accuracy of pattern recognition that switches arbitrarily over time, increases relaxation, boosts accuracy of processing of rapidly delivered visual information and reduces susceptibility to distracting information during memory tests. May improve aspects of cognitive performance when delivered with caffeine, as in tea.

Glucose

Enhances memory of recent words or images, increases verbal fluency, improves pace of some types of serial subtraction, speeds decision times, enhances facial recognition and, among children, limits vulnerability to distraction when working alone.

Guarana

Increases alertness and the ability to recall words and images at a later point in time.

Emerging Substances

Ginkgo biloba

Improves pattern recognition and sustained attention, enhances delayed recall and memory of faces, and improves pace of serial subtraction and executive decision making.

Chinese ginseng

Enhances speed of recall, improves performance on simple arithmetic tasks and decreases false alarms on tests that require rapid processing of visual information.

Cocoa flavanols

Increase processing of rapid visual information and improve the ability to count backward (though have led to more errors in some serial subtractions).

— *Janet Raloff*

Researchers report that American ginseng (*P. quinquefolius*) also shows promise. Compared with a placebo, all doses improved some aspect of cognition, Swinburne's Andrew Scholey and colleagues report in October in *Psychopharmacology*. One difference: This herbal supplement had no effect on blood glucose.

The Northumbria researchers are also exploring the idea that some natural products bolster brain function by affecting blood flow. For instance, if they dilate vessels, the products might allow more fuel—glucose—in to power brain activities. Kennedy and colleagues tested the idea by giving 30 students a cup of cocoa on three mornings. Each day's formulation contained a different amount—46, 520 or 994 milligrams per serving—of cocoa flavanols, natural agents that have antioxidant and sometimes heart-healthy properties.

The cocoa packages used in the study were prepared by Mars, a candy company that has been exploring health attributes of some chocolate products.

Both higher-dose formulations, especially the middle one, improved performance during mentally challenging tests involving math and the visual processing of information, the scientists report. At the same time, the college students receiving the middle dose reported a reduction in mental fatigue. Maximum benefits showed up two hours into testing, which roughly corresponds to the expected peaks in concentrations of flavanols in the blood and in blood flow to the brain, Kennedy's team reported in the October *Journal of Psychopharmacology*.

Buyer Beware

The concept of mental energy is hardly new; recognition of it, on some level, dates back to Aristotle. But only during the last two decades has a steady trickle of studies begun quantifying how various dietary constituents battle fatigue and the fuzzy thinking that may accompany it.

The food industry has paid rapt attention to study findings (and, as is the case with Unilever and Mars, has even helped pay for some of the research). Indeed, O'Connor observes, hundreds of new products claim to boost mental energy. And their appeal is understandable since mental energy helps motivate people not only to work but also to stick with it when the going gets hard.

"Unfortunately," he adds, product claims "rarely are supported by compelling, unbiased scientific evidence."

Michael Falk and colleagues at the Life Sciences Research Organization in Bethesda, Md., recently conducted a major review of supplements and ingredients (other than caffeine) that purport to boost attentiveness and mental performance in people. The researchers identified 265 research reports in the scientific literature that met certain criteria.

Falk's team focused on 35 dietary constituents or factors, such as meal timing and the number of calories consumed. Promising data exist for ginkgo, ginseng, glucose and a few others, Falk says. But overall, his team concluded, for most "insufficient evidence is available to evaluate mental energy claims."

Hundreds of products claim to boost mental energy, but few claims are supported by evidence.

Much of the problem may reflect how the testing was conducted, he points out. For about three-fourths of the substances, there were no more than 10 qualifying studies; for more than half, there were five or fewer, the team reported in the December 2010 *Nutrition Reviews*. And for any given nutrient, Falk notes, different trials often applied different tests to assess mood, motivation and mental prowess—which made comparisons difficult.

Many of the reports also tested very different populations (young adults in some, the elderly in others), had different criteria for whether subjects were healthy, and failed to establish baseline measures of mood and mental proficiency before administering a potential brain booster. Further complicating the picture: "You're looking at what are relatively small effects and hard to measure," he says. "And these are against a background of high methodological and statistical noise." Such variations "undermine our ability to make strong conclusions."

But Falk suspects that may change fairly soon. Researchers have been investigating what to measure and how to do it. And they've determined that agents with promise don't always point to common benefits. Some may aid memory. Others may sharpen mental focus or speed up reaction times. Still others might make decision making easier.

When scientists begin standardizing tests, "I'm betting they'll come out with stronger, more narrowly focused and more [scientifically] supportable conclusions," Falk says. Findings that he says should point to whom these dietary supplements will benefit—and under which real-world conditions.

Explore More

H.E. Gorby, A.M. Brownawell and M.C. Falk. "Do specific dietary constituents and supplements affect mental energy? Review of the evidence." *Nutrition Reviews,* December 2010.

Critical Thinking

1. Identify the challenges of evaluating the "brain boosting power" of dietary substances.

2. Compare the effects of the dietary substances that are touted to increase brain function.

3. List the three factors that are commonly evaluated when considering brain function.

Influencing Food Choices
Nutrition Labeling, Health Claims, and Front-of-the-Package Labeling

For nearly 2 decades, nutrition labeling and health claims found on food packaged in the United States have supplied consumers with information based on a food's nutritional content and the potential health benefits from consuming the food. To further assist consumers in making food choices based on nutrient content, a number of organizations—professional and trade associations, grocery chains, and food manufacturers— have developed a variety of tools and labeling programs to supplement the Food and Drug Administration– regulated nutritional labeling effort. This article highlights Web resources that address nutritional labeling, health claims, in-store nutrition navigation, and several front-of-the-pack labeling programs.

KATHLEEN L. CAPPELLANO, MS, RD, LDN

Nutrition Labeling

The United States is one of 7 nations that require nutrition labeling on food packaging. The Nutrition Labeling and Education Act, signed into law in 1990, authorized the Food and Drug Administration (FDA) to require food manufacturers to include nutrition labeling in the form of a Nutrition Facts label on the packaging of most domestic and imported prepared foods. The law also requires that all nutrient content and health claims meet FDA regulations. Foods exempt from this requirement include meat, poultry, and eggs, which are regulated by the US Department of Agriculture, and alcoholic beverages containing more than 7% alcohol. The Nutrition Facts panel discloses the caloric, total fat, saturated and unsaturated fat, cholesterol, sodium, sugar, fiber, and carbohydrate content of the food. As of January 1, 2006, manufacturers are required to include the *trans*-fatty acid content per serving on the Nutrition Facts label.[1]

Food and Drug Administration

The FDA's website furnishes information about food labeling regulations, label claims, food allergens, and links to food labeling and packaging survey reports and to print resources such as its comprehensive Food Labeling Guide (www.fda.gov/Food/GuidanceComplianceRegulatory Information/GuidanceDocuments/FoodLabelingNutrition/ FoodLabelingGuide/default.htm).[2] By following the FDA's Nutrition Labeling Consumer Information link: www .fda.gov/Food/LabelingNutrition/ConsumerInformation/ default.htm, one can access pages that describe how to use the Nutrition Facts label (www.fda.gov/Food/Labeling Nutrition/ConsumerInformation/ucm078889.htm) and a description of *trans*-fat labeling in English (www.fda .gov/Food/LabelingNutrition/ConsumerInformation/ ucm109832.htm) and Spanish (www.fda.gov/Food/ LabelingNutrition/ConsumerInformation/ucm110019 .htm).[3-6] Another page, www.fda.gov/Food/Labeling Nutrition/ConsumerInformation/ucm121642.htm, leads to food labeling and nutrition education tools.[7] Colorful posters containing nutrition information for the 20 most frequently consumed fresh fruits, vegetables, and fish in the United States are available in multiple-size PDF format. These materials can be displayed or distributed by retailers participating in the voluntary point-of-purchase program.[8]

Make Your Calories Count

A user-friendly interactive program for learning about the Nutrition Facts label includes an overview and diagram of a sample label and explanations on how to interpret information pertaining to serving size; calorie and protein content; nutrients to limit such as fat, saturated and *trans* fat, cholesterol, sugar, and sodium; and guidance to purchase foods containing nutrients that are typically lacking in American diets such as vitamins A and C, calcium, iron, and fiber (www.fda.gov/Food/LabelingNutrition/ConsumerInformation/ucm114022.htm).[9]

Health Claims

Explanation of the 3 types—health, nutrient content, and structure/function claims allowed on packaging of food and dietary supplements—can be found at www.fda.gov/Food/LabelingNutrition/LabelClaims/ucm111447.htm.[10] A summary of health claims approved for use on food and dietary supplement labels is accessible in Appendix C of the Food Labeling Guide at www.fda.gov/Food/Guidance ComplianceRegulatoryInformation/GuidanceDocuments/FoodLabelingNutrition/FoodLabelingGuide/ucm064919 .htm.[11]

Nutrient Content Claims

The Nutrition Labeling and Education Act allows the use of nutrient content claims that describe nutrient levels by using terms such as *free, high,* and *low* and/or *lite* on food packaging. Most nutrient content claim regulations pertain to nutrients for which there is an established daily value—reference points for intakes based on a 2,000-calorie diet. Appendix A: Definitions of Nutrition Content Claims,[12] www.fda .gov/Food/GuidanceComplianceRegulatoryInformation/GuidanceDocuments/FoodLabelingNutrition/Food LabelingGuide/ucm064916.htm, and Appendix B: Additional Requirements for Nutrient Content Claims to the Food Labeling Guide,[13] www.fda.gov/Food/GuidanceComplianceRegulatoryInformation/GuidanceDocuments/FoodLabelingNutrition/Food LabelingGuide/ucm064916.htm, provide examples of nutrient content claims.[12,13] The FDA Modernization Act of 1997 permits manufacturers to submit notification of a nutrient content claim based on scientific evidence typically supported by the Food and Nutrition Board of the Institute of Medicine at the National Academy of Sciences to the FDA. Health claims may be used on product packaging 120 days after receipt of notification if the FDA takes no action to modify or prohibit the claim.[14]

Structure/Function Claims

Structure/function claims on packaged foods, dietary supplements, and pharmaceuticals describe how a nutrient or ingredient may benefit normal function in humans.

Guidance regarding compliance to the regulations on structure/function claims can be accessed at www.fda .gov/Food/GuidanceComplianceRegulatoryInformation/GuidanceDocuments/DietarySupplements/ucm103340 .htm.[15]

Nutrition Labeling—Too Much or Too Little?

There has been much debate about the shortcomings of FDA's nutrition labeling program. Critics believe that the Nutrition Facts panel is too confusing—shoppers are rushed or distracted with little time to decipher the label and ingredients list. Calorie and total fat information reportedly is most useful to consumers in selecting food. However, the nutritional information appearing on labels varies across product categories given the differences in nutrient content among foods and is often inconsistent, particularly with respect to portion sizes even within the same product category. The percentage of daily value is a difficult concept for some to comprehend. Furthermore, the small font size used on the packaging is hard to read for some people. Nutrition labeling may be of limited use to the increasing number of Americans for which English is not the primary language.

Voluntary Labeling Programs— Stars, Stamps, and Checkmarks

Hannaford Guiding Stars

The Hannaford Guiding Stars program (www.hannaford .com/Contents/Healthy_Living/Guiding_Stars/index .shtml) is the first storewide navigation system to offer at-a-glance nutrition information for more than 25,000 foods including fresh produce, meat, seafood, deli items, and packaged foods. Bottled waters and foods with less than 5 calories per serving are not rated.[16]

The Guiding Stars scoring system, which is based on a "good, better, and best" approach was developed by nutrition scientists and an advisory panel of nutrition and medical experts. The nutrient data are analyzed from the information on the Nutrition Facts label and the US Department of Agriculture's nutrient database. A food with a poor nutritional score is given a "no star" ranking; a product with a 3-star score contains more micronutrients and/or whole grains and less *trans* and saturated fats, cholesterol, added sugars, and/or sodium. The scoring does not distinguish between foods that are organically or conventionally produced. The stars are placed on the unit price tags on grocery shelves, on produce signs, and those appearing on meat, poultry, and seafood cases.[17]

Front-of-Pack Nutrition Labeling

Professional and trade associations, grocers, and food manufacturers have developed a number of nutrition labeling tools to educate consumers and influence food purchasing. Nutrition scientists and food industry representatives hypothesize that a single, credible front-of-the pack labeling system that is recognizable and uniform across categories will benefit consumers greatly. They welcome a quick and easy means to bring attention to the caloric content of foods and to identify those rich in certain nutrients and/or food groups.

Nutrition scientists and food industry representatives hypothesize that a single, credible front-of-the pack labeling system that is recognizable and uniform across categories will benefit consumer greatly.

American Heart Association

The American Heart Association's (AHA's) food certification program, established in 1995, is designed to provide guidance for healthy people older than 2 years (www.americanheart.org/presenter.jhtml?identifier=2115).[18]

The heart-check program has 3 levels of certification: standard, for those products meeting the criteria for saturated fat and cholesterol; whole-grains certification, for foods meeting saturated fat, cholesterol, and whole-grains criteria; and whole-oat soluble fiber certification, for foods that meet the saturated fat and cholesterol criteria and contain 0.75 g of β-glucan per serving. A list of approximately 800 AHA-certified foods arranged by food category and manufacturer can be accessed at http://checkmark.heart.org. Foods ineligible for heart-check certification include bottled water, alcoholic beverages, meal replacements, certain beef cuts, nuts, products containing stanol-sterols, foods manufactured by tobacco companies, and those that do not align with AHA science.[19]

Whole Grains Council

The Whole Grains Council (www.wholegrainscouncil.org/find-whole-grains) is a nonprofit consumer advocacy group that works to increase consumption of whole grains for better health by encouraging manufacturers to create products using whole grains; help consumers find whole-grain foods and understand their health benefits; and ensure accurate reporting about whole grains among the media. In 2002, food manufacturers, scientists, and chefs convened at a Whole Grains Summit to outline a number of goals, one being the development of a packaging symbol—the Whole Grain Stamp—to help American shoppers easily select and purchase whole products as a means to reach the goal of consuming the recommended 3 daily servings of whole grains.[20]

The Whole Grain Stamp program participants must file information about each qualifying product and be a member of the Whole Grains Council. Manufacturers are bound by a legal agreement to abide by all the rules and guidelines of the program, thus providing a safeguard to consumers. The Whole Grain Stamps first appeared on grocery shelves in 2005 when stamps displayed on packaging described a food as a "good source" with a minimum of 8 g per serving; an "excellent source" containing 16 g of fiber; or "100% excellent" for products that contained all whole grains and at least 16 g of fiber for serving. The phase 2 program launched in June 2006 uses the Basic Stamp on the packaging for foods that contain at least 8 g of whole grain but may also contain refined grains, extra bran, germ, or refined flour. A product bearing the 100% Stamp must contain all whole grains as grain ingredients and 16 g of whole grain per serving. The stamps also include a number indicating the number of whole grains per serving.[21]

With recent expansion to Canada, Mexico, the Dominican Republic, and the United Kingdom, more than 2,100 products have used the Whole Grain Stamps on their packaging as of September 2008. A list of these products searchable by country and/or category, that is, granola and snack bars, beverages, breads and cereals, pasta, pizzas, entrees, and side dishes, is accessible at www.wholegrainscouncil.org/find-whole-grains/stamped-products.[22] Frequently-asked-questions pages for consumers and manufacturers can be found at www.wholegrainscouncil.org/whole-grain-stamp/stamp-faq-consumers and www.wholegrainscouncil.org/whole-grain-stamp/stamp-faq-manufacturers.[23,24]

Smart Spot

Pepsico's Smart Start program (www.pepsico.com/Purpose/Health-and-Wellness/Smart-Spot.html), launched in 2004, marks products with the Smart Spot symbol that are nutritious and contribute fiber and at least 10% of the daily value for nutrients such as protein, calcium, and vitamins A and C; meet limits for fat, saturated and *trans* fat, cholesterol, sodium, and added sugar; or are reduced in calories, fat, saturated or total fat, sodium, and sugar.[25]

Smart Choices Program

Led by the nonprofit Keystone Center, a partnership of scientists, university faculty, and representatives from the food and beverage industry and health and research organizations convened in 2007 to establish a comprehensive voluntary front-of-the pack labeling initiative to help consumers make smart food selections. This effort they hoped would improve shoppers' nutrition knowledge and encourage selection of healthful foods and would subsequently positively impact the health of the U.S. public.

The Smart Choices program (http://smartchoicesprogram .com) launched in August 2009 marked products in 19 food product categories with a symbol displayed on the front of the package to guide shoppers in making quick and smarter food and beverage selections within a product category.[26] To help consumers make fast calorie comparisons, Smart Choices products also included calorie information on the front of the package indicating the number of calories per serving and servings per container.

The Smart Choices program was voluntarily suspended in late October pending an FDA ruling on package-front nutrition labeling.[27]

References

1. American Heart Association nutrition labeling. www .americanheart.org/presenter.jhtml?identifier=4631. Accessed June 16, 2009.

2. Food labeling guide guidance for industry. April 2008. www .fda.gov/Food/GuidanceComplianceRegulatoryInformation/ GuidanceDocuments/FoodLabelingNutrition/ FoodLabelingGuide/default.htm. Accessed July 2, 2009.

3. FDA nutrition labeling consumer information. www.fda.gov/ Food/LabelingNutrition/ConsumerInformation/default.htm. Accessed July 2, 2009.

4. How to understand and use the nutrition facts label. www .fda.gov/Food/LabelingNutrition/ConsumerInformation/ ucm078889.htm. Accessed July 2, 2009.

5. *Trans* fat now listed with saturated fat and cholesterol on the nutrition facts label. www.fda.gov/Food/ LabelingNutrition/ConsumerInformation/ucm109832.htm. Accessed July 2, 2009.

6. Los Ácidos Grasos Trans Ahora Serán Listados Junto con las Grasas Saturadas y el Colesterol en la Etiqueta de Información Nutricional. www.fda.gov/Food/LabelingNutrition/ ConsumerInformation/ucm110019.htm. Accessed July 2, 2009.

7. Label Education Tools. Food labeling and nutrition education tools. www.fda.gov/Food/LabelingNutrition/ ConsumerInformation/ucm121642.htm. Accessed July 2, 2009.

8. Nutrition Information for Raw Fruits, Vegetables and Fish www.fda.gov/Food/LabelingNutrition/ FoodLabelingGuidanceRegulatoryInformation/ InformationforRestaurantsRetailEstablishments/ucm063367 .htm. Accessed July 3, 2009.

9. Make Your Calories Count. www.fda.gov/Food/ LabelingNutrition/ConsumerInformation/ucm114022.htm. Accessed July 3, 2009.

10. Claims that can be made for conventional foods and dietary supplements. www.fda.gov/Food/LabelingNutrition/ LabelClaims/ucm111447.htm. Accessed July 3, 2009.

11. Appendix C: Health claims April 2008 guidance for industry. A food labeling guide. www.fda.gov/ Food/GuidanceComplianceRegulatoryInformation/ GuidanceDocuments/FoodLabelingNutrition/ FoodLabelingGuide/ucm064919.htm. Accessed July 3, 2009.

12. Appendix A: Definitions of nutrition content claims April 2008. Guidance for industry, a food labeling guide. www.fda.gov/Food/ GuidanceComplianceRegulatoryInformation/GuidanceDocuments/ FoodLabelingNutrition/FoodLabelingGuide/ucm064911.htm. Accessed July 3, 2009.

13. Appendix B: Additional requirements for nutrient content claims guidance for industry, a food labeling guide. www.fda.gov/Food/ GuidanceComplianceRegulatoryInformation/GuidanceDocuments/ FoodLabelingNutrition/FoodLabelingGuide/ucm064916.htm. Accessed July 3, 2009.

14. Nutrient content claims notification for choline containing foods. www.fda.gov/Food/LabelingNutrition/LabelClaims/ FDAModernizationActFDAMAClaims/ucm073599.htm. Accessed July 3, 2009.

15. Guidance for industry: structure/function claims, small entity compliance. www.fda.gov/Food/ GuidanceComplianceRegulatoryInformation/ GuidanceDocuments/DietarySupplements/ucm103340.htm. Accessed July 3, 2009.

16. Hannaford Guiding Stars. www.hannaford.com/Contents/ Healthy_Living/Guiding_Stars/index.shtml. Accessed June 16, 2009.

17. Hannaford Guiding Stars frequently asked questions. www .hannaford.com/Contents/Healthy_Living/Guiding_Stars/faqs .shtml. Accessed June 16, 2009.

18. American Heart Association. www.americanheart.org/presenter .jhtml?identifier=2115. Accessed June 16, 2009.

19. American Heart Association food certification program list of foods. http://checkmark.heart.org. Accessed June 16, 2009.

20. WholeGrains Council.org. www.wholegrainscouncil.org/ find-whole-grains. Accessed June 16, 2009.

21. Whole Grains Stamp program. www.wholegrainscouncil.org/ whole-grain-stamp. Accessed June 16, 2009.

22. Whole Grains Stamp Products. www.wholegrainscouncil.org/ find-whole-grains/stamped-products. Accessed June 16, 2009.

23. Whole Grains Council consumer FAQs. www .wholegrainscouncil.org/whole-grain-stamp/ stamp-faq-consumers. Accessed June 16, 2009.

24. Whole Grains Council FAQ manufacturers. www .wholegrainscouncil.org/whole-grain-stamp/ stamp-faq-manufacturers. Accessed June 16, 2009.

25. Smart Spot. www.pepsico.com/Purpose/Health-and-Wellness/ Smart-Spot.html. Accessed October 28, 2009.

26. Smart Choices Program™. http://smartchoicesprogram.com. Accessed October 28, 2009.

27. Food label program to suspend operations. The New York Times business section, October 24, 2009. www.nytimes .com/2009/10/24/business/24food.html?_r=2. Accessed October 26, 2009.

Critical Thinking

1. What is the Food and Nutrition Labeling Act of 1990?
2. Which nutrients are required to be included on the nutrition facts panel?
3. What is the difference between health claims, nutrient content claims, and structure/function claims on product labels?

KATHLEEN L. CAPPELLANO, MS, RD, LDN, is an instructor at the Friedman School of Nutrition Science and Policy, Tufts University, Boston, Massachusetts, and former Nutrition Information Manager at the Jean Mayer United States Department of Agriculture Human Nutrition Research Center on Aging at Tufts University. A member of the American Dietetic Association and Dietitians in Business and Communications practice group, Cappellano has over a decade of experience in evaluating and writing about medical, health, and food and nutrition websites.

From *Nutrition Today,* 44(6), November/December 2009, pp. 269–273. Copyright © 2009 by Lippincott, Williams & Wilkins/Wolters Kluwer Health. Reprinted by permission via Rightslink.

UNIT 7

Food Safety and Technology

Unit Selections

Learning Outcomes

After reading this Unit, you will be able to:

- Describe the responsibilities of the USDA in ensuring our food supply is safe.

- Identify foods that have been the culprits in the spread of *E. coli* 0157.

- Discuss the advantages and disadvantages of genetically modified crops.

- What percentage of corn, cotton, and soybeans grown in the United States are genetically modified?

- Discuss the advantages and disadvantages to growing meat in a lab.

- Explain how the world's food supply and agriculture change if we could harvest meat in a petri dish.

- List the four most common biological contaminants (bacteria and viruses) found in our water supply.

- Explain how you can decrease the number of bacteria that you have on the surface of your faucets.

Student Website

www.mhhe.com/cls

Internet References

American Council on Science and Health (ACSH)
www.acsh.org
Centers for Disease Control and Prevention (CDC)
www.cdc.gov
FDA Center for Food Safety and Applied Nutrition
www.fda.gov/food/foodsafety/default.htm
Food Safety Project (FSP)
www.extension.iastate.edu/foodsafety
USDA Food Safety and Inspection Service (FSIS)
www.fsis.usda.gov

Food-borne disease constitutes an important public health problem in the United States. The U.S. Centers for Disease Control has reported 76 million cases of food-borne illness each year, out of which 5,000 end in death. The annual cost of losses in productivity ranges from $20 to 40 billion. Food-borne disease results primarily from microbial contamination (bacteria, viruses, and protozoa) and also from naturally occurring toxins, environmental contaminants, pesticide residues, and food additives.

The first Food and Drug Act was passed in 1906 and was followed by tighter control on the use of additives as possible carcinogens. In 1958, the Delaney Clause was passed and a list of additives that were considered as safe for human consumption (GRAS list) was developed.

The Food and Drug Administration (FDA) controls and regulates procedures dealing with food safety, including food service and production. The FDA has established rules (Hazard Analysis and Critical Control Points) to improve the control of food safety practices and to monitor the production of seafood, meat, and poultry.

Agricultural trade between nations has led to a truly globalized food supply. This globalization meets the demand of wealthy nations for year-round access to foods grown in tropical environments and strengthens the economies of poorer, underdeveloped countries. One detriment of the global food supply is the translocation of biological contaminants via food. Less than 1 percent of foods imported into the United States are inspected each year. Although U.S. demand for a variety of foods has driven the worldwide food trade, our nation has not established an effective method to regulate the safety of foods shipped in from other countries. The current regulatory agency for U.S. food, the Food and Drug Administration, is faced with many challenges of trying to regulate the U.S. food and pharmaceutical industries, much less the newly introduced challenges of the safety of food imports.

Imported foods are not the only concern for biological contaminants. Changes in food production and farming in the United States have led to an increase in the spread of bacterial contamination of our foods. Many conventional poultry and livestock farms raise their animals in crowded, unsanitary conditions. The crowded conditions make the spread of bacteria very likely; therefore, conventional farmers must inoculate their animals with antibiotics to prevent bacteria from spreading throughout the entire stock. An example of the poor regulation of foods grown in the United States is the dramatic increase in *Salmonella* and *Campylobacter* bacteria in chickens over the past few years. Possible explanations for the increase in these two microorganisms could be due to the U.S. Department of Agriculture having no standards for *Campylobacter* and testing for *Salmonella* in a very small proportion of animals.

Surveys show that over 95 percent of the time people do not follow proper sanitation methods when working with food. Thus our best defense is to have safe food-handling practices at home. The U.S. government, therefore, launched the Food Safety Initiative program to minimize food-borne disease and to educate the public about safe-handling practices. An emphasis on improving food safety practices at home is also seen in the 2010 Dietary Guidelines. In these latest guidelines the subcommittees of the USDA and HHS recommend creating and offering food safety education programs for children in schools and preschools, along with improving education efforts with adults.

Genetically modifying our food crops is a controversial topic. The topic has gained much attention from people who perceive the

© PhotoLink/Getty Images

possible threats of genetically altered crops. The positions of people who oppose the practice are fueled by the actions of large agricultural companies that have genetically altered seeds to be resistant to herbicides, which allows for easier and heavy use of the herbicide on the crops. However, there are benefits to using genetically modified crops, but usually involve research conducted in academia rather than by the industry seeking a profit. Genetically modified crops can be used to increase the world's food supply to meet the demand of its growing population and increase the nutrient density of crops to provide the key nutrients missing in underdeveloped countries' food supply.

The final controversial, some think bizarre, topic that is covered in this unit is the concept of growing meat for human consumption in a lab. Harvesting meat tissue grown in petri dishes to be grilled, sauteed, or broiled along with your favorite sauce, is an ingenious idea to some and odd to others. Several labs are working to perfect techniques to grow beef, chicken, and lamb tissue in a chemistry lab. The concept would significantly impact agriculture and food supply. The article by Jeffrey Bartholet addresses this concept and provides a historical perspective of this practice.

Genetic Engineering for Good

A researcher modifies crops to feed the hungry and cut pesticide use.

ERIK VANCE, FROM *CONSERVATION*

In the mid-1940s, Norman Borlaug started the Green Revolution on a small farm in Mexico. His idea was simple. As the human population skyrocketed, he would grow a new kind of wheat with a thicker stem and bigger seed heads, thus increasing yield and allowing farmers to grow more wheat—and feed more people—per acre.

The results were staggering. Within two decades, Mexico's wheat harvest had swollen sixfold, thanks to crops descended from Borlaug's modified wheat. Borlaug then turned his talents toward rice in the Philippines, and high-yield crops spread into almost every major food staple. All told, Borlaug's revolution helped feed millions of people in poor and developing countries—an achievement that earned him the 1970 Nobel Peace Prize.

But the Green Revolution wasn't "green" in the modern sense of the word. In fact, it exacted a huge environmental toll. Its crops require liberal use of fertilizer and pesticides that bleed into the land and sea, poisoning wildlife and creating nitrogen-rich dead zones in the oceans. Now, with climate change threatening to upend many of the world's crops, a new generation of researchers is poised to correct some of the original revolution's flaws.

Pam Ronald, a University of California, Davis, researcher, sees a future dominated not by Monsanto-like corporations but by small partnerships between farmers and scientists. By combining genetically modified crops with organic farming and other eco-friendly practices, Ronald believes, we can create a system that slashes pesticide use, insulates crops against floods and drought, and protects the livelihoods of poor farmers in the developing world. Using genetic engineering as a conservation tool sounds like an oxymoron to many people, but the scales may finally be tipping in Ronald's favor.

Her ideas have become a favorite of opinion makers such as Michael Pollan and Bill Gates. What's more, they serve as a stark reminder that genetically modified foods are here, whether we like it or not. Which means that, at a time when we need to reinvent the world's food supply, the critical question may be: Can we get it right?

Ronald is an unlikely genetic-engineering advocate. Pulling into her driveway, I see that her yard looks like that of any eco-foodie. Her pesticide-free garden—a tangled mix of herbs and native plants—has a happy, new age feel. Her barn sports a mural that she describes as "Diego Rivera meets Cesar Chavez." And her husband, Raoul Adamchak, is an organic farmer.

But Ronald, a plant geneticist, is also an unabashed supporter of genetically modified (GM) crops. Her book on the benefits of bioengineered organic crops, *Tomorrow's Table* (Oxford University Press, 2008), which she wrote with Adamchak, has started reshaping the way we look at GM foods.

While debate traditionally has been focused on genetically modified corn and other lucrative foodstuffs, Ronald has been doing pioneering work on a crop that is largely ignored: rice. In fact, while companies such as Monsanto pour billions into GM crops, rice research is almost solely the province of publicly funded academics. "The big companies aren't working on broccoli or carrots—there's just not enough profit in that," she says. "And they don't work on rice. It feeds half the world, but not the wealthy half."

Rice could be the ideal proving ground for genetic engineering to improve the environment while preparing for a warmer world, she says.

Take flooding, for instance. No one knows for certain how much flooding will increase as the planet warms, but scientists believe it will become more frequent and last longer in places such as Southeast Asia, where it already causes around $1 billion in annual damage to rice crops.

That's why Ronald's lab teamed up with colleague Dave Mackill in the late 1990s to create a species of rice that could be submerged for weeks and survive. Unlike many crops, rice has a dizzying number of varieties (as many as 140,000), all with distinct genetic codes. Mackill found one variety from eastern India with an unusual ability to live underwater for long spans. Ronald's team undertook the painstaking task of sorting through the genome until they found a single gene that seemed to act as a "master switch" for flood tolerance.

It was a neat trick, but the researchers wanted something that could be used easily by poor rice farmers. One method would have been to slice the gene out and simply slide it into a commercial crop, making it "genetically modified." However, they finally decided to simply breed the old with the new while targeting that specific place in the gene that held the precious submergence trait. This so-called marker-assisted breeding blends genetic work with old school, dirty-finger-nails farming. Because the actual genetic transfer was done in rice fields, the new strain is not considered modified and is thus under less scrutiny from government agencies than lab-modified strains are.

In a 2006 paper in *Nature,* the team announced a new strain of rice that could survive two weeks totally underwater. And it was easy to grow. By the end of 2010, the floodproof rice was expected to cover 125,000 acres in four countries. That's projected to jump tenfold this year.

This is just the beginning, Ronald says. Flooding is one of climate change's three key threats to agriculture. Drought and pest outbreaks are the other two, and Ronald believes lab-aided rice can be designed to resist them all. She is just beginning to work on drought-tolerant rice, and she believes a bug- and weed-resistant rice could slash the amount of pesticides used by rice farmers.

It's an example of how genetic engineering has accomplished exactly what many environmentalists and organic farmers want, Ronald says. Genetically modified cotton is a prime example. Little more than a decade ago, farmers in China started using "Bt cotton," a genetically engineered variety containing a protein that kills pests but is not toxic to mammals. (The Bt protein is a favorite insecticide among organic farmers.) Within four years, the Chinese cotton farmers reduced their annual use of poisonous insecticides by 70,000 metric tons—almost as much as is used in all of California each year.

The line between "genetically engineered" and "traditional" crops exists only in the media and politics. For scientists, it's more of a continuum.

Opponents worry that GM food carries some still-undiscovered health risks or that it's just a tool that helps big corporations sell more pesticides. And Doug Gurian-Sherman of the Union of Concerned Scientists worries that expensive GM research siphons money from less-sexy techniques. He likes marker-led breeding, he says, but he wants to see more money spent on organic techniques that reduce sprawling monocultures.

The danger of pesticides far outweighs that of switching a few base pairs in the DNA, Ronald says. She frequently notes that there's no record of anyone ever becoming sick from a GM crop.

Ronald also points out that the debate revolves around several false dichotomies. While naysayers declare genetic modification to be a new and evil practice, Ronald says the line between "genetically engineered" and "traditional" crops really exists only in the media and politics. For scientists, she says, it's more of a continuum—with traditional breeding on one end and crops with genes borrowed from vastly different creatures on the other.

Another false tradeoff is the idea that embracing genetic engineering means doing away with other environmentally friendly agriculture practices. If we are to feed the world without destroying the planet, Ronald believes, we must incorporate not just genetic modification but also crop rotations, crop diversity, and other ideas promoted by organic farmers.

To explain what might finally tip the scales, Ronald points to the developing world. As global warming intensifies, poor subsistence farmers will be devastated by food insecurity far more than the wealthy West.

"If farmers don't change the seed they're planting now, in 25 years they're going to be getting half the yield," Ronald says. She believes altering rice and other crops—such as strains of bananas—could help prevent future famine, much in the way that Borlaug's wheat spared millions of people from starvation. If we're going to accomplish that, environmentalists need to think more broadly. "You don't have to choose between productivity and sustainability," she says. "You can have both."

Critical Thinking

1. Evaluate the benefit of the initial work of Norman Borlaug.
2. Explain why agriculture research on rice is primarily conducted by academics, whereas wheat, corn, and soy are heavily researched by agriculture companies.
3. Justify the need for the current research on flood-resistant rice.
4. Critique the following statement: "The line between genetically engineered traditional crops really exist in the media and politics."

Plant geneticist Pamela Ronald blogs about agriculture and genetics issues at scienceblogs.com/tomorrowstable. Reprinted from *Conservation* (July–Sept. 2010), "the magazine for environmental intelligence" published by the Society for Conservation Biology. www.conservationmagazine.org.

Food Fight

Genetically modified crops, says agro-research czar Roger Beachy, receive an unjustified shellacking from environmentalists.

BRENDAN BORRELL

Roger Beachy grew up in a traditional Amish family on a small farm in Ohio that produced food "in the old ways," he says, with few insecticides, herbicides or other agro-chemicals. He went on to become a renowned expert in plant viruses and sowed the world's first genetically modified food crop—a tomato plant with a gene that conferred resistance to the devastating tomato mosaic virus. Beachy sees no irony between his rustic, low-tech boyhood and a career spent developing new types of agricultural technologies. For him, genetic manipulation of food plants is a way of helping preserve the traditions of small farms by reducing the amount of chemicals farmers have to apply to their crops.

In 2009 Beachy took the helm of the National Institute of Food and Agriculture, a new research arm of the U.S. Department of Agriculture, where he controls a $1.5-billion budget for pursuing his vision of the future of agriculture. In the past year Beachy's institute has funded ambitious agricultural research, such as a massive genomic study of 5,000 lines of wheat and barley, alongside unexpected projects: a $15-million behavioral study on childhood obesity in rural states, for one.

Beachy's appointment sparked controversy among environmentalists because his work helped to kick-start the $11-billion global agricultural biotechnology industry. Seed companies never commercialized his virus-resistant plants, but their success—tomato plants that showed near-complete resistance to multiple virus strains—underlined the potential for a technology that was ultimately widely embraced by U.S. farmers. Today in the U.S. more than 90 percent of soybean and cotton crops and more than 80 percent of corn plants are genetically engineered to resist herbicides and insects using methods similar to the ones developed by Beachy. Organic farmers and locavores worry about Beachy's ties to big agriculture—much of his tomato work received funding from Monsanto—and his advocacy of genetic modification of food crops. Beachy, though, remains unrepentant. Although he believes seed companies can do more to improve food security in the developing world, he insists that genetic manipulation is essential to feed the earth's growing population

In Brief

A pioneer in developing genetically modified foods has assumed an influential role as head of the U.S. Department of Agriculture's research agency.

Roger Beachy continues to advocate for a prominent place for genetic engineering of crops, which he claims provides a basis for chemical-free, sustainable agriculture that will prove more of a boon for the environment than have conventional weed and pest control.

Detractors of GM foods, meanwhile, have expressed their chagrin at Beachy's appointment.

Without GM crops, Beachy contends that farmers would need to return to older practices that would produce lower crop yields, higher prices and an increase in the use of agrochemicals inimical to health.

sustainably. Edited excerpts of a phone conversation with Beachy follow.

*SCIENTIFIC AMERICAN: **Did you actually get to see the first GM tomatoes when they were planted in the field in Illinois in 1987?***
BEACHY: Oh, my goodness, I planted them. I went out and hoed them. I was out there once a week looking at everything in the field, and my daughter K. C. even helped me weed the tomato patch one time. I really wanted to observe the patch and see how it was progressing.

Were you surprised by how effective the virus-resistance gene was?
Absolutely. As the parental plants without the resistance gene were getting sicker and sicker, the ones that had the gene looked just dynamite. I still have the original photos from 25 years ago, and it's pretty remarkable even now to look at them and say, "By George, our stuff really works!" Other people have seen the same kind of technology work in cucumbers and papaya and squash and green peppers; many are surprised at

how relatively simple the concept was and yet how much of an impact it can have.

That effectiveness does not last forever, of course. Today we are seeing the resistance these technologies provide against pests and disease being overcome. Do you think the industry has relied too much on GM as a "silver bullet"?

No, these things happen in plant breeding of all kinds, whether it's traditional breeding or molecular breeding like we're doing now. In the 1960s and 1970s new types of wheat rust spread up from Mexico on the wind, and the plant breeders would hustle and hustle to find resistance to one strain of rust, and then, several years later, another strain would come, so they would have to be looking ahead to find any new resistance.

Durable, permanent resistance is almost unheard of, which brings up the question of why did we create GM crops in the first place? What we've gotten over the past 15 to 20 years is a considerable amount of insecticides not being used in the environment. That's remarkable. What we're wondering now is if we will go back to using only chemicals or if we will be able to find new genes that will capture the diversity of pests that we're seeing around the world.

Unlike in the U.S., tropical regions of the world, including parts of China, face constant pressure from multiple insects. To control the variety of crop-damaging insects, scientists will need a variety of different genetic technologies, or it may be necessary to apply nongenetic technologies, such as different proven insecticides to control them. Overall, we'll find the kinds of genes that will protect against white flies in one country and aphids in another country. If we manage this right, we'll have the genetic solutions to these questions and not chemical solutions and will therefore, in my opinion, be more sustainable.

Critics of the agricultural biotechnology industry complain that it has focused on providing benefits to farmers rather than improving foods for consumers. What do you say to them?

In the early years many of us in the university community were looking at using genetic engineering to enhance vitamin content of foods, improve the quality of seed proteins and develop crops that don't require use of pesticides—all things we thought would benefit agriculture and consumers. The process for approval of a biotechnology product was onerous, expensive and unknown for academics. It would take the private sector to make the new technologies successful and find an opportunity to give farmers crops with higher productivity. But the food companies that purchased these crops—General Mills, Kellogg's—were not used to paying more for wheat or oats that had more nutritional content or for vegetables that were higher in minerals.

Why not?

Because the American public would not be willing to pay more for those products.

Today consumers are willing to pay more for crops that are labeled "organic" or even "GM-free" because they view them as more sustainable. How do you think GM crops can help make agriculture more sustainable?

In my opinion, the GM crops we have today already contributed to sustainable agriculture. They have reduced the use of harmful pesticides and herbicides and the loss of soils because they promote the use of no-till methods of farming. Nevertheless, there is much more that can be done. As you know, agriculture and forestry account for approximately 31 percent of global greenhouse gas emissions, larger than the 26 percent from the energy sector. Agriculture is a major source of emissions of methane and nitrous oxides and is responsible for some of the pollution of waterways because of fertilizer run-off from fields. Agriculture needs to do better.

We haven't reached the plateau of global population and may not until 2050 or 2060. In the interim, we must increase food production while reducing greenhouse gas emissions and soil erosion and decrease pollution of waterways. That's a formidable challenge. With new technologies in seeds and in crop production, it will be possible to reduce the use of chemical fertilizers and the amount of irrigation while maintaining high yields. Better seeds will help, as will improvements in agricultural practices.

Environmentalists have been reluctant to embrace GM crops because of concerns about genes flowing to non-GM crops and also to wild native plants. That's one reason a federal judge in California recently ordered genetically modified sugar beets to be destroyed.

You are correct. Nevertheless, it is important to note that the court ruling is not about the safety of the sugar beets or the plants that result from cross-pollination. The farmers who brought suit charge a premium for their crops because they are branded as organic—a definition that does not include genetic engineering. They are worried that their non-GM crops will be pollinated by pollen from GM crops, reducing their value. In this case, it is not an issue of food safety but of product marketing.

On the other hand, it's true that there are reasons why we want to preserve wild populations of crop plants: they act as a reservoir for genetic diversity. Here in the U.S., we are not, for instance, planting GM corn alongside wild maize, which is from Mexico. There are some native species for which there is a cross-pollination possibility, for example, squashes and melons, where there are some wild progenitors out in the field. It will be important to ensure that such germplasm is preserved.

In some quarters it might actually be seen as positive if a trait for disease or pest resistance, whether or not it was of GM origin, was transferred to weedy relatives, because it will reduce pests or pathogens in the area.

It may be a positive thing for agriculture, but not necessarily for wild ecosystems. What are the consequences if you create a vitamin A–rich rice and that gene spreads into an environment where vitamin A is scarce?

Most scientists do not predict any negative consequences if the genes used to develop Golden Rice [vitamin A–rich rice] are transferred to other varieties or to wild relatives. In contrast, the payoff for making Golden Rice widely available to those with vitamin A–poor diets is enormous. Imagine if we further delayed the release of such improved foods, leaving many hundreds of thousands of children with blindness and impaired vision and early deaths because of deficiency of vitamin A. What is the value of sight in children? What is the potential damage should the genetic trait be transferred to wild or feral rice? You're right—you can't say that every place in the country or every place in the world or every environment, hot or cold, that it won't have an impact, but we need to weigh the risks and benefits.

Some scientists have complained that biotech companies have stymied research on GM crops. Aren't these studies needed to get accurate answers about the risks of these crops?

That's a complex question with many different factors at play. In my opinion, the field would be more advanced if more academic scientists were involved in testing and other types of experimentation. We've had too little involvement of the academic sector in some of these cases. Many of us urged early on that there be more sharing, and I can understand the concerns of the academics.

On the other hand, I've asked companies why seed isn't made readily available for academic scientists' use. Some point out that there have been a number of academic studies in the past 20 years about using GM crops that were incomplete or poorly designed. And as a result, there was a lot of wasted effort by many other scientists that follow up on such studies.

Take the case of the report that pollen from insect-resistant corn harms larvae of Monarch and other butterflies, which led many to conclude that GM corn would have a devastating effect on Monarch populations. This finding was widely quoted in the media, and the USDA spent a great deal of energy and investment on follow-up research, which in the end showed that Monarch larvae were likely to be affected under very restricted conditions: for example, if the pollination of a crop occurs at the same time and place as the larval growth of the butterfly—a very, very rare occasion.

Furthermore, because the use of insect-resistant corn reduced the use of chemical pesticides, the outcome increased the population of butterflies and other insects. From this and other examples, companies were justifiably concerned about the quality of some academic studies and felt that they had more to lose than to gain in such cases. Yet there is much to be gained from academic scientists conducting well-designed studies with GM crops, and I hope that the future brings greater collaboration and less suspicion between public-sector and private-sector scientists in agriculture biotechnology.

What would be the consequence if GM crops were suddenly removed from the market?

Here in the U.S., there would likely be a modest increase in food prices because the efficiency of food production is currently high as a consequence of using GM traits, resulting in low food prices. We would have to go back to older types of production that would result in lower density of planting and likely lower per-acre outputs. We would likely see an increase in acreage planted, including the use of some marginal lands to increase total output. In the U.S. and other countries, there would be a significant increase in the use of agrochemicals, and the related health issues associated with such use would increase. Although there have been great advances in plant breeding during the past 20 years, the yields of the major commodity crops, such as maize, soybeans and cotton, would be less in the absence of biotechnology than with it. If total global crop production drops, the impacts would, of course, be greater on poorer nations than on those that are wealthier. The agriculturally poor countries would certainly suffer more than those that have a strong foundation of food agriculture production.

More to Explore

Genetically Modified Foods: Debating Biotechnology. Edited by Michael Ruse and David Castle. Prometheus Books, 2002.

Safe Food: The Politics of Food Safety. Marion Nestle. University of California Press, 2010.

Critical Thinking

1. Describe the first genetically modified crop. Who designed it and why?

2. Explain why Roger Beachy's appointment as the head of the National Institute of Food and Agriculture is controversial.

3. What percentage of corn, cotton, and soybeans grown in the United States are genetically modified?

4. Discuss the advantages and disadvantages of genetically modified crops.

BRENDAN BORRELL is based in New York City and frequently writes about science and the environment for *Scientific American* and *Nature*.

H₂ Uh–Oh

Do You Need to Filter Your Water?

NUTRITION ACTION NEWSLETTER

"For years, people said that America has the cleanest drinking water in the world," William K. Reilly, the Environmental Protection Agency's administrator under President George H. W. Bush, told *The New York Times* last year.

"That was true 20 years ago. But people don't realize how many new chemicals have emerged and how much more pollution has occurred. If they did, we would see very different attitudes."

Part of the problem: "The regulatory system is, frankly, slow to respond to emerging threats to water safety," says Shane Snyder, a water-contaminant expert and professor of environmental engineering at the University of Arizona.

Here's some of what may be lurking in your tap water . . . and why you may not be able to rely on your local water utility to keep you safe.

Germs

"We estimate that 19.5 million illnesses occur each year in the United States that are caused by microorganisms in drinking water," says University of Arizona microbiologist Kelly Reynolds. Particularly vulnerable are older adults, young children, and people with weakened immune systems.

The culprits: viruses (primarily Norovirus), bacteria (like *Campylobacter*, *E. coli*, and *Shigella*), and cysts that are produced by protozoa like *Cryptosporidium* and *Giardia*. They can cause diarrhea, headaches, and, in rare cases, chronic conditions like reactive arthritis.

How do germs get into drinking water?

- **Contaminated surface water.** About two-thirds of Americans get their water from surface water sources like reservoirs, lakes, and rivers. "And all surface waters, no matter how pristine, contain water-borne pathogens from birds and animals, such as *Campylobacter* and *Salmonella*," notes Reynolds.

 Surface water can also harbor gastrointestinal germs that are flushed down the toilet by humans

when they're sick. How do they get into waterways? Blame it, at least in part, or the weather.

The water systems that serve some 40 million Americans—often older systems in the Northeast, the Great Lakes region, and the Pacific Northwest—carry sewage and storm water in the same pipes. When water from heavy or sustained rains overloads a system, the overflow—wastewater along with rainwater—is discharged into rivers and creeks to prevent it from backing up.

At least 40,000 sewage overflows occur each year in the United States. And that wastewater could become your drinking water after it's been treated by your local water utility. Since treatment plants can't eliminate 100 percent of the germs, some can get through to your tap.

Climate change will likely add to the stress on water utilities in the Northeast and Midwest if, as predicted, it results in more and heavier precipitation there. Researchers at Johns Hopkins University in Baltimore found that heavy downpours preceded half of the 548 reported water-borne disease outbreaks in the United States from 1948 to 1994.[1]

- **Contaminated groundwater.** "Historically, groundwater supplies were thought to be free of disease-causing microorganisms because the soil naturally filters them out," says Reynolds. But viruses and other microbes from contaminated septic tanks, landfill leaks, or inadequate disposal of animal waste or wastewater can end up in water beneath the surface.

 The Environmental Protection Agency now requires utilities to disinfect ground-water that has a history of contamination.

- **Leaks in the distribution pipes.** Disease-causing microorganisms can also get into drinking water after it leaves the treatment plant. About a quarter of the nation's water distribution pipes are in poor condition, with leaks, cracks, and corrosion. On average, a city loses 18 to 44 percent of its water from leaking pipes, notes Yale University microbiologist Stephen Edberg.

Those pipes are often buried in the same trenches as sewer pipes. Changes in water pressure can allow contaminants in the soil to be sucked into the water pipes, fouling the drinking water.

"The proportion of disease outbreaks linked to breaches in the water distribution has increased over the past decade," says Reynolds, "and it's going to be a continuing problem."

- **Plumbing.** In 2004, University of Arizona researchers measured bacteria in the tap water of seven Tucson homes. The EPA limits the amount of these bacteria—which in most cases are harmless—to no more than 500 per milliliter of drinking water. Tucson's public water averaged only about 50, so it was relatively clean.

Not so most of the homes. Water from kitchen and bathroom faucets in the seven houses averaged more than 3,000 bacteria per milliliter. Levels varied among homes (one had virtually none, while another had 13,000 bacteria), and from day to day within the same house. Bathroom tap water in two homes averaged 2,400 bacteria first thing in the morning, then dropped to 140 after running the water for 30 seconds.[2]

Where do the bacteria come from?

"If you have pets that lick the faucet, or children with dirty hands who play with the faucet, or if you handle raw meats arid then touch the faucet, bacteria can enter the pipes and grow," says Reynolds. "They get back-washed into the pipes, where they can form a layer, or biofilm."

Another potential source of bacteria is stagnant water sitting in pipes. "Maybe you're on vacation or maybe you have a second home," says Reynolds. "Bacteria can grow in pipes while you're gone, and then you can get a big dose when the water is turned back on again."

The antidote: "Flush out the system by letting the water run until it's as cold as it gets," suggests Reynolds. "That will certainly rinse out bacteria that haven't established a biofilm on the inside of the pipes."

If a bacteria biofilm has developed, it could loosen over time as the water faucet is used, says Reynolds, "and a chunk can break off and you can suddenly get exposed to a big dose of bacteria. It could be a significant health risk."

What to Do

Use a filter that has been certified for microbiological purification by the Water Quality Association (WQA), NSF International, or Underwriters Laboratories (UL).

Lead

It's clear that lead can damage the brains and nervous systems of children. But it may also cause high blood pressure, cataracts, decline in mental abilities, and kidney problems in adults. (See *Nutrition Action,* March 2005, cover story.)

"We're learning that older adults should also be concerned about lead poisoning," says researcher Marc Edwards, a professor of civil and environmental engineering at Virginia Tech University in Blacksburg.

"Recent studies have shown that low levels of lead in the blood that we once considered safe are causing health problems in adults. No one thinks to ever look for it in older people." (The most common symptoms are abdominal pain, headache, fatigue, muscular weakness, and pain, numbness, or tingling in the extremities.)

The evidence that lead affects the brain is troubling. In one study of nearly 600 women aged 47 to 74, those with higher levels of lead in their bones scored worse on memory and other cognitive tests than those with lower levels.[3] The women with higher lead had scores comparable to women who were three years older.

Where does lead in water come from?

"The lead or brass service lines that connect the community water supply from streets to homes in older cities can leach lead," says Edwards. So can the lead solder or brass and lead plumbing fixtures inside many buildings.

"Sometimes just one tap in a house might be providing water loaded with lead," notes Edwards. "It could be because some plumber had a bad day and did some sloppy soldering 40 years ago when your house was being built."

A case in point: The ex-mayor of a North Carolina town had suffered from chronic fatigue for years. "The kitchen tap in her apartment was perfectly clean," Edwards reports. "It was her bathroom faucet that had just outrageously high amounts of lead." All it took was an occasional drink of water from the bathroom tap.

Another potential source: hot tap water, which can contain high levels of dissolved lead.

"We're finding that there's quite a heavy use of hot tap water by the elderly to make tea, coffee, soup, and other foods," says Edwards. "And some devices that are used to heat water—like coffeemakers and those electric heating coils that are submerged directly into a cup of water—can dissolve high levels of lead into the water. It's safer to take cold water and heat it in a teapot on the stove."

What to Do

"People shouldn't panic, because the vast majority of taps in this country are safe," says Edwards. "Maybe only one out of 100 faucets is dispensing hazardous levels of lead into the water." That may not seem like many, says Edwards, "but if that's your family and that's your house, it's not good."

For about $20 per sample, you can have your water tested for lead. But testing isn't 100 percent reliable.

"We're discovering that little pieces of lead particles or solder, or lead rust that has corroded, can flake off the insides of pipes," says Edwards. "And that can deliver very, very high doses of lead" that a one-time test can miss.

The solution: a filter that removes lead at the faucet for all the water you use for cooking and drinking. "If there's a lead problem; it's probably coming from your plumbing, so you've got to treat it right at the end of the system," says Edwards.

Disinfection Byproducts

"Chlorine is an extremely good disinfectant for killing disease-causing bacteria and viruses in drinking water," says Paul Westerhoff director of Arizona State University's School of Sustainable Engineering and the Built Environment. "Plus, it's cheap."

That's why more than half the country's water treatment plants use chlorine. Another 30 percent use chloramine, a combination of chlorine and ammonia. Others use ozone. But there's a downside to those disinfectants.

"Chlorine combines with organic matter that is naturally found in water to form hundreds of compounds called disinfection byproducts, or DBPs," says Westerhoff. Chloramine and ozone produce smaller amounts of DBPs.

The EPA regulates the 11 most common and best-studied DBPs. Nine of the 11 cause cancer in laboratory animals.[4]

"This is an absolutely clear-cut case of humans' being exposed to chemicals that are known to be toxic in high doses," says David Savitz of the Mount Sinai School of Medicine in New York. "We all drink this water." (The EPA estimates that 94 percent of Americans consume foods and beverages that are made with chlorinated water.)

"The question is whether the DBPs are present at high enough levels to have measurable adverse effects on our health," Savitz explains. Researchers have focused on bladder cancer and pregnancy.

- **Bladder cancer.** "Using water with elevated levels of DBPs over years or decades does appear to be associated with a small increased risk of bladder cancer," says Savitz.

  A 2004 meta-analysis of studies pooled from the United States, Canada, France, Italy, and Finland found that men—but not women—whose tap water contained an average of more than 1 part per billion of DBPs (the legal limit is 80 ppb) had a 24 percent greater risk of being diagnosed with bladder cancer than men who had no more than 1 ppb in their water.[5]

  The EPA estimates that from 2 to 17 percent of the 56,000 new cases of bladder cancer each year in the United States may be caused by DBPs in

---

Is Bottled Water Better?

Is bottled water safer than tap water?

"There are not a lot of outbreaks associated with bottled water," notes the University of Arizona's Kelly Reynolds. But it's not clear whether that's because bottled water is less contaminated, or because it's harder to pin outbreaks on it.

"Bottled water gets distributed all over the country," says Reynolds. "If it caused an outbreak, that might be hard to identify."

In theory, *purified* bottled water should be safer. "Many bottled water companies start with tap water that has met all federal standards," notes Reynolds. "And the companies often add an additional treatment"—something like ultraviolet light or ozone to further disinfect the water or reverse osmosis to remove chemicals. "So you do sometimes get a higher standard of treatment."

The two big differences between tap and bottled water:

- The EPA, which regulates tap water, requires utilities to notify consumers when their water fails to meet legal standards. The FDA, which regulates bottled water, doesn't require bottlers to do the same. (The EPA's and FEA's standards are essentially the same.) So bottled-water drinkers are unlikely to know about any violations.
- Tap water doesn't come in plastic bottles that can end up in landfills.

BOTTLE BASICS

Purified Water: Most likely municipal tap water that has been distilled or treated with a process like deionization or reverse osmosis to remove impurities. The two major bottled drinking waters, Dasani and Aquafina, are purified water.

Spring Water: Comes from an underground formation from which water flows naturally to the surface of the earth. May be collected only at the spring or through a borehole tapping the underground formation that feeds the spring.

Mineral Water: Contains not less than 250 parts per million total dissolved mineral solids when it emerges from its source. No minerals can be added.

Sparkling Bottled Water: Contains the same amount of carbon dioxide that it had as it emerged from its source. (Companies sometimes add CO_2 to replace what's lost during bottling.) Depending on the source, it may be labeled something like "sparkling drinking water," "sparkling mineral water," or "sparkling spring water."

Source: Adapted from the International Bottled Water Association (bottledwater.org/content/labeling-0).

drinking water. When the agency slightly lowered the maximum levels of some DBPs permitted in water in 2006, it estimated that the move would prevent about 275 cancer cases a year.

New research suggests that breathing in some DBPs and absorbing them through the skin could be more harmful than swallowing DBPs. Roughly half of our exposure to chlorinated water comes from washing with it and being near running water and flushing toilets, notes Savitz.

- **Pregnancy.** "Tap Water can Increase Risk of Miscarriages During First Trimester," warned the Associated Press headline in 1998. In a study of roughly 5,000 pregnant women in northern California, those who lived where the tap water contained more than 75 parts per billion of disinfection byproducts were nearly twice as likely to miscarry, but only if they drank at least five glasses of water a day.[6]

But a later study by Savitz found no link between DBPs and miscarriage in 2,400 pregnant women in Texas, Tennessee, and North Carolina.[7] "It was a pretty sophisticated study and it didn't corroborate the California research," says Savitz, then at the University of North Carolina in Chapel Hill.

Levels of the 11 regulated DBPs in drinking water have dropped by 60 to 90 percent since the early 1970s. "Their regulation has led to a huge improvement in drinking water quality," notes Westerhoff.

But there are more than 600 DBPs in water, and "new research over the last decade suggests that some of the unregulated ones that occur at very low concentrations are actually more genotoxic than the 11 regulated ones," he adds.

Genotoxic compounds damage DNA and can cause cancer. Among the metropolitan areas with the highest levels of the 11 regulated DBPs: Baltimore, Boston, Little Rock, Phoenix, and Washington, DC.

What to Do

Use a water filter that's certified to reduce volatile organic compounds (VOCs), which include DBPs.

Other Chemicals

"There's growing evidence that numerous chemicals in water are more dangerous than previously thought, but the EPA still gives them a clean bill of health," Linda Birnbaum, director of the government's National Institute of Environmental Health Sciences, told *The New York Times* in December 2009.

"These chemicals accumulate in body tissue. They affect developmental and hormonal systems in ways we don't understand." Some examples:

- **Atrazine.** It's the pesticide most often found in drinking water, especially in the Midwest, where it's applied to cornfields to kill weeds. It's also widely used on lawns, in parks, and on golf courses.

All of the watersheds monitored by the EPA, and some 40 percent of groundwater samples from agricultural areas, test positive for atrazine, according to the Natural Resources Defense Council.

In some studies, women living in areas with higher levels of atrazine in the drinking water were more likely to have lower-birth-weight babies. And in two studies, women in those areas were at higher risk of having babies with gastroschisis, a birth defect in which the intestines, stomach, or liver push through a hole in the abdominal wall.[8]

The EPA limits atrazine in drinking water to 3 parts per billion when averaged over an entire year. But people in agricultural areas may be exposed to much higher levels when use of the pesticide spikes during the growing season. The EPA says that it is reevaluating the safety of atrazirte, and will decide "whether new restrictions are necessary to better protect health and the environment."

- **Perchlorde.** It's an ingredient in solid fuels used for explosives, fireworks, road flares, and rocket motors. It also occurs naturally and is a byproduct that forms in bleach. And it can be detected in drinking water and groundwater in 35 states and in the urine of just about every American.[9]

In large amounts, perchlorate blocks iodine from reaching the thyroid gland, which can make it harder to produce thyroid hormone. Perchlorate may also block the transfer of iodine from mother to fetus, which can hinder normal growth.

California, Massachusetts, and New Jersey limit perchlorate levels in drinking water. In 2008, the EPA concluded that national perchlorate regulations wouldn't produce a great enough public health benefit. The agency now says that it's reevaluating its decision.

"It's extremely difficult for water utilities to remove perchlorate," says University of Arizona water expert Shane Snyder. "The only technologies available are ion exchange, which is extremely rare in water treatment systems, or a reverse osmosis system that's also rarely used because it is energy-intensive."

How to Choose a Water Filter

Point-of-use filters remove contaminants at the faucet, so they protect you from lead and other pollutants that may have gotten into your water after it left the treatment plant.

How do you go about choosing one for your home? "There's no one technology that takes everything out of water," says Joseph Harrison, former technical director at the Water Quality Association, a trade group of water filter manufacturers. Your choice generally narrows down to one or a combination of these basic types of filters:

Activated carbon: When water passes over the granular activated carbon or powdered carbon block, the negative ions of the contaminants are attracted to the slight positive charge of the carbon.

Reverse osmosis: A semipermeable membrane traps contaminants that activated carbon can't. Chlorine degrades the membranes, so most units contain activated carbon prefilters. Reverse osmosis is inefficient; it typically wastes three to five gallons of water for every gallon filtered. And it filters out good minerals like calcium and fluoride along with the contaminants.

Ion exchange: As water percolates through bead-like resins, ions in the water are swapped for ions on the beads. The system is used mostly to soften water.

Which filtration system is for you? That depends on what kind of protection you want and how much you're willing to spend:

1. **For basic protection.** Get an activated carbon filter that's certified to reduce lead, cysts, and volatile organic compounds (VOCs). Filtering VOCs should help protect you from disinfection byproducts (DBPs), atrazine and some other pesticides, and several dozen other contaminants. The filter should also be certified to eliminate the taste and smell of chlorine.

   Check the filter's box or literature to make sure that the claims for lead, VOCs, and any other contaminants have been certified using NSF/ANSI Standard 53. Claims that the filter eliminates "aesthetic" contaminants (like taste, odor, or chlorine) should be certified using NSF/ANSI Standard 42. The non-profit

NSF International establishes standards for consumer goods and certifies products.

2. **To filter out bacteria and viruses.** Get a system that has been certified for micro-biological purification by the Water Quality Association (WQA), NSF International, or Underwriters Laboratories (UL). It could consist of an ultraviolet light to disinfect the water or a filter with pores so fine that microorganisms can't get through them.
3. **To target contaminants you know are in your water.** Have your tap water tested. Or get a copy of the Consumer Confidence Report that most water utilities are required to mail out by July 1 of every year. Many utilities also post the reports on their website. If your water has elevated levels of any contaminants, look for a filter that has been certified to reduce them.
4. **For the cleanest water on your block.** "Get a reverse osmosis system plus an activated carbon system," says Harrison. Then add a filter that has been certified for microbiological purification.

Before You Buy Any Filter

Check the website of the California Department of Public Health (cdph.ca.gov/certlic/device/Pages/WTD2009Directory .aspx). If the filter you're looking at is sold in California, the website will tell you whether its claims have been verified by independent, state-approved laboratories.

The website lists all approved models and what they are certified to remove, and has separate lists of filters that have been certified to remove arsenic, *Cryptosporidium* and *Giardia* cysts, fluoride, chromium, lead, bacteria and viruses, MTBE (a gasoline additive), nitrates, perchlorate, radium, and volatile organic compounds (VOCs) like disinfection byproducts (DBPs) and atrazine.

For basic information on the water supply and the effectiveness of different kinds of filters, see the EPA's booklet "Water on Tap" (www.epa.gov/safewater/wot/pdfs/ book_waterontap_full.pdf). For questions about your drinking water, you can call the EPA's Safe Drinking Water Hotline (800-426-4791).

- **Drugs.** When you take an aspirin, or birth control pills, or Lipitor, or another drug, tiny amounts end up in the toilet bowl, where they're flushed into the sewage system and, eventually, into a wastewater treatment plant.

"Conventional wastewater plants typically remove more than 90 percent of these compounds," explains Snyder. "But even if you have 99.99 percent removal, that still leaves parts per trillion in the water which is subsequently discharged into rivers and streams." And that water, with its drug residues, can eventually end up coming out of your tap.

While the traces of drugs in drinking water are one-ten-thousandth to one-hundred-thousandth the amount in any therapeutic dose, "I don't know that we can completely dismiss the impact on human health," says Snyder, "because we don't know much about the toxicity of mixtures of drugs. But based on the concentrations of the individual compounds, harm to humans doesn't appear to be likely."

What to Do

- **Atrazine.** Use a filter that's certified to reduce levels of volatile organic compounds (VOCs), which include atrazine.

- **Perchlorate.** Only reverse osmosis and ion exchange filters reduce perchlorate.
- **Drugs.** Claims that filters reduce drug residues are based on the manufacturers' own tests. Official standards to verify the tests are in the works, though.

Notes

1. *Am. J. Public Health 91:* 1194, 2001
2. *Int. J. Food Microbiol. 92:* 289, 2004.
3. *Environ. Health Perspect. 117:* 574, 2009.
4. *Mutation Research 636:* 178, 2007.
5. *Epidemiology 15:* 357, 2004.
6. *Epidemiology 9:* 134, 1998.
7. *Epidemiology 19:* 729 and 738, 2008.
8. *Am. J. Obstet. Gynecol. 202:* 241, 2010.
9. *J. Expo. Sci. Environ. Epidemiol. 17:* 400, 2007.

Critical Thinking

1. What are the four most common biological contaminants (bacteria and viruses) found in our water supply?
2. How can water from household faucets be contaminated with bacteria by humans or pets?
3. What are the detrimental effects of consuming lead, other than the well-known effects on the brain and nervous system?

Inside the Meat Lab

A handful of scientists aim to satisfy the world's growing appetite for steak without wrecking the planet. The first step: grab a petri dish.

Jeffrey Bartholet

It is not unusual for visionaries to be impassioned, if not fanatical, and Willem van Eelen is no exception. At 87, van Eelen can look back on an extraordinary life. He was born in Indonesia when it was under Dutch control, the son of a doctor who ran a leper colony. As a teenager, he fought the Japanese in World War II and spent several years in prisoner-of-war camps. The Japanese guards used prisoners as slave labor and starved them. "If one of the stray dogs was stupid enough to go over the wire, the prisoners would jump on it, tear it apart and eat it raw," van Eelen recalls. "If you looked at my stomach then, you saw my spine. I was already dead." The experience triggered a lifelong obsession with food, nutrition and the science of survival.

One obsession led to another. After the Allies liberated Indonesia, van Eelen studied medicine at the University of Amsterdam. A professor showed the students how he had been able to get a piece of muscle tissue to grow in the laboratory. This demonstration inspired van Eelen to consider the possibility of growing edible meat without having to raise or slaughter animals. Imagine, he thought, protein-rich food that could be grown like crops, no matter what the climate or other environmental conditions, without killing any living creatures.

If anything, the idea is more potent now. The world population was just more than two billion in 1940, and global warming was not a concern. Today the planet is home to three times as many people. According to a 2006 report by the Food and Agriculture Organization, the livestock business accounts for about 18 percent of all anthropogenic greenhouse gas emissions—an even larger contribution than the global transportation sector. The organization expects worldwide meat consumption to nearly double between 2002 and 2050.

Under normal conditions, 10 cells could grow into 50,000 metric tons of meat in just two months. One such cell line would be sufficient to feed the world.

Meat grown in bioreactors—instead of raised on farms—could help alleviate planetary stress. Hanna Tuomisto, a Ph.D. candidate at the University of Oxford, co-authored a study last year on the potential environmental impacts of cultured meat. The study found that such production, if scientists grew the muscle cells in a culture of cyanobacteria hydrolysate (a bacterium cultivated in ponds), would involve "approximately 35 to 60 percent lower energy use, 80 to 95 percent lower greenhouse gas emissions and 98 percent lower land use compared to conventionally produced meat products in Europe."

As it is, 30 percent of the earth's ice-free land is used for grazing livestock and growing animal feed. If cultured meat were to become viable and widely consumed, much of that land could be used for other purposes, including new forests that would pull carbon out of the air. Meat would no longer have to be shipped around the globe, because production sites could be located close to consumers. Some proponents imagine small urban meat labs selling their products at street markets that cater to locavores.

The Only Choice Left

Even Winston Churchill thought in vitro meat was a good idea. "Fifty years hence, we shall escape the absurdity of growing a whole chicken in order to eat the breast or wing by growing these parts separately under suitable medium," he predicted in a 1932 book, *Thoughts and Adventures*. For most of the 20th century, however, few took the idea seriously. Van Eelen did not let it go. He worked all kinds of jobs—selling newspapers, driving a taxi, making dollhouses. He established an organization to help underprivileged kids and owned art galleries and cafes. He wrote proposals for in vitro meat production and eventually plowed much of his earnings into applying for patents. Together with two partners, he won a Dutch patent in 1999, then other European patents and, eventually, two U.S. patents. In 2005 he and others finally convinced the Dutch Ministry of Economic Affairs to pledge €2 million to support in vitro meat research in the Netherlands—the largest government grant for such research to date.

By that time, an American scientist had already succeeded in growing a piece of fish filet in a lab. Using a small grant from NASA, which was interested in developing food sources for deep-space voyages, Morris Benjaminson removed skeletal muscle from a common goldfish and grew it outside the fish's body. Then an associate briefly marinated the explants in olive oil, chopped garlic, lemon and pepper, covered them in bread crumbs and deep-fried them. "A panel of female colleagues gave it a visual and sniff test," says Benjaminson, now an emeritus professor at Touro College in Bay Shore, N.Y. "It looked and smelled pretty much the same as any fish you could buy at the supermarket." But NASA, apparently convinced there were easier ways to provide protein to astronauts on long deep-space voyages, declined to further fund Benjaminson's research.

The Dutch money was used by van Eelen and H. P. Haagsman, a scientist at Utrecht University, to fund a consortium that would aim to show that stem cells could be taken from farm animals, cultured and induced to become

GLOBAL TRENDS

Meaty Problems

The rich world already eats a lot of meat; the developing world is catching up. One reason is that as more people move to cities, improved infrastructure means that meat can be kept cold throughout its journey from the slaughterhouse to the kitchen. Yet as demand for meat increases, so will the environmental consequences. Livestock farming already accounts for 17.8 percent of all anthropogenic greenhouse gas emissions.

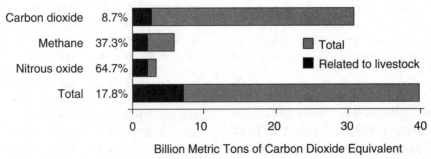

skeletal muscle cells. The team included a representative from meat company Meester Stegeman BV, then part of Sara Lee Corporation in Europe, and top scientists at three Dutch universities. Each university studied different aspects of in vitro meat production. Scientists at the University of Amsterdam focused on producing efficient growth media; a group at Utrecht worked on isolating stem cells, making them proliferate and coaxing them into muscle cells; and those at Eindhoven University of Technology attempted to "train" the muscle cells to grow larger.

The scientists made some progress. They were able to grow small, thin strips of muscle tissue in the lab—stuff that looked like bits of scallop and had the chewy texture of calamari—but several obstacles remained to commercial-scale production. "We gained knowledge; we knew a lot more, but we still didn't have [something that tasted like] a T-bone steak that came from a petri dish," says Peter Verstrate, who represented Meester Stegeman in the consortium and now works as a consultant. In time, the Dutch money ran out.

Van Eelen now fumes that one scientist involved was "stupid" and others just milked him and the Dutch government for money. "I don't know what they did in four years—talking, talking, talking—every year taking more of the money," he says. For their part, the scientists say that van Eelen never understood the scale of the challenge. "He had a naive idea that you could put muscle cells in a petri dish and they would just grow, and if you put money into a project, you'd have meat in a couple of years," says Bernard Roelen, a cell biologist who worked on the project at Utrecht.

Van Eelen was not the only one who imagined a revolution. In 2005 an article in *The New York Times* concluded that "in a few years' time there may be a lab-grown meat ready to market as sausages or patties." A couple of months before the story appeared, researchers had published the first peer-reviewed article on cultured meat in the journal *Tissue Engineering*. The authors included Jason G. Matheny, co-founder of the lab-produced meat advocacy group New Harvest. He understands the challenges better than most. "Tissue engineering is really hard and extremely expensive right now," he says. "To enjoy market adoption, we mainly need to solve the technical problems that increase the cost of engineered meat." That will take money, he notes, and few governments or organizations have been willing to commit necessary funding.

To the scientists involved, that failure seems short-sighted. "I think [in vitro meat] will be the only choice left," says Mark J. Post, head of the physiology department at Maastricht University. "I'm very bold about this. I don't see any way you could still rely on old-fashioned livestock in the coming decades."

Assembly Required

In theory, an in vitro meat factory would work something like this: First, technicians would isolate embryonic or adult stem cells from a pig, cow, chicken or other animal. Then they would grow those cells in bioreactors, using a culture derived from plants. The stem cells would divide and redivide for months on end. Technicians would next instruct the cells to differentiate into muscle (rather than, say, bone or brain cells). Finally, the muscle cells would need to be "bulked up" in a fashion similar to the way in which animals build their strength by exercising.

For now there are challenges at every stage of this process. One difficulty is developing stem cell lines that can proliferate for long periods without suddenly deciding they want to differentiate on their own. Another challenge is to be sure that when stem cells are prompted to differentiate, the overwhelming majority of them turn into muscle as instructed. "If 10 cells differentiate, you want at least seven or eight to turn into muscle cells, not three or four," Roelen says. "We can achieve 50 percent now."

The Utrecht scientists tried to extract and develop embryonic stem cell lines from pigs. Such cells would, in normal conditions, be able to duplicate every day for long periods, meaning 10 cells could grow into a staggering amount of potential meat in just two months—more than 50,000 metric tons. "Culturing embryonic stem cells would be ideal for this purpose since these cells have an (almost) infinite self-renewal capacity," according to a 2009 report by the Utrecht team. "In theory, one such cell line would be sufficient to literally feed the world."

Until now, however, such cell lines have been developed only from mice, rats, rhesus monkeys and humans. Embryonic cells from farm animals have had a tendency to differentiate quickly—and of their own accord—into specialized cells. In the report, Utrecht team's porcine cells often veered toward "a neural lineage"—brains, not bacon.

The Utrecht group also worked with adult stem cells, which have the advantage of being largely preprogrammed. These cells exist within skeletal muscle (as well as other parts of the body) with a specific mission: to do repair work when tissue is injured or dies off. So if you are making in vitro meat and want stem cells that will almost surely turn into muscle tissue, adult stem cells from skeletal muscle tissue should work very well. Until now, however, scientists have not been able to get these cells to proliferate as readily as they can embryonic cells.

Cost is another barrier. The culture used to grow stem cells of any kind is very expensive. With currently available media, it might cost $50,000 to produce a pound of meat, according to Roelen, and the most efficient nutrient bath is derived from fetal calf or horse serum taken from slaughtered animals. In recent years scientists have developed their own recipes for "chemically defined media" that include no animal products. By using recombinant-DNA technology, they have also been able to get plant cells to produce animal proteins that could be used to grow the meat. But both these types of media are, for now, prohibitively expensive. An algae-based medium may eventually work best because algae can produce the proteins and amino acids necessary to sustain cell life, but that, too, is costly—at least for now.

Once the researchers get a big supply of muscle cells, they will need to keep them alive and bulk them up. It is possible now to engineer a thin strip of tissue, but if it gets thicker than a few cell layers, parts of it start to die off. The cells need a constant flow of fresh nutrients to stay alive. In the body, these nutrients are delivered by the bloodstream, which also removes waste. Post is working on how to develop a three-dimensional system that delivers such nutrients.

He is also exploring bulking up the muscle cells. "If you take your cast off after a bone break, it scares you: the muscles are gone," he says. "But within a couple of weeks they're back. We need to replicate that process." The body achieves this in several ways, including exercise. In a lab setting, scientists can stimulate the tissue with electrical pulses. But that is costly and inefficient, bulking up the cells by only about 10 percent. Another method is simply to provide anchor points: once the cells are able to attach to different anchors, they develop tension on their own. Post has made anchors available by providing a scaffold of sugar polymers, which degrades over time. But at this stage, he says, "We're not looking at Schwarzenegger muscle cells."

He has one more method in mind, one he thinks might work best. But it is also more complex. The body naturally stimulates muscle growth with tiny micropulses of chemicals such as acetylcholine. These chemicals are cheap, which is part of what makes this approach appealing. "The trick is to do it in very, very short pulses," Post says. The hurdles to that are technological, not scientific.

Breakthroughs in all these areas will take money, of course. In 2008 People for the Ethical Treatment of Animals (PETA) offered $1 million to the first person or persons who could grow commercially viable chicken in a lab by 2012. But that was mainly a publicity stunt and no help to scientists who need money to get research done now. More seriously, the Dutch government recently pledged roughly €800,000 toward a new four-year project that would continue the stem cell research at Utrecht—and also initiate a study on the social and moral questions related to in vitro meat.

The Ick Factor

Some see social acceptance as the biggest barrier of all to producing in vitro meat on a commercial scale. "I've mentioned cultured meat to scientists, and they all think, 'great idea,'" says Oxford's Tuomisto. "When I talk to nonscientists, they are more afraid of it. It sounds scary. Yet it's basically the same stuff: muscle cells. It's just produced differently."

Cor van der Weele of Wageningen University is heading up the philosophical aspects of the new Dutch study (for example, is cultured meat a moral imperative or morally repugnant, or some combination of the two?). She has been intrigued by the emotional reactions that some people have toward the idea. "We call it the 'yuck response,'" she says. "People initially think that it might be something contaminated or disgusting."

But that perception can change quickly, van der Weele observes. She notes that people often associate cultured meat with two other ideas: genetically modified foods—which are often seen, particularly in Europe, as a dangerous corporate scheme to dominate or control the food supply—and negative perceptions of the meat industry in general, with its factory farms, disease and mistreatment of animals. Once people realize that cultured meat is not genetically modified and could be a clean, animal-friendly alternative to factory farms, she says, "the scared, very negative response is often very fleeting."

Such observations are only anecdotal, of course. The study will assess popular responses to in vitro meat in detail—comparing reactions across different regions and cultures—and will determine ways to frame the issue that might enhance consumer interest. Proponents imagine a day when governments will levy special environmental taxes on meat produced from livestock or when consumers will be able to opt for in vitro meat that is labeled "cruelty-free."

"I don't think you want to know about the hygienic conditions in the majority of slaughterhouses in the U.S. or the efficiency of euthanasia," says Post, who spent six years at Harvard University and Dartmouth College before returning home to the Netherlands in 2002. Another outbreak of disease—like mad cow or bird flu—could make cultured meat seem all the more appetizing. "We are far from what we eat," Roelen says. "When we're eating a hamburger, we don't think, 'I'm eating a dead cow.' And when people are already so far from what they eat, it's not too hard to see them accepting cultured meat."

Post has a bold scheme to attract new funding: he aims to create an in vitro sausage just to demonstrate that it is possible. He estimates that it will cost €300,000 and take six months of work by two doctoral students using three incubators. "We'll take two or three biopsies of a pig—say, 10,000 stem cells," Post says. "After 20 population doublings, we'll have 10 billion cells." The students will use 3,000 petri dishes to produce many tiny bits of porcine muscle tissue, which then will be packed into a casing with some spices and other nonmeat ingredients to give it taste and texture. In the end, scientists will be able to display the sausage next to the living pig from which it was grown.

"It's basically a stunt to generate more funds," Post says. "We're trying to prove to the world we can make a product out of this." But will it taste like a sausage? "I think so," Roelen says. "Most of the taste in a chicken nugget or a sausage is artificially made. Salt and all kinds of other things are added to give it taste."

Van Eelen, who regards himself as "the godfather of in vitro meat," is not a fan of the sausage proposal. He is a diehard idealist and thinks it is important to launch the in vitro revolution with meat that looks, smells and tastes just like anything you would buy off the farm. Van Eelen probably also realizes that time is running out to realize a dream that he has pursued nearly his entire life. "Every time you talk to him, he's speaking about someone else he's found who will be the top scientist who will solve his problems," Roelen says. "I can understand his point of view. But I can't change the laws of the universe."

More to Explore

Production of Animal Proteins by Cell Systems. H. P. Haagsman, K. J. Hellingwerf and B. A. J. Roelen. University of Utrecht, October 2009.

Livestock Production: Recent Trends, Future Prospects. Philip K. Thornton in *Philosophical Transactions of the Royal Society B*, vol. 365, no. 1554, pages 2853–2867; September 27, 2010.

Food: A Taste of Things to Come? Nicola Jones in *Nature,* vol. 468, pages 752–753; 2010.

Animal-Free Meat Biofabrication. B. F. Bhat and Z. Bhat in *American Journal of Food Technology,* vol. 6, no. 6, pages 441–459; 2011.

New Harvest: www.new-harvest.org.

Critical Thinking

1. What life events led Willem van Eelen to pursue a career of producing meat in a lab?

2. Discuss the advantages and disadvantages to growing meat in a lab.

3. Critique the concept of meat grown in a petri dish going mainstream.

4. Explain how the world's food supply and agriculture change if we could harvest meat in a petri dish

JEFFREY BARTHOLET is a veteran foreign correspondent and former Washington bureau chief for *Newsweek* magazine.

UNIT 8

Hunger, Nutrition, and Sustainability

Unit Selections

Learning Outcomes

After reading this Unit, you will be able to

- Define the Thrifty Food Plan (TFP) and evaluate whether the TFP is an effective way to determine the lowest cost for a healthy diet in the United States.

- Evaluate the advantages and disadvantages of using synthetic fertilizers.

- Explain why a plant-based diet will lead to less destruction of the atmosphere and pollutants of our water supplies.

- Define food insecurity.

- Evaluate the causes of the nutrition and health disparities among native people.

- List the factors that impact the price of the global food supply.

- Identify the barriers to international food assistance and education programs.

- Explain how double vouchers could be used to increase the fruit and vegetable intake of SNAP participants.

- Define perennial grain crops and explain how perennial grain crops differ from annual grain crops.

- Identify the three grain crops that provide 70 percent of the calories for human consumption worldwide.

Student Website

www.mhhe.com/cls

Internet References

Food and Agriculture Organization of the United Nations (FAO)
   www.fao.org
Population Reference Bureau
   www.prb.org
U.S. Sustainable Agriculture Research and Education Program, University of California-Davis
   www.sarep.ucdavis.edu/concept.htm
World Health Organization (WHO)
   www.who.int/en

Considering the economic instability of the past years, more Americans are living at or below the poverty level. The changes in our economy and employment rates lead many Americans in general to spend less money on food for themselves and their families. It is possible to consume fresh and nutritious foods on a tight budget, but it is challenging in our current food culture. Several articles in this unit describe some of the challenges that low-income populations face in obtaining nutritious foods and what can be done to improve the accessibility of nutritious foods for those that struggle to feed their families.

Malnutrition is the main culprit for lowered resistance to disease, infection, and death, especially in children. The malnutrition-infection combination results in stunted growth, lowered mental development in children, lowered productivity, and higher incidence of degenerative disease in adulthood. This directly affects the economies of developing countries. Over 1 billion people globally suffer from micronutrient malnutrition frequently called "hidden hunger." In addition, partnerships between the public and private sectors may prove valuable in combating malnutrition. Solutions to these problems such as building sustainable systems through indigenous knowledge and practices that are community based and environmentally friendly with emphasis on biofortification and dietary diversification may combat hunger and nutrient deficiencies in the future.

Malnutrition not only affects children and adults in developing countries, but it is also prevalent in the United States. Thirty million Americans (including 11 million children), experience food insecurity and hunger. In a country where one-fifth of the food is wasted and 130 pounds of food per person is disposed of, it is unacceptable that Americans go hungry. Food security is now critical to consumers worldwide.

Nutrient deficiencies magnify the effect of disease, resulting in more severe symptoms and greater complications in countries with developing economies. For example, vitamin A deficiency leads to blindness in about 250,000–300,000 children annually and exacerbates the symptoms of measles. Iron deficiency, which is widespread among pregnant women and those in the child-bearing years in developing countries, increases the risk of death from hemorrhage in their offspring and reduces physical productivity and learning capacity. Finally, iodine deficiency causes brain damage and mental retardation. It is estimated that 1.5 billion people are at risk for iodine deficiency disorders.

The final two articles are about sustainable agriculture versus conventional agricultural practices. Current conventional

© Dimitri Vervitsiotis/Getty Images

agricultural techniques depend on nitrogen-based fertilizers for crop production; however, as the use of these chemical fertilizers spreads to other countries, it is posing threats to our health and the health of our ecosystems. The article by Townsend and Howarth describes the history of nitrogen-based fertilizers and the damage that results from too much nitrogen in our atmosphere. The other agriculture article addresses food security through genetically modifying grain crops to be perennial crops rather than annual crops. Our agricultural grain crops are annuals, meaning the plants must be planted each year from seed and the plants are cleared from the fields at the end of the growing season. Plant geneticists are now able to develop perennial grain plants that could have significant ecological, environmental, and health benefits to the world's food supply.

Many of the articles in this unit focus on food insecurity, hunger, and food/health disparities. This topic was emphasized in this unit because of the growing number of food insecure households in the United States as a result of the economy. The topic of hunger has always been a central focus in international nutrition; however, more people in the United States are affected by food insecurity, even with the abundant amount of food that is wasted here. Food assistance programs are needed domestically as well as for the millions of undernourished people living in developing countries.

Divided We Eat

As more of us indulge our passion for local, organic delicacies, a growing number of Americans don't have enough nutritious food to eat.
How we can bridge the gap.

LISA MILLER

For breakfast, I usually have a cappuccino—espresso made in an Alessi pot and mixed with organic milk, which has been gently heated and hand-fluffed by my husband. I eat two slices of imported cheese—Dutch Parrano, the label says, "the hippest cheese in New York" (no joke)—on homemade bread with butter. I am what you might call a food snob. My nutritionist neighbor drinks a protein shake while her 5-year-old son eats quinoa porridge sweetened with applesauce and laced with kale flakes. She is what you might call a health nut. On a recent morning, my neighbor's friend Alexandra Ferguson sipped politically correct Nicaraguan coffee in her comfy kitchen while her two young boys chose from among an assortment of organic cereals. As we sat, the six chickens Ferguson and her husband, Dave, keep for eggs in a backyard coop peered indoors from the stoop. The Fergusons are known as locavores.

Alexandra says she spends hours each day thinking about, shopping for, and preparing food. She is a disciple of Michael Pollan, whose 2006 book *The Omnivore's Dilemma* made the locavore movement a national phenomenon, and believes that eating organically and locally contributes not only to the health of her family but to the existential happiness of farm animals and farmers—and, indeed, to the survival of the planet. "Michael Pollan is my new hero, next to Jimmy Carter," she told me. In some neighborhoods, a lawyer who raises chickens in her backyard might be considered eccentric, but we live in Park Slope, Brooklyn, a community that accommodates and celebrates every kind of foodie. Whether you believe in eating for pleasure, for health, for justice, or for some idealized vision of family life, you will find neighbors who reflect your food values. In Park Slope, the contents of a child's lunchbox can be fodder for a 20-minute conversation.

Over coffee, I cautiously raise a subject that has concerned me of late: less than five miles away, some children don't have enough to eat; others exist almost exclusively on junk food. Alexandra concedes that her approach is probably out of reach for those people. Though they are not wealthy by Park Slope standards—Alexandra works part time and Dave is employed by the city—the Fergusons spend approximately 20 percent of their income, or $1,000 a month, on food. The average American spends 13 percent, including restaurants and takeout.

And so the conversation turns to the difficulty of sharing their interpretation of the Pollan doctrine with the uninitiated. When they visit Dave's family in Tennessee, tensions erupt over food choices. One time, Alexandra remembers, she irked her mother-in-law by purchasing a bag of organic apples, even though her mother-in-law had already bought the nonorganic kind at the grocery store. The old apples were perfectly good, her mother-in-law said. Why waste money—and apples?

The Fergusons recall Dave's mother saying something along these lines: "When we come to your place, we don't complain about your food. Why do you complain about ours? It's not like our food is poison."

"I can't convince my brother to spend another dime on food," adds Dave.

"This is our charity. This is my giving to the world," says Alexandra, finally, as she packs lunchboxes—organic peanut butter and jelly on grainy bread, a yogurt, and a clementine—for her two boys. "We contribute a lot."

According to data released last week by the U.S. Department of Agriculture, 17 percent of Americans—more than 50 million people—live in households that are "food insecure," a term that means a family sometimes runs out of money to buy food, or it sometimes runs out of food before it can get more money. Food insecurity is especially high in households headed by a single mother. It is most severe in the South, and in big cities. In New York City, 1.4 million people are food insecure, and 257,000 of them live near me, in Brooklyn. Food insecurity is linked, of course, to other economic measures like housing and employment, so it surprised no one that the biggest surge in food insecurity since the agency established the measure in 1995 occurred between 2007 and 2008, at the start of the economic downturn. (The 2009 numbers, released last week, showed little change.) The proportion of households that qualify as "hungry"—with what the USDA calls "very low food security"—is small, about 6 percent. Reflected against the obsessive concerns of the foodies in my circle, and the glare of attention given to the plight of the poor and hungry abroad, even a fraction of starving children in America seems too high.

Mine seems on some level like a naive complaint. There have always been rich people and poor people in America and, in a capitalist economy, the well-to-do have always had the freedom to indulge themselves as they please. In hard times, food has always marked a bright border between the haves and the have-nots. In the earliest days of the Depression, as the poor waited on bread lines, the middle and upper classes in America became devoted to fad diets. Followers of the Hollywood 18-Day Diet, writes Harvey Levenstein in his 1993 book *Paradox of Plenty,* "could live on fewer than six hundred calories a day by limiting each meal to half a grapefruit, melba toast, coffee without cream or sugar, and, at lunch and dinner, some raw vegetables."

What you eat for dinner has become the definitive marker of social status.

But modern America is a place of extremes, and what you eat for dinner has become the definitive marker of social status; as the distance between rich and poor continues to grow, the freshest, most nutritious foods have become luxury goods that only some can afford. Among the lowest quintile of American families, mean household income has held relatively steady between $10,000 and $13,000 for the past two decades (in inflation-adjusted dollars); among the highest, income has jumped 20 percent to $170,800 over the same period, according to census data. What this means, in practical terms, is that the richest Americans can afford to buy berries out of season at Whole Foods—the upscale grocery chain that recently reported a 58 percent increase in its quarterly profits—while the food insecure often eat what they can: highly caloric, mass-produced foods like pizza and packaged cakes that fill them up quickly. The number of Americans on food stamps has surged by 58.5 percent over the last three years.

Corpulence used to signify the prosperity of a few but has now become a marker of poverty. Obesity has risen as the income gap has widened: more than a third of U.S. adults and 17 percent of children are obese, and the problem is acute among the poor. While obesity is a complex problem—genetics, environment, and activity level all play a role—a 2008 study by the USDA found that children and women on food stamps were likelier to be overweight than those who were not. According to studies led by British epidemiologist Kate Pickett, obesity rates are highest in developed countries with the greatest income disparities. America is among the most obese of nations; Japan, with its relatively low income inequality, is the thinnest.

Adam Drewnowski, an epidemiologist at the University of Washington, has spent his career showing that Americans' food choices correlate to social class. He argues that the most nutritious diet—lots of fruits and vegetables, lean meats, fish, and grains—is beyond the reach of the poorest Americans, and it is economic elitism for nutritionists to uphold it as an ideal without broadly addressing issues of affordability. Lower-income families don't subsist on junk food and fast food because they lack nutritional education, as some have argued. And though many poor neighborhoods are, indeed, food deserts—meaning that the people who live there don't have access to a well-stocked supermarket—many are not. Lower-income families choose sugary, fat, and processed foods because they're cheaper—and because they taste good. In a paper published last spring, Drewnowski showed how the prices of specific foods changed between 2004 and 2008 based on data from Seattle-area supermarkets. While food prices overall rose about 25 percent, the most nutritious foods (red peppers, raw oysters, spinach, mustard greens, romaine lettuce) rose 29 percent, while the least nutritious foods (white sugar, hard candy, jelly beans, and cola) rose just 16 percent.

"In America," Drewnowski wrote in an e-mail, "food has become the premier marker of social distinctions, that is to say—social class. It used to be clothing and fashion, but no longer, now that 'luxury' has become affordable and available to all." He points to an article in *The New York Times,* written by Pollan, which describes a meal element by element, including "a basket of morels and porcini gathered near Mount Shasta." "Pollan," writes Drewnowski, "is drawing a picture of class privilege that is as acute as anything written by Edith Wharton or Henry James."

I finish writing the previous paragraph and go downstairs. There, in the mail, I find the Christmas catalog from the luxury retail store Barneys. HAVE A FOODIE HOLIDAY, its cover reads. Inside, models are covered—literally—with food. A woman in a red $2,000 Lanvin trench has an enormous cabbage on her head. Another, holding a green Proenza Schouler clutch, wears a boiled crab in her bouffant. Most disconcerting is the Munnu diamond pendant ($80,500) worn by a model who seems to have traded her hair for an octopus. Its tentacles dangle past her shoulders, and the girl herself wears the expression of someone who's stayed too long at the party. Food is no longer trendy or fashionable. It is fashion.

Tiffiney Davis, a single mom, lives about four miles away from me, in subsidized housing, in a gentrifying neighborhood called Red Hook. Steps from her apartment, you can find ample evidence of foodie culture: Fairway, the supermarket where I buy my Dutch cheese, is right there, as is a chic bakery, and a new-fangled lobster pound. Davis says she has sometimes worried about having enough food. She works in Manhattan, earning $13 an hour for a corporate catering company (which once had a contract with NEWSWEEK), and she receives food stamps. She spends $100 a week on food for herself and her two kids. Sometimes she stretches her budget by bringing food home from work.

Davis is sheepish about what her family eats for breakfast. Everybody rises at 6, and there's a mad rush to get the door, so often they eat bodega food. Her daughter, Malaezia, 10, will have egg and cheese on a roll; her son, 13-year-old Tashawn, a muffin and soda. She herself used to pop into a Dunkin' Donuts for two doughnuts and a latte, but when New York chain restaurants started posting calories on their menus, she stopped. "I try my best to lessen the chemicals and the fattening stuff," she says, "but it's hard."

Time is just part of the problem, Davis explains, as she prepares Sunday dinner in her cheerful kitchen. Tonight she's making fried chicken wings with bottled barbecue sauce; yellow rice from a box; black beans from a can; broccoli; and carrots, cooked in olive oil and honey. A home-cooked dinner doesn't happen every night. On weeknights, everyone gets home, exhausted—and then there's homework. Several nights a week, they get takeout: Chinese, or Domino's, or McDonald's. Davis doesn't buy fruits and vegetables mostly because they're too expensive, and in the markets where she usually shops, they're not fresh. "I buy bananas and bring them home and 10 minutes later they're no good. . . Whole Foods sells fresh, beautiful tomatoes," she says. "Here, they're packaged and full of chemicals anyway. So I mostly buy canned foods."

In recent weeks the news in New York City has been full with a controversial proposal to ban food-stamp recipients from using their government money to buy soda. Local public-health officials insist they need to be more proactive about slowing obesity; a recent study found that 40 percent of the children in New York City's kindergarten through eighth-grade classrooms were either overweight or obese. (Nationwide, 36 percent of 6- to 11-year-olds are overweight or obese.) Opponents of the proposal call it a "nanny state" measure, another instance of government interference, and worse—of the government telling poor people what to do, as if they can't make good decisions on their own. "I think it's really difficult," says Pickett, the British epidemiologist. "Everybody needs to be able to feel that they have control over what they spend. And everybody should be able to treat themselves now and again. Why shouldn't a poor child have a birthday party with cake and soda?"

But Davis enthusiastically supports the proposal. A 9-year-old boy in her building recently died of an asthma attack, right in front of his mother. He was obese, she says, but his mom kept feeding him junk. "If these people don't care at all about calorie counts, then the government should. People would live a lot longer," she says.

Claude Fischler, a French sociologist, believes that Americans can fight both obesity and food insecurity by being more, well, like the French. Americans take an approach to food and eating that is unlike any other people in history. For one thing, we regard food primarily as (good or bad) nutrition. When asked "What is eating well?" Americans generally answer in the language of daily allowances: they talk about calories and carbs, fats, and sugars. They don't see eating as a social activity, and they don't see food—as it has been seen for millennia—as a shared resource, like a loaf of bread passed around the table. When asked "What is eating well?" the French inevitably answer in terms of "conviviality": togetherness, intimacy, and good tastes unfolding in a predictable way.

Even more idiosyncratic than our obsession with nutrition, says Fischler, is that Americans see food choice as a matter of personal freedom, an inalienable right. Americans want to eat what they want: morels or Big Macs. They want to eat where they want, in the car or alfresco. And they want to eat when they want. With the exception of Thanksgiving, when most of us dine off the same turkey menu, we are food libertarians. In surveys, Fischler has found no single time of day (or night) when Americans predictably sit together and eat. By contrast, 54 percent of the French dine at 12:30 each day. Only 9.5 percent of the French are obese.

America is one of the most obese nations; japan, with low income inequality, is the thinnest.

When I was a child I was commanded to "eat your eggs. There are starving children in Africa." And when I was old enough to think for myself, I could easily see that my own eaten or uneaten eggs would not do a single thing to help the children of Africa. This is the Brooklyn conundrum, playing out all over the country. Locally produced food is more delicious than the stuff you get in the supermarket; it's better for the small farmers and the farm animals; and, as a movement, it's better for the environment. It's easy—and probably healthy, if you can afford it—to make that choice as an individual or a family, says the New York University nutritionist Marion Nestle. Bridging the divide is much harder. "Choosing local or organic is something you can actually do. It's very difficult for people to get involved in policy."

Locavore activists in New York and other cities are doing what they can to help the poor with access to fresh food. Incentive programs give food-stamp recipients extra credit if they buy groceries at farmers' markets. Food co-ops and community-garden associations are doing better urban outreach. Municipalities are establishing bus routes between poor neighborhoods and those where well-stocked supermarkets exist.

Joel Berg, executive director of the New York City Coalition Against Hunger, says these programs are good, but they need to go much, much further. He believes, like Fischler, that the answer lies in seeing food more as a shared resource, like water, than as a consumer product, like shoes. "It's a nuanced conversation, but I think 'local' or 'organic' as the shorthand for all things good is way too simplistic," says Berg. "I think we need a broader conversation about scale, working conditions, and environmental impact. It's a little too much of people buying easy virtue."

Even the locavore hero Pollan agrees. "Essentially," he says, "we have a system where wealthy farmers feed the poor crap and poor farmers feed the wealthy high-quality food." He points to Walmart's recent announcement of a program that will put more locally grown food on its shelves as an indication that big retailers are looking to sell fresh produce in a scalable way. These fruits and vegetables might not be organic, but the goal, says Pollan, is not to be absolutist in one's food ideology. "I argue for being conscious," he says, "but perfectionism is an enemy of progress." Pollan sees a future where, in an effort to fight diabetes and obesity, health-insurance companies are advocates for small and medium-size farmers. He dreams of a broad food-policy conversation in Washington. "The food movement," he reminds me, "is still very young."

Berg believes that part of the answer lies in working with Big Food. The food industry hasn't been entirely bad: it developed the technology to bring apples to Wisconsin in the middle of winter, after all. It could surely make sustainably produced fruits and vegetables affordable and available. "We need to bring social justice to bigger agriculture as well," Berg says.

My last stop was at Jabir Suluki's house in Clinton Hill, about two miles from my home. Suluki has toast for breakfast, with a little cheese on top, melted in the toaster oven. He is not French—he was born and raised in Brooklyn—but he might as well be. Every day, between 5 and 7, he prepares dinner for his mother and himself—and any of his nieces and nephews who happen to drop by. He prepares food with the confidence of a person descended from a long line of home cooks—which he is.

Both Suluki and his mother are diabetic. For them, healthy, regular meals are a necessity—and so he does what he can on $75 a week. "To get good food, you really got to sacrifice a lot. It's expensive. But I take that sacrifice, because it's worth it." Suluki uses his food stamps at the farmers' market. He sorts through the rotten fruit at the local supermarket. He travels to Queens, when he can get a ride, and buys cheap meat in bulk. He is adamant that it is the responsibility of parents to feed their children good food in moderate portions, and that it's possible to do so on a fixed income.

For dinner he and his mother ate Salisbury steak made from ground turkey, with a little ground beef thrown in and melted cheese on top "because turkey doesn't have any taste"; roasted potatoes and green peppers; and frozen green beans, "heated quickly so they still have a crunch." For dessert, his mother ate two pieces of supermarket coffeecake.

Suluki thinks a lot about food, and the role it plays in the life of his neighbors. He doesn't have soda in his refrigerator, but he opposes the New York City soda proposal because, in light of the government's food and farm subsidies—and in light of all the other kinds of unhealthy cheap foods for sale in his supermarket—he sees it as hypocrisy. "You can't force junk on people and then criticize it at the same time." Suluki is a community organizer, and sees the web of problems before us—hunger, obesity, health—as something for the community to solve. "We can't just attack this problem as individuals," he tells me. "A healthy community produces healthy people." That's why, on the weekends, he makes a big pot of rice and beans, and brings it down to the food pantry near his house.

Critical Thinking

1. How much does the average American spend on food, including restaurants and take out?

2. What is the latest estimate of the number of Americans who live in a food insecure environment?

3. Define food insecurity.

4. Discuss the different food philosophies of the people who were included in this article.

Address Health Disparities in American Indians

Cultivating traditions and promoting nutrition can make a difference.

ELAINE KOVACS, MA, AND MELISSA IP, MA, RD

As children, we may learn about the Three Sisters—squash, corn, and beans—during elementary school explorations into American Indian life. The cultivation of the Three Sisters represented ingenuity in sustainable agricultural practices. For the Iroquois, the Three Sisters were the spiritual sustainers of life, providing complete vegetarian protein.

Yet, despite a tradition of physically active lifestyles and a diet of whole, unprocessed foods, American Indian and Alaska Native communities today are experiencing some of the worst nutrition disparities in the United States. In 2009, 67 percent of American Indians and Alaska Natives were overweight or obese.[1] (Not easily simplified, the term "American Indian and Alaska Native" describes more than 560 federally recognized tribes spread across the United States, making up 1.6 percent of the U.S. population today.[2])

With an understanding of the challenges facing this population and an awareness of the programs that are making a difference by emphasizing traditional foods and physical activity, nutrition professionals can help address the health disparities affecting American Indians.

Contextualizing American Indian Health

In addressing health disparities such as obesity, diabetes, and food insecurity, context always matters. Traditionally speaking, American Indians regard food as more than just sustenance; it is a way of life. But as American Indians face limited resources, geographic isolation, and a failing government food aid system, particularly for those living on rural reservations, they are more likely to experience malnutrition and food insecurity than the general U.S. population.[3] Food aid provided to the tribes continues to be insufficient and often of low quality, ignoring the addition of traditional American Indian foods in federal nutrition assistance programs.[4]

The spiritual value of food, as well as its use as positive reinforcement, has both positive and negative impacts on many American Indian communities. Food is respected as nourishment, but it may also be used for "rewarding children with foods such as candy, bakery sweets, pop, and ice cream that were restricted when the parents themselves were young children in extreme poverty and didn't have access to such foods and beverages," notes Karen Strauss, MS, a retired dietitian with 20 years of experience in the Indian Health Service.

These issues of poor diet and lack of resources did not happen overnight. As the 2004 U.S. Commission on Civil Rights Report "Broken Promises: Evaluating the Native American Health Care System" notes, "The nation's lengthy history of failing to keep its promises to Native Americans, including the failure of Congress to provide the resources necessary to create and maintain an effective health care system for Native Americans," has been deeply detrimental to the long-term health of many American Indian and Alaska Native populations. Current funding appropriated for the Indian Health Service provides only 55 percent of what is needed to ensure standard mainstream personal health-care services for American Indians.[5] In addition, more than one-quarter of American Indians are living in poverty, a rate that is more than double that of the general U.S. population.[6]

Given this reality of severely underfunded healthcare services, the need to focus on preventive healthcare measures (eg, healthful eating, exercise, routine care) becomes all the more vital in American Indian communities. Strauss recommends that public health strategies "involve the community via coalitions or similar organizations in developing and implementing interventions" rather than imposing a vision of public health from an outsider's perspective. Local culture and traditions should be integrated into any public health policy by accounting for the diversity of beliefs and traditions among American Indians.

Nutrition Transitions in American Indian Communities

Like many communities in the United States, many American Indian tribes have undergone nutrition transitions whereby chronic diseases are becoming more prevalent. According to one study in the August 2006 issue of *Diabetes Care*, when comparing two groups of Pima Indians with similar genetic makeup—one in traditional environments in Mexico and the other in Western environments in the United States—the prevalence of type 2 diabetes was overwhelmingly higher among Pima Indians in the United States. With many American Indians adopting a sedentary lifestyle typical of rural America, the lack of physical activity and oversupply of fatty, sugary foods has become a recipe for disaster.

With American Indian families ill equipped with financial resources, parenting support, and access to healthful foods, current generations of American Indians are struggling with obesity and prediabetes. Despite categorizing American Indians as part of the same racial or ethnic group, American Indian tribes are not all the same—not in culture or even in diabetes rates (with some at 5 percent and others at 33 percent).[7] Therefore, interventions must be uniquely planned and implemented with the individual situations in mind. The focus should be on prevention with cultural competency at the heart of these programs.

Promoting Health and Heritage

Many efforts have focused on preventing diabetes and obesity in American Indian communities by promoting the consumption of local and traditional foods. In her book *Recovering Our Ancestors' Gardens: Indigenous Recipes and Guide to Diet and Fitness*, Devon Abbott Mihesuah, PhD, a historian and member of the Choctaw Nation of Oklahoma, asserts that fry bread and Indian tacos are not traditional fare. While many American Indians have grown up eating these foods, Mihesuah points out that traditional American Indian diets did not include wheat or dairy products. Fry bread, like other foods made from wheat, came from the federal commodity food program, which provided surplus white flour, cheese, sugar, lard, and canned foods to American Indian reservations.

By contrast, traditional American Indian diets featured a wide range of meats, vegetables, fruits, and herbs. Some traditional foods popularly appeared in Thanksgiving dinners—for example, turkey, corn, green beans, potatoes, squash, cranberries, pumpkin, and beans—and the variety of foods did not end there. Walnuts, avocados, red and yellow bell peppers, strawberries, cactus, guava, papaya, and artichokes are all indigenous to the Americas. American Indian tribes also included wild plants such as dandelion, elderberry, mint, purslane, and watercress in their diet.

Community-based organizations such as Tohono O'odham Community Action in Sells, Ariz., are taking steps to promote healthful lifestyles among American Indians. In 2000, Tohono O'odham Community Action helped organize the Desert Walk for Health and Heritage, a march that lasted more than a week and took participants more than 200 miles from El Desemboque, a Mexican village on the Sea of Cortez, across the Sonoran Desert to Tucson, Ariz. The aim was to raise awareness of healthful, traditional foods, particularly as a solution to the diabetes epidemic that has affected one-half of Tohono O'odham adults,[8] through the revival of a heritage walk traditionally undertaken by young Tohono O'odham men. During the event, walkers ate stewed nopalitos (cactus pads), mesquite and amaranth pancakes with prickly pear syrup, and punch made with ocotillo flowers.

Tohono O'odham Community Action is currently working with the Indian Oasis-Boboquivari School District to improve the nutritional quality of meals by serving students healthful, local, and traditional foods. Teachers are also trained to use lesson plans that promote traditional foods and healthful eating through garden-based activities.

Urban health centers are also addressing nutrition disparities among American Indians. (Contrary to popular belief, almost two-thirds of American Indians and Alaska Natives reside off reservation in metropolitan areas.[9]) One urban effort to improve American Indian health is the Running Is My High event hosted by the Native American Health Center in Oakland, Calif. The annual event celebrates sobriety and wellness by bringing back the tradition of running among American Indians. In addition, the American Indian Health Service of Chicago offers The Healing Circle, a community diabetes program for urban American Indians. The program provides outreach screenings, educational sessions, and home visits to promote the prevention and management of diabetes while linking community members to medical care at the clinic.

Nutrition Professionals' Role

Dietitians can also do their part to make a difference in improving the health of American Indians.

Strauss recalls an overweight patient in his late 20s who had recently been diagnosed with diabetes. "As a clinical dietitian, I always looked for one, maybe two often-eaten foods that could quickly make a difference to blood sugar levels," she says. Following a now-common practice in American Indian communities, this man consumed a large amount (1 liter) of soda per day. "My only recommendation that day was for him to switch to water or diet soda." On his return visit, his blood sugar had dropped to normal levels.

The young man continued to meet with Strauss weekly, and she became his friend and partner in nutrition care. On subsequent visits, he seemed thrilled to show Strauss his progressively smaller waistline.

Strauss offers some advice: Dietitians considering offering consultant nutrition services to American Indian communities should become involved in the community and get to know its people. "Clients may be reluctant to keep appointments with a dietitian they consider an outsider," she says. RDs should also learn about the history and the challenges in the community in which they are working. While serving as the nutrition authority, they should take a collaborative rather than an authoritarian approach, serving as an advisor and friend, not the all-knowing professional. Dietitians can best work with the American Indian community by advising or loosely leading community coalitions and advisory groups. They should also withhold judgment when the social and cultural characteristics of a community or family are not consistent with their own personal experiences and ideals.

Diversifying Dietetics Practice

In trying to explain the disproportionate burden of obesity and diabetes in American Indian communities, Mihesuah asserts in Recovering Our Ancestors' Gardens that there are "not enough native nutritionists. If more people were nutritionists, then Native people would be more inclined to listen to health advice." Indeed, in 2005, less than 1 percent of American Dietetic Association members and dietetics students were American Indian, Alaska Native, or Hawaiian Native.[10]

In attempts to bridge this gap, the Southwestern Dietetic Internship Consortium prepares dietetics professionals to work in both urban and rural American Indian communities. Its goals are to improve American Indians' access to nutrition care with a qualified dietetics professional and increase the number of American Indian dietitians. In addition, the Multicultural Scholars in Dietetics Program at the University of North Dakota offers financial assistance to undergraduate students majoring in dietetics or community nutrition.

Coming Full Circle

Addressing health disparities takes a socioecological approach. Culturally appropriate food services, nutrition education and medical nutrition therapy, school gardens, and farm-to-school initiatives all have important roles to play in tackling the epidemic of obesity and chronic disease among American Indians, as they do in all communities across the United States.

While many see a return to tradition as the best way to combat diabetes and obesity, Mihesuah and others advocate for combining the best of the old and new, such as choosing traditional American Indian ingredients and adding healthful foods and flavors from other continents. Someone could put a twist on the Three Sisters stew by combining the traditional lima beans, yellow squash, and hominy corn and adding a bit of olive oil, thyme, and fresh homegrown cilantro. Such a tasty meal both preserves long-held traditions and allows new ingredients to make a healthful impact.

References

1. Henry J. Kaiser Family Foundation. Overweight and obesity rates for adults by race/ethnicity, 2009. Available at: www.statehealthfacts.org/comparetable.jsp?ind=91& cat=2&sort=137. Accessed April 10, 2011.

2. Centers for Disease Control and Prevention. American Indian & Alaska Native populations. Updated November 30, 2010. Available at: www.cdc.gov/omhd/populations/aian/aian.htm. Accessed March 1, 2011.

3. Gundersen C. Measuring the extent, depth, and severity of food insecurity: An application to American Indians in the USA. *J Popul Econ.* 2008;21:191–215.

4. Edwards K, Patchell B. State of the science: A cultural view of Native Americans and diabetes prevention. *J Cult Divers.* 2009;16(1):32–35.

5. Indian Health Service. Facts on Indian health disparities. January 2006. Available at: http://info.ihs.gov/Files/ DisparitiesFacts-Jan2006.pdf. Accessed March 1, 2011.

6. Sarche M, Spicer P. Poverty and health disparities for American Indian and Alaska Native children: Current knowledge and future prospects. *Ann N Y Acad Sci.* 2008;1136:126–136.

7. Centers for Disease Control and Prevention. National diabetes fact sheet: National estimates and general information on diabetes and prediabetes in the United States, 2011. Available at: www.cdc.gov/diabetes/pubs/pdf/ndfs_2011.pdf.

8. *Unnatural Causes: Is Inequality Making Us Sick* [DVD/VHS]. San Francisco: California Newsreel; 2008.

9. Urban Indian Health Commission. Invisible tribes: Urban Indians and their health in a changing world. 2007. Available at: www.rwjf.org/files/research/uihc2007report.pdf.

10. University of North Dakota College of Nursing. Multicultural scholars into dietetics program (MSDP). Available at: www.nursing.und.edu/nutrition-dietetics/msdp.cfm. Accessed April 10, 2011.

Critical Thinking

1. What percentage of American Indians and Alaska Natives are overweight or obese?

2. Evaluate the causes of the nutrition and health disparities among native people.

3. Summarize the findings of the Commission on Civil Rights Report Broken Promises: Evaluating the Native American Health Care System.

ELAINE KOVACS, MA, is currently pursuing her master's degree in social work while working in Austin, Tex. MELISSA IP, MA, RD, is a health educator in New York City.

Rising Prices on the Menu

Higher Food Prices May Be Here to Stay

Thomas Helbling, and Shaun Roache

Around the world, poor weather has reduced harvests and driven up food prices, fueling inflation risks and hitting the most vulnerable. Floods in Australia, Pakistan, and parts of India have helped push up the cost of food, as have droughts in China, Argentina, and Eastern Europe. Energy prices are again on the rise, with likely knock-on effects for food.

Many countries—especially developing and emerging economies—are struggling with the implications of high food prices, given their effects on poverty, inflation, and, for importing countries, the balance of payments. Higher food prices may also have contributed to social unrest in the Middle East and North Africa.

International food prices were broadly stable through the first half of 2010, but they surged in the second half of 2010, and have continued rising in 2011. The IMF's food price index (see box) is now close to the previous spike in June 2008.

The increase in food prices is, of course, bad news for all consumers. But the poor—as well as consumers in developing and emerging economies in general—are hit harder by higher food costs because food represents a much larger share of their overall spending (IMF, 2011). At the same time, rapidly rising food prices pose important macroeconomic policy challenges for decision makers in emerging and developing economies.

International Food Markets

Food, more than perhaps any other product, is laden with both symbolic and practical value. Concerns about food security, sufficient domestic production, and relative incomes in agriculture mean that food is not traded as readily as manufactured goods, because of protectionist agricultural policies. Despite these trade barriers, some major food items—especially major grains and oilseeds—are traded internationally. In this article we focus on the international prices of such products. Much food is not traded, so international food prices are only one determinant of domestic food inflation.

The world grew accustomed to relatively low international food prices in the 1980s and the 1990s, when prices adjusted for inflation were below those recorded during the Great Depression. But since the turn of the century, food prices have been rising steadily—except for declines during the global financial crisis in late 2008 and early 2009—and this suggests that these increases are a trend and don't just reflect temporary factors.

Expensive Tastes

Perhaps the most important explanation for the trend increase in food prices is that consumers in emerging and developing economies are becoming richer and changing their diet as a result. In particular, consumers in these economies are eating more high-protein foods such as meat, dairy products, edible oils, fruits and vegetables, and seafood. These products are more "income elastic" than staple grains. In other words, as people get richer, they demand more of these high-protein foods, whereas their consumption of grains may grow more slowly or even decline.

This increases the demand for scarce agricultural resources—for example, more land might be devoted to cattle grazing instead of crop planting, while more crops are used for animal feed. Reflecting these changes, emerging and developing economies have accounted for about three-quarters of the total growth in global demand for major crops since the early 2000s.

Food and Fuel

Another influence on the markets for food products over the past decade has been the boom in biofuels. High oil prices and policy support have boosted demand for biofuels, which are used as supplements in transportation fuels, particularly in the advanced economies and also in some emerging economies, including Brazil. This demand, in turn, has buoyed the demand for feedstock crops. In 2010, for example, the production of corn-based ethanol absorbed some 15 percent of the global corn crop. Other crops whose demand is correlated with that of biofuels are cane sugar, palm kernels, and rapeseed.

In addition to these indirect effects, high oil prices also have a direct effect on the cost of producing food because fuel—including natural gas—is used to produce inputs, such as fertilizers. Fuel is also used in all stages of the agricultural production cycle—from sowing to harvesting to distribution. Food prices are partly dependent on oil prices, and biofuels have likely strengthened this link.

Tracking Food

The IMF food price index tracks the spot prices of the 22 most commonly internationally traded agricultural food items.

These include major grains—wheat, rice, and corn; oil seeds—soybeans; edible oils—palm oil; basic meats—beef carcasses; some basic seafood items—fish meal; some tropical fruits—bananas; and sugar.

The index was created to facilitate assessment of food market developments and prospects for the IMF's *World Economic Outlook*. The commodities it follows are those with the largest shares in international trade, and those shares determine the weight of each commodity in the index. These items generally have an international reference price—for example, the price of U.S. corn exports at Gulf of Mexico ports.

Yielding Crops

With the structural increases in the demand for many crops and other foods, prices can only remain stable over the medium term if there is a matching structural increase in supply. In other words, average prices have to increase to provide the incentives for increased supply. While farmers have responded to the opportunities from rising demand, their response has only been gradual. The interplay between productivity and acreage growth is key to understanding the supply response. Traditionally, rapid productivity growth in agriculture helped drive down food prices. But over the past decade, global productivity growth—as measured by the amount of crop produced per hectare—has fallen for rice and wheat compared with the 1980s and 1990s and has been broadly stagnant for corn and soybeans. Less productivity growth means higher prices, everything else being equal.

With lower yield growth, production increases have had to be achieved by using more land. But increasing the amount of land devoted to producing more of a crop comes at a cost, which is reflected in higher prices. The higher cost is due to two main factors.

First, crops compete for land. Since there are geographical limits to where crops can be produced, higher acreage for one crop often means lower acreage for another. Farmers decide what to plant depending on crops' relative prices. Second, because demand for many crops has been rising at the same time, overall acreage also had to increase. To encourage farmers to plant and harvest more acreage, particularly on marginal land that is less productive, crop prices need to rise.

From a longer-term perspective, the recent decline in yield growth is worrying. It means that continued growth in demand for food will require further increases in acreage. But some of the additional land will be less productive than that now being used, whether due to lack of irrigation in arid areas, poor infrastructure, or simply lower soil fertility. In areas with rapid urbanization, fertile land is being used for purposes other than agriculture. And soil degradation and climate change have hampered yield growth.

Low yield growth and limited land availability amid rapid demand growth in an economy can lead to shifts in international trade patterns. In China, for example, rising demand for animal feed has turned that country into a net importer of corn and soybeans. Because international food markets are still relatively shallow—that is, only a small share of global production is exported, as most production is consumed locally—such developments can have large effects on world prices.

Weathering Production Cuts

The ongoing structural change in international food markets is clearly one factor behind the trend increase in food prices. But trends usually don't result in abrupt price movements. To really understand recent price surges, we have to look at other factors. Indeed, the catalyst of the food price surge since mid-2010 has been a series of weather-related supply shocks. The sequence of events is well known by now.

First, drought and wildfires caused a decline in wheat production in Russia, Ukraine, and Kazakhstan. As a result, the global wheat harvest for the current crop year is now estimated to have declined by over 5 percent. Then, a hot and wet summer led to a lower-than-expected corn harvest in the United States. Finally, starting in fall 2010, one of the strongest La Niña weather episodes in the past 50 years began to hit harvests—including rice—in Asia. The damage to harvests in Asia not only caused rises in the price of international food commodities but also affected local food markets, notably through the negative impact on local fruit and vegetable production.

The global price response to a supply shortfall depends not only on the size of the shortfall but also on other factors. One amplifying factor was the imposition of grain export restrictions in Russia and Ukraine. This helps to keep domestic prices low and stable but leads to higher world prices. A pattern of protectionist trade policy responses to supply shocks have also been observed during past price surges for food commodities, including in the 1973–74 and the 2006–08 booms (see Martin and Anderson, 2011).

Stocking Up

Food prices are also affected by the level of stocks. Many of the major food commodities—as opposed to perishable food—are storable and, when there are harvest shortfalls, stocks can add to supply. The lower stocks are relative to consumption—the so-called stock-use ratio—the more reluctant inventory holders will be to release parts of their stocks at any given price, assuming they are maintaining them partly to protect against future shortages. So the effect of supply shocks on prices goes up as stock-use ratios fall.

Low stock-use ratios have amplified the effects on prices of recent supply disappointments and have contributed to an uptick in food price volatility. Stock levels relative to consumption decreased substantially over the past decade. At the previous food price peak in 2008, they had reached a low comparable to that recorded during the 1973–74 commodity and food price boom. Favorable harvest outcomes in the second half of 2008 and early 2009 allowed for only minor rebuilding of stocks. So when supply shocks started to hit in mid-2010, food markets were still vulnerable.

The effects of supply shocks tend to be short lived. Crop production usually returns to trend quickly as weather normalizes. Indeed, periods with production shortfalls and large price spikes are usually bracketed by long periods of relative price stability (Deaton and Laroque, 1992, among others, have emphasized this pattern). In the absence of further weather disturbances, the recent food price surge can be expected to ease when the new Northern Hemisphere crop season begins later this year. But the upward trend in prices is unlikely to reverse soon because the supply adjustment to the structural increases in demand for major food commodities will take time.

Impact

The surge in international food prices has already caused higher domestic food inflation and headline consumer price inflation as of early 2011 in many economies. Such direct effects are referred to as "first-round," and are part of the normal pass-through of prices. As in 2007–08, these effects have been greater in emerging and developing economies, where the share of food items in the consumer basket is higher than in advanced economies (IMF, 2008).

Just as poorer countries and households spend a higher proportion of their budget on food, so too the actual cost of food makes up a larger proportion of the cost of food products in poor countries than in rich countries, where the cost of labor, transportation, marketing, and packaging add value that are not in the form of calories.

But if international food prices stabilize, the first-round effects fade unless underlying, or core, inflation is affected. Economists call these indirect or "second-round" effects and they occur if the food price increases affected expectations of future inflation. If people expect food to continue to go up in price, they begin to demand higher wages, leading to increased core inflation.

The experience of the past two decades has been that risks of a pass-through from rising food prices to core inflation are low for advanced economies, but are significant for emerging and developing economies.

The main reasons for this difference are twofold (IMF, 2008). First, with the much larger expenditure shares for food and larger cost shares of raw food in the latter group of countries, food price spikes are more likely to unhinge inflation expectations and trigger increases in wage demands. Second, monetary policy credibility in emerging and developing economies remains lower despite recent improvements, implying that economic actors will be less confident in a strong central bank response to emerging inflation pressures and will thus be more likely to adjust their medium-term inflation expectations.

The IMF has traditionally advised countries to accommodate the first-round, direct effects of rising commodity prices on inflation, but to be prepared to tighten monetary policy to avoid second-round effects. At the same time, such policies have to be complemented by measures that strengthen social safety nets and protect the poor from the ravages of rising grocery bills.

Higher Food Prices—Here to Stay?

The world may need to get used to higher food prices. A large part of the recent surge is related to temporary factors, such as the weather. Nevertheless, the main reasons for rising demand for food reflect structural changes in the global economy that will not be reversed.

Over time, supply growth can be expected to respond to higher prices, as it has in previous decades, easing pressures on food markets, but this will take time counted in years rather than months. There is also the prospect that the world may face increasing scarcity in inputs important for food production, including land, water, and energy. Technology and higher yield growth could compensate for such scarcity.

In the meantime, policymakers—particularly in emerging and developing economies—will likely have to continue confronting the challenges posed by food prices that are both higher and more volatile than the world has been used to.

References

Deaton, Angus, and Guy Laroque, 1992, *"On the Behavior of Commodity Prices," Review of Economic Studies,* vol. 59, no. 1, pp. 1–23.

Grilli, Enzo, and Maw Cheng Yang, 1988, *"Primary Commodity Prices, Manufactured Goods Prices, and the Terms of Trade of Developing Countries: What the Long Run Shows," The World Bank Economic Review,* vol. 2, no. 1, pp. 1–47.

International Monetary Fund, 2008, *World Economic Outlook,* Chapter 3, *"Is Inflation Back? Commodity Prices and Inflation"* (Washington, October).

_____, 2011, *World Economic Outlook* (Washington, April).

Martin, Will, and Kym Anderson, 2011, *"Export Restrictions and Price Insulation During Commodity Price Booms"* Revised version of a paper presented at the World Bank-UC Berkeley Conference on Agriculture for Development—Revisited, Berkeley, October 1–2, 2010.

Pfaffenzeller, Stephan, Paul Newbold, and Anthony Rayner, 2007, *"A Short Note on Updating the Grilli and Yang Commodity Price Index," The World Bank Economic Review,* vol. 21, no. 1, pp. 151–63.

Critical Thinking

1. List the factors that impact the price of the global food supply.
2. How has the economic growth in emerging and developing countries impacted the price and supply of food?
3. Explain why growing crops for biofuels impacts the supply and price of food crops.

Thomas Helbling is an Advisor and **Shaun Roache** is an Economist, both in the IMF's Research Department.

Can Low-Income Americans Afford a Healthy Diet?

Many nutritional professionals believe that all Americans, regardless of income, have access to a nutritious diet of whole grains, lean meats, and fresh vegetables and fruits. In reality, food prices pose a significant barrier for many consumers who are trying to balance good nutrition with affordability. The Thrifty Food Plan, commonly cited as a model of a healthy, low-cost diet, achieves cost goals by relaxing some nutrition constraints and by disregarding the usual eating habits of the American population. Diet optimization techniques, when sensitive to cost and social norms, can help identify affordable, good-tasting, nutrient-rich foods that are part of the mainstream American diet. *Nutr Today.* 2009;44(6):246–249.

ADAM DREWNOWSKI, PhD, AND PETRA EICHELSDOERFER, ND, MS, RPh

When incomes drop and family budgets shrink, food choices shift toward cheaper but more energy-dense foods. The first items dropped are usually healthier foods—high-quality proteins, whole grains, vegetables, and fruits. Low-cost, energy-rich starches, added sugars, and vegetable fats represent the cheapest way to fill hungry stomachs.[1,2]

Lower diet quality separates lower-income from the more affluent Americans.[3] Higher-income households are more likely to buy whole grains, seafood, lean meats, low-fat milk, and fresh vegetables and fruits. Lower-income households purchase more cereals, pasta, potatoes, legumes, and fatty meats. Their vegetables and fruits are often limited to iceberg lettuce, potatoes, canned corn, bananas, and frozen orange juice.

Many nutritionists insist that all Americans have equal access to healthy fresh foods; if only they made the effort.[4] In reality, energy-dense sweets and fats are tasty, cheap, readily available, and convenient. Where kitchen facilities, cooking skills, money, or time is limited or absent, they offer satisfying, but nutrient-poor, options. They also help reduce waste, spoilage, and cooking costs. Not surprisingly, they are often chosen in preference to fresh produce and other more nutrient-rich foods by lower-income groups.[5]

Nutritious Diets at Low Cost

The US Department of Agriculture food plans are cited to support arguments that healthy diets can be inexpensive.[6] The computer-generated Thrifty, Low-Cost, Moderate-Cost, and Liberal Food Plans were designed to illustrate how nutritious diets can be obtained at different income levels.

In June 2008, the lowest-cost Thrifty Food Plan (TFP) was estimated at $588.30 per month, or around $20 per day, for a reference family of 4. Cost estimations of nutritious diets are significant because the TFP cost is used to set maximal benefits available from the Supplemental Nutrition Assistance Program (SNAP, previously called "food stamps").[7]

One way that the TFP achieves its cost objectives is by using inexpensive foods. In the 1999 TFP, most of the energy came from oil, shortening and mayonnaise, white bread, sugar, potatoes, and beans. The only fresh fruit choices were low-cost oranges, apples, bananas, and grapes. Although vegetable servings technically met the guidelines, the amounts of fresh tomatoes or lettuce in the TFP were very small.

Another way that the TFP achieves its low-cost objectives is by ignoring the current eating habits of the American population. In its 2006 revision, the TFP was dramatically different from the observed patterns of consumption. The goals of the TFP could be achieved only by pushing the consumption of rarely eaten foods (eg, legumes or whole-grain pasta) to unacceptable amounts, sometimes exceeding current amounts by a factor of 20 or more. By contrast, the consumption of other food groups (eg, citrus juices and whole milk) would need to drop to zero. There is nothing in the food marketing or nutrition education literature to indicate that such massive shifts from existing eating habits are even feasible. Keeping the TFP closer to the actual eating habits of the population would, of course, entail higher costs.

Time poverty presents an additional problem. Decades ago, many American households included at least one person with sufficient time to shop for and prepare meals "from scratch."

The 2006 TFP recognized that workforce demographic shifts necessitated more convenience foods, yet after modifications, the estimated time required to purchase, prepare, and cook the TFP foods is still higher than the American norm.

In other words, low-cost nutritious diets can be created, in principle, by the TFP framework. However, such diets may be low in palatability and variety, require dramatic shifts in eating habits, and be time intensive to prepare. Working mothers can follow TFP guidelines and prepare low-cost nutritious foods or can have a paying job outside the home but may find it difficult to do both.

The benefits of SNAP are intended to provide low-income families with sufficient food purchasing power to obtain a nutritious diet. However, good nutrition does go beyond mere survival and should include taste, convenience, and variety and be consistent with societal norms. Some suggestions on how low-income families can improve their diets have lost track of these basic facts. Low-income families face a bad situation, which is worsening in the present economic climate.[8]

The "Dinner Plate of Healthy Foods"

A November 2008 article in the Economic Research Service/ US Department of Agriculture publication[4] asserted that SNAP provided low-income households with ample purchasing power to afford healthy diets. A prominent photograph, composed mostly of steamed and fresh vegetables, was entitled "a dinner plate of healthy foods." The suggestion was that low-income food assistance recipients move them to the "center of their plates and budgets."

We purchased the pictured foods from a local chain supermarket in the smallest quantities necessary (see Table 1). Purchased were 3 brussels sprouts, 12 green beans, 3 olives, 1 mushroom, 1 red pepper, and 1 head of romaine lettuce, exactly as pictured by the Economic Research Service. Purchases of grated carrots, pasta, and grapes were limited by the smallest purchasable size. Produce preparation included washing, trimming, coring, slicing, boiling, and draining while the noodles were boiled. Estimated preparation time totaled 40 minutes. Reported consumption frequencies were obtained from the 1999–2002 National Health and Nutrition Examination Survey (NHANES) database. Nutrient composition analysis was performed using the Food Processor for Windows program (version 8.5.0; ESHA Research, Salem, Oregon).

The minimum purchase price for one person was $9.28. Because some foods had to be purchased in minimum quantities, the per-person cost of the described dinner dropped to $4.17 per person for a reference family of four. That amount exceeded 80% of that family's maximal SNAP benefits for one day, with the foods selected falling far short of a full day's total nutrient needs.

Table 1 USDA/ERS "Dinner Plate of Healthy Food": Ingredients, Weights, Preparation Time, Prices, and Frequency of Consumption

Food	Net Purchase Weight, g	Purchase Price, $	Total Preparation Time, min	Portion Shown, g	Kcal per Portion Shown	Cost per Portion Shown, $	Total Price/4 Servings, $	Cost/100 kcal, $	Frequency of Consumption[a]
Romaine lettuce	440	1.79	4	33	6	0.13	1.79	2.39	312
Brussels sprouts	78	0.54	8	76	27	0.51	2.16	1.87	5
Green beans, whole	77	0.50	8	70	25	0.47	2.00	1.91	71
Mushroom, crimini	28	0.36	2	9	2	0.12	0.72	5.84	100
Carrots, shredded	233	1.79	1	30	12	0.23	1.79	1.87	1265
Whole-wheat thin spaghetti, boxed	371	1.50	8	132	164	0.18	1.50	0.11	2
Red pepper	200	1.50	6	48	12	0.36	3.00	2.88	69
Grapes, green seedless[b]	120	1.03	2	74	51	0.65	2.65	1.27	823
Olives	13	0.27	1	13	37	0.27	1.08	0.74	138
Total		9.28	40	485	335	2.92	16.69		

Abbreviations: ERS, Economic Research Service; NHANES, National Health and Nutrition Examination Survey; USDA, US Department of Agriculture.

[a]Reported frequency of consumption, listed in NHANES, as purchased and consumed, without added salt or fat.

[b]Grapes from Metropolitan Market, where they could be purchased in small quantities.

The healthy dinner weighed 458 g (1 lb) yet supplied just 335 kcal, mostly from carbohydrates. Protein content was inadequate (13 g), whereas percentage energy from fat was 13% (5 g). Overall energy density was 0.7 kcal/g, less than half that of the typical American diet without beverages (1.6 kcal/g). The pictured low-income "dinner" was nutritionally unbalanced and based on expensive and rarely eaten foods. Of the foods shown, only shredded carrots, grapes, and romaine lettuce were consumed with any regularity by NHANES study adults. Reported consumption of whole-wheat pasta or brussels sprouts in NHANES was close to zero.

What Are the Affordable Nutrient-Rich Foods?

More realistic dietary guidelines would do well to emphasize nutrient-rich foods that are affordable, appealing, and part of the mainstream American diet. This may require 2 novel research tools. First, nutrient profiling techniques can help calculate nutrients per calorie and nutrients per unit cost for individual foods or food groups.[9] Second, diet optimization techniques, similar to the TFP framework, but more sensitive to consumption constraints, can help translate dietary guidelines into more concrete food plans for consumers at every income level.[10]

Nutrient profiling involves systematically ranking or classifying foods on the basis of nutrient content, through calculation of key nutrient content, relative to dietary energy. Nutrient-rich foods provide relatively more nutrients than calories. For example, the Nutrient-Rich Foods index (NRF) is based on 9 nutrients that should be encouraged: protein; fiber; vitamins A, C, and E; calcium; iron; potassium; and magnesium, and on 3 nutrients that should be limited: saturated fat, added sugar, and sodium, with all amounts calculated per 100 kcal of food or per serving size.

Combining nutrient profiling with food price analyses allows researchers to directly evaluate nutrients per calorie and nutrients per unit cost, allowing "energy cost" comparisons across foods and food groups. Preliminary data already suggest that milk, yogurt, eggs, beans, potatoes, carrots, cabbage, citrus juices, and fortified cereals offer high nutrient density at low cost, as do many canned and frozen foods. Dietary guidelines ought to combine sound nutritional advice with analysis of cost.

Diet optimization models can be used to translate dietary recommendations into food plans at different levels of nutritional quality and cost. Such models should minimize the difference between the observed and the recommended diets by setting consumption limits based on the eating habits of the referent population. To prevent the food plan from including excessive amounts of any one food group, lower and upper bounds for consumption are included in the model. Food plans based on dietary guidelines can then be designed for different population subgroups. For those with good dietary habits, the recommended dietary changes may be small and achievable. On the other hand, those with poor baseline diets may find it difficult to achieve the recommended goals. The

development of dietary guidelines ought to be accompanied by a feasibility analysis.

Toward 2010 Dietary Guidelines for All Americans

Reducing food expenditures below a certain amount virtually ensures an energy-dense diet with low nutrient content. With affordable good nutrition the theme of the day, identifying affordable nutrient-rich foods becomes a matter of prime concern to dietary guidelines.

Affordable good nutrition requires reconciling nutrient density, nutrient cost, and current consumption patterns or social norms. These diverse factors must be considered to develop dietary guidelines truly applicable to all segments of American society. The current economic situation demands that the 2010 Dietary Guidelines Advisory Committee take food prices and the food choices made by real people into account.

References

1. Darmon N, Briend A, Drewnowski A. Energy-dense diets are associated with lower diet costs: a community study of French adults. *Public Health Nutr.* 2004;7:21–27.
2. Andrieu E, Darmon N, Drewnowski A. Low cost diets: more energy, fewer nutrients. *Eur J Clin Nutr.* 2006;60:434–436.
3. Drewnowski A, Specter SE. Poverty and obesity: the role of energy density and energy costs. *Am J Clin Nutr.* 2004;79:6–16.
4. Golan E, Stewart H, Kuchler F, Dong D. Can low-income Americans afford a healthy diet? *Amber Waves.* 2008;5:26–33.
5. Drewnowski A, Darmon N. The economics of obesity: dietary energy density and energy cost. *Am J Clin Nutr.* 2005;82(suppl):265S–273S.
6. Carlson A, Lino M, Juan W-Y, Hanson K, Basiotis PP. Thrifty Food Plan, 2006. US Department of Agriculture, Center for Nutrition Policy and Promotion, CNPP-19. 2007. www.cnpp.usda.gov/Publications/FoodPlans/MiscPubs/TFP2006Report.pdf. Accessed December 8, 2008.
7. Hanson K, Andrews M. Rising food prices take a bite out of food stamp benefits. US Department of Agriculture, Economic Research Service, EIB–41. December 2008. www.ers.usda.gov/Publications/EIB41/. Accessed December 23, 2008.
8. Tillotson J. Why does my food suddenly cost so much? *Nutr Today.* 2009;44:31–37.
9. Drewnowski A, Fulgoni V III. Nutrient profiling of foods: creating the nutrient rich foods index. *Nutr Rev.* 2008; 66(I):23–39.
10. Masset G, Monsivais P, Maillot M, Darmon N, Drewnowski A. Diet optimization methods can help translate dietary guidelines into a cancer prevention food plan [published online ahead of print June 17, 2009]. *J Nutr.*

Critical Thinking

1. According to the Thrifty Food Plan, what is the lowest cost required to feed a healthy diet to a family of four in the United States?
2. Explain how time poverty affects the dietary intake of lower-income U.S. households.

3. How does the Thrifty Food Plan affect U.S food assistance programs such as SNAP?

4. What is nutrient profiling?

ADAM DREWNOWSKI, PHD, is director of the Nutritional Sciences Program, the Center for Public Health Nutrition, and the University of Washington Center for Obesity Research. He is a professor of epidemiology and medicine and a joint member of the Fred Hutchinson Cancer Research Center. **PETRA EICHELSDOERFET, ND, MS, RPH,** is a postdoctoral research fellow funded through the National Centers for Complementary and Alternative Medicine. A naturopathic physician, certified nutritionist, and pharmacist, she is affiliated with the Bastyr University Research Institute. Her research interests include public health, obesity, and the gut microbiota.

Adam Drewnowski, PhD, was supported by the US Department of Agriculture grant CSREES 2004-35215-14441 on "Poverty and Obesity: The Role of Energy Density and Cost of Diets" and by The Nutrient Rich Food Coalition. Petra Eichelsdoerfer, ND, MS, RPh, was supported by National Centers for Complementary and Alternative Medicine grant 2 T32AT000815. Corresponding author: Adam Drewnowski, PhD, University of Washington, 305 Raitt Hall, Box 353410, Seattle, WA 98195 (adamdrew@u.washington.edu).

From *Nutrition Today,* 44:6, November/December 2009, pp. 246–249. Copyright © 2009 by Lippincott, Williams & Wilkins/Wolters Kluwer Health. Reprinted by permission via Rightslink.

Tackling Undernutrition the Right Way

Gary R. Gleason, PhD

While many problems facing nutritionists in the United States today involve overnutrition, undernutrition affects more than 360 million undernourished children in more than 36 of the world's poorer countries. Undernutrition contributes to more than 3.5 million related child deaths each year.[1] Despite this tragic situation, improving nutrition is often neglected and given low priority among national development policies. Nutrition is rarely listed as one of the key elements of international assistance.

Neglect of nutrition may change if a recent major international effort by a broad coalition of the United Nations (UN) and multilateral organizations, bilateral agencies, civil society organizations, and developing country partners takes hold. The coalition is growing and strengthens a movement aimed at placing undernutrition toward a central position in international assistance and national planning in poorer countries. The main product of this broad and growing coalition is a powerful global "Policy Brief, Scaling Up Nutrition: A Framework for Action" released in March 2010 and posted on the World Bank Web site and published in the Food and Nutrition Bulletin.[2] The document was written by a team of experts targeting political and opinion leaders rather than nutrition specialists. It is being broadly disseminated and promoted by many large international donors, UN, and organizations in the international nutrition community. The policy brief is in the hands of leaders of the G8 group of countries including Canada, France, Germany, Italy, Japan, Russia, the United Kingdom, and the United States.

The policy brief on scaling up nutrition reflects a broad international consensus that a multisectoral approach with adoption and scale-up of high-impact nutrition interventions are needed to make UN's Millennium Development Goals a reality (see Box 1). Clear justification for moving nutrition into the central core of international assistance and national development strategies of sectors responsible for food security and agriculture, health, and social protection sectors has been well documented in the more detailed preliminary drafts of the policy brief (personal correspondence with Meera Shekar, lead health and nutrition specialist, Human Development Network, World Bank, November 2009) that draws substantially from a major position paper of the World Bank with the bold title "Repositioning Nutrition as Central to Development."[3]

The first of the 8 Millennium Development Goals calls for elimination of extreme poverty and hunger by 2015 (see Box 1). Despite global and national commitments to this goal, nutrition has been a neglected policy area in many of the poorer developing countries and also in the context of international aid. Management of malnutrition in children is clearly the responsibility of the health sectors in these countries, but the broader areas of nutritional improvement and the prevention of malnutrition usually lack a clear organizational home in governments structures. This is because multiple interventions are required to improve nutrition, and these are often spread across the responsibilities of several different sectors such as agriculture, education, social protection, health, light industry, and, in many cases, trade. Even within the UN organizations, the various factors that contribute to adequate nutrition for children are spread across the mandates of several agencies. Thus, the multisector policies needed to prevent undernutrition lack clear ownership, the necessary legislation to implement them, and coordination to make the programs realities.

In 2004, economists working with the Copenhagen Consensus Center, a world-renowned development aid think tank, concluded that poverty would not be easily addressed without concurrent interventions targeting malnutrition among the poor.[4] They also found that nutrition interventions such as vitamin and mineral supplementation, food fortification, and breast-feeding promotion were among the most cost-effective in terms of development assistance. The World Bank report noted above as calling for moving nutrition toward the center of international and national development agendas was complemented in 2008, by a special series in the *Lancet,* with 5 substantial papers focused on maternal and child nutrition. The *Lancet* series provided evidence supporting a set of potentially high-impact interventions that would improve child nutrition because of their effectiveness in improving health and development[5] and also showed their potential to improve nutrition to an extent where there would be positive impact on national economies.[6] These interventions mainly target pregnant women and young children and aim to ensure normal growth and development during fetal development and from birth to 24 months of age (see Box 2).

Box 1
Millennium Development Goals

The Millennium Development Goals are 8 international development goals set in 2001 that all 192 UN member states and at least 23 international organizations have agreed to achieve by the year 2015

1. Eradicate extreme poverty and hunger
2. Achieve universal primary education
3. Promote gender equality and empower women
4. Reduce child mortality
5. Improve maternal health
6. Combat HIV/AIDS, malaria, and other diseases
7. Ensure environmental sustainability
8. Develop a global partnership for development

Box 2
Major Intervention Areas and Key Interventions for Scale-up to Act Against Malnutrition

1. Prepregnancy and maternal nutrition
   a. Adequate maternal nutrition and prevention of low birth weight
      i. Maternal protein/calorie supplementation
      ii. Iron-folate supplementation
      iii. Multiple micronutrient supplements
      iv. Iodized salt and oil
      v. Food fortification; biofortification
   b. Prevention and management of infection
      i. Deworming during pregnancy
      ii. Use of insecticide-treated bed nets and intermittent preventive treatment of malaria
2. The infant and young child nutrition
   a. Adequate infant nutrition
      i. Promotion and protection of breast-feeding
      ii. Promotion of appropriate and safe complementary foods
3. Micronutrient investments
   a. Supplementation
      i. Vitamin A supplementation
      ii. Iron supplementation
      iii. Therapeutic zinc supplements
      iv. Multiple supplements for children
   b. Fortification
      i. Salt fortified with iodine
      ii. Fortification of different vehicles with multiple micronutrients (wheat flour, cooking oils, rice condiments)
4. Management and prevention of severe acute malnutrition
   a. Prevention of acute undernutrition in emergency situations
   b. Prevention of acute undernutrition in nonemergency situations
      i. Facility-based treatment of severe acute undernutrition
      ii. Community-based management of severe acute undernutrition
5. Prevention and management of infection
   a. Hygiene measures and hand washing
   b. Deworming
   c. Use of insecticide-treated bed nets

The harm, both acute and permanent to health and cognitive development from undernutrition during this critical "human development window" of −9 to 24 months continues well beyond those ages and has substantial adverse impacts across the full life cycle. This overall impact of poor nutrition during pregnancy and early childhood includes lost productivity, a massive burden on educational systems, and excess costs in the health services that will be needed to deal with the effects many years later.

On an organizational note, the *Lancet* series also concluded that the field of nutrition was fraught with problems, including a breakdown in international guidance, low organizational priorities, and lack of leadership.[7]

International agencies and other donors often provide assistance for a limited range and type of interventions, such as food fortification, improved crops, micronutrient supplements (food aid, etc), without requiring linkage to alternative or complementary interventions. They need to move nutrition toward a more central and integrated position on their development assistance agendas.

On the positive side, a number of potent new nutrition interventions have been developed during the past decade. For example, small, inexpensive packets of encapsulated micronutrients, often called "sprinkles" (see Sprinkles Global Health Initiative at www.sghi.org), can be safely and effectively added to all home-prepared complementary foods for young children. This type of product is an effective alternative to both commercially fortified complementary foods and to micronutrient supplement syrups. Another example is "Ready-to-Use Therapeutic Foods" (see www.fantaproject.org/downloads/pdfs/D3.S8Jarrett.pdf), which provide a specific dose of key nutrients in highly convenient packages that are easy to keep clean and can be squeezed directly into a young child's mouth. Ready-to-Use Therapeutic Food greatly curtails the need for hospital-based care for children with severe acute malnutrition and allows many to be managed by their families in their homes.

Multi-intervention, community-based nutrition programs are vital with multisectoral participation and coordination with community participation and ownership as key elements. Their number and quality are growing in several developing countries and that some international assistance agencies are helping to move such programs toward effective reality.

Positive signs of greater national commitment to eliminate malnutrition among young children are also evident in acceleration of efforts in some countries to complete national nutrition policies and work out cross-sector coordinating procedures. Rwanda, for example, launched a national "Emergency Plan to Eliminate Malnutrition" in May 2009. More than 1.4 million young children were screened in their villages and neighborhoods, and more than 84 000 were treated for moderate or severe acute malnutrition. The country held its first National Nutrition Summit in November 2009 and called for developing District Malnutrition Elimination Plans across the country that target children younger than 5 years. These plans are likely to be cross-sector strategies that involve collaboration among district officials in local government, health, agriculture, social protection, education, and a number of nongovernmental, private, and voluntary aid organizations. To be effective such plans will need to focus on both treatment and prevention of childhood undernutrition and the interventions will need to involve organizing communities to improve both food security at the household level and the nutrition security of children.

Community-organized growth monitoring systems can provide an early warning system on nutrition problems for families with children. Families in which acute malnourishment is found will need to be better linked into social safety net programs such as free health insurance, income generating activities, and household gardens and livestock.

Other counties including Namibia, Kenya, Malawi, Swaziland, and Zimbabwe have recently completed various stages in producing national nutrition policies, strategies, and plans of action. Some have phases that cover several years and include sections as diverse as micronutrient nutrition, land reform, and emergency nutrition in the case of natural disasters and civil disturbances. All of the newer nutrition policies in African countries include a substantial section on Nutrition and HIV/AIDS.

The "Food, Fuel and Finance" crisis that had such a great adverse effect on nutrition in 2008 was a wake-up call to nutrition planners in many countries.[8] It made them realize the need for much stronger linkage between agricultural policies, food security programs, and nutrition improvement. Efforts are now under way to link nutrition improvement more directly with the rapidly accelerating and well-resourced programs to improve agricultural productivity of small African farmers. The best plans also tackle household food security with interventions to better ensure nutrition security of the women and young children in farm families and in rapidly growing town and urban populations.

The new policy brief on Scaling Up Nutrition is a solid, evidence-based resource from which to advocate for greater and more focused international and national investments in nutrition interventions that protect the growth and development of young children. Critical information on costs is drawn from economic analysis of implementing the interventions. In late 2009, a World Bank meeting centered around discussions of "Scaling Up Nutrition: What Will It Take."[8] A detailed analysis of the costs and benefits of scaling up key interventions needed to eliminate undernutrition among young children estimated US $10.3 billion would be needed annually from international and national sources. A positive rate of return should result from lower needs of heath care, lower level of chronic disease during adulthood, and improved productivity across the life cycle.

Multiple interventions across multiple governmental sectors are needed.

Despite the progress on nutrition policy development, greater emphasis on multiple intervention packages, and cross-sectoral and community nutrition programs is needed in a number of African countries, powerful advocacy to catalyze major new international action and national commitments at the needed levels.

Scaling Up Nutrition provides an action framework supporting greater investment in scale-up of proven investments that can eliminate undernutrition in young children. The impact of effective scale-up goes beyond ameliorating the impact of undernutrition on individual lives to include national social and economic development and greater likelihood of achieving the Millennium Development Goals. Economic modeling has generated models that clearly demonstrate the national costs and benefits of young child nutrition.

There is a political window of opportunity for nutrition programs if they can attract key decision makers in governments.

These factors point to a powerful "political window of opportunity" for success with nutrition program advocacy that targets national leaders and heads of major donor organizations. Advocacy efforts for an increased focus and resources for nutrition of young children and pregnant women are bolstered by linkage of child nutrition to human rights. Thus, there is much promise for generating greater investment in effective interventions and promoting the capacity building needed to support their effective scale-up.

Advocacy at the level of senior political and opinion leaders requires targeting of experts as well. National experts and researchers must agree on the technical side and also come together to support cross-sectoral collaboration, community participation, and involvement of the private sector and civil society.

Box 3
Scale-Up Challenges for Nutrition Interventions

Despite growing acceptance of the high potential impact of key interventions affecting maternal and child nutrition, there are many challenges to their promotion, introduction, and, particularly, to their effective and sustainable scale-up to national levels. Constraints to sustainable, national scale-up success are common even with what seem to be simple and inexpensive child nutrition interventions. For example:

- Exclusive breast-feeding promotion can be constrained by private sector promotion of breast milk substitutes, by unsupportive peer pressure, work environment circumstances, or limited support from medical professionals.
- Micronutrient supplementation interventions, ranging from periodic vitamin A supplementation, to use of "packets" for in-home fortification of common complementary foods, can be constrained by logistics, commodity costs, regulations, health worker training, marketing, community awareness, and concern about potential adverse effects.
- Lack of donor-supplied commodities and "invisible symptoms" contribute to why few sub-Saharan African countries implement effective anemia prevention and control programs at national scale despite international guidelines.
- Decades of successful implementation in North America, powerful international advocacy, and availability of technical and funding support have brought salt iodization to universal production or access levels in many countries where iodine deficiency disease remains prevalent. However, major populations are still missed. In China, for example, despite major international and national investments and achieving universal salt iodization levels, more than 130 million Chinese citizens remain without access to iodized salt.
- Deworming, treated bed nets, hand washing, and other straightforward infection control interventions are synergistic with child nutrition but large-scale implementation and sustainability face many constraints.
- Community nutrition programs incorporating growth monitoring and other nutrition interventions, community ownership, and participation are known to be effective in principle and on a large sale in some countries. When taken beyond well supported effective pilot efforts, most comprehensive community nutrition strategies models prove difficult to scale up in broader settings.
- New experiences in operational linking and community nutrition activities with poverty alleviation programs, social safety nets, and cross-sector district and community level planning processes are expanding but lack ongoing documentation or active sharing of lessons learned.

Intervention challenges occur, and they should be expected (see Box 3). Many of the needed and potentially effective nutrition interventions programs aim toward the most disadvantaged populations and often seek change in deeply embedded social norms and behavioral practices. Some require significant levels of community or individual involvement and/or time or cash expenditures. Others interventions compete with major private sector interests and may involve substantial commodity costs borne by consumers, product manufacturers, governments, and/or donors.

Many nutrition interventions are also affected by relationships between household food security and income. Nutrition and the nutrition security of young children and women may differ significantly among households, within communities, and among different regional and cultural groups. All of these factors add to the problems of advocacy. They also increase the complexity of improving and expanding interventions known to improve maternal and child nutrition. In many cases, introduction of nutrition interventions that are well accepted in one region is stymied for long periods or progresses slowly in other regions.

Despite these constraints and challenges, "Scaling Up Nutrition: A Framework for Action," holds great promise and offers a new level of support for advocacy toward greater political commitment and larger investment in the interventions known to be effective in protecting and improving nutrition during pregnancy and early childhood. If these commitments and investments are coupled and linked to guidelines, obtain adequate technical support, and include the capacity building needed, there is reason to predict that the prevalence of undernutrition in young children in poorer countries will be greatly reduced in the decade ahead.

References

1. Black RE, Allen, LH, Bhutta ZA, et al. Maternal and child undernutrition: global and regional exposures and health consequences. *Lancet.* 2008;371(80):243–260. www.who.int/nutrition/topics/Lancetseries_Undernutritionl.pdf.
2. Policy brief: scaling up nutrition: a framework for action *Food Nutr Bull.* 2010;31(1):178–186.
3. Shekar M, Heaver R, Lee YK. *Repositioning Nutrition as Central to Development.* Washington, DC: International Bank for Reconstruction and Development/The World Bank; 2006. http://siteresources.worldbank.org/NUTRITION/Resources/281846-1131636806329/NutritionStrategy.pdf. Accessed January 14, 2010.
4. Behrman JR, Alderman H, Hoddinott J. *Challenges and Opportunities: Hunger and Malnutrition.* Copenhagen, Denmark: Copenhagen Consensus Center; 2004.
5. Bhutta ZA, Ahmed T, Black RE, et al. What works? Interventions for maternal and child undernutrition and survival, www.thelancet.com/journals/lancet/article/PIIS0140-6736(07)61693-6/fulltext. Accessed January 14, 2010.
6. Horton R. Maternal and child undernutrition. *Lancet.* 2008;371 (special):9608. www.who.int/nutrition/topics/lancetseries_maternal_and_childundernutrition/en/index.html. Accessed January 14, 2010.
7. Morris SS, Cogill B, Uauy R. Effective international action against undernutrition: why has it proven so difficult and what can be done to accelerate progress. *Lancet.* 2008; 371(special):9612.
8. Horton S, Shekar M, McDonald C, Mahal A, Brooks JK. *Scaling Up Nutrition: What Will It Cost.* Washington, DC: World Bank; 2009. Report of International Conference at the World Bank, November 2009, Washington, DC. http://siteresources.worldbank.org/HEALTHNUTRITIONANDPOPULATION/Resources/ScalingUpNutritionMeetingReport.pdf. Accessed January 14, 2010.

Critical Thinking

1. Discuss the challenges of strengthening global nutrition policy and food assistance programs.
2. Identify the most cost-effective global nutrition interventions.
3. Define "human development window" and "scaling up to national standards"
4. Identify the barriers to international food assistance and education programs.

GARY R. GLEASON, PhD, is working primarily on "Fork to Fuel," a large-scale exhibition on human food and nutrition, international technical assistance on nutrition policies against child undernutrition, micronutrient deficiencies, improved management of nutrition research and communication, and social change strategies for prevention and control of HIV/AIDS. He is communication director for the International Nutrition Foundation and an adjunct associate professor at the Friedman School of Nutrition Science and Policy at Tufts University, Boston, Massachusetts.

From *Nutrition Today*, vol. 45, no. 5, September/October 2010, pp. 202–206. Copyright © 2010 by Lippincott, Williams & Wilkins/Wolters Kluwer Health. Reprinted by permission via Rightslink.

Food Stamps for Good Food

Should the program target hunger *and* obesity by promoting consumption of fruits and veggies?

MELANIE MASON

Coretta Dudley's monthly grocery shopping strategy is as finely calibrated as a combat plan. Armed with $868 in Supplemental Nutrition Assistance Program (SNAP) benefits (the fancy new name for food stamps), she stops first at FoodMaxx, a discount supermarket in East Oakland, where she stocks up on four weeks' worth of nonperishables: cases of noodles, cans of vegetables and boxes of the sugary cereals her kids like. She also buys fresh fruit—apples and pears and bananas and grapes—but those will be gone in a week. Then she swings by Wal-Mart for bread, eggs and milk. Later, she'll hit the family-owned meat market, where she chooses hamburger and cube steaks. Other than $100 she sets aside to replenish the milk, eggs and cheese later in the month, that first multipronged attack will last her and her six children, ages 4 to 16, the whole month. That's the idea, anyway.

"At the end of the month, we'll still need something," she says. "It never fails."

Almost 500 miles away, in the City Heights neighborhood of San Diego, Tsehay Gebere has developed her own shopping plan at the Saturday farmers' market. The lines are long, and the ten-pound sacks of oranges, plentiful at 9 AM, will have disappeared by noon. But Gebere, a weekly fixture at the market, has the inside track. She persuades farmer Bernardino Loera to sock away four bags in his van. Forty-five minutes later, she gets back to Loera's stall and collects her hoarded prize.

Like Dudley, Gebere receives food stamp benefits, for herself and her four children. Like Dudley, Gebere shops at discount supermarkets like Food 4 Less for most of her groceries. But while Dudley buys four bags of fruit every month, Gebere buys at least four bags every week—made possible by the free money she gets at the farmers' market.

Yes, free money—though the technical name is "double voucher." The market matches a certain amount of money from a customer's federal food assistance benefits, essentially doubling the customer's purchasing power. City Heights was one of the first double voucher markets in the country; there are now more than 160 participating farmers' markets in twenty states. They reach just a tiny fraction of the more than 43 million Americans receiving food stamps. But their very existence raises questions about SNAP's identity: is it a welfare program or, as its recent name change suggests, a nutrition program?

These questions are the subject of lively debate in USDA offices and advocacy circles, where the idea of giving extra money for fruits and veggies, innocuous as it may seem, is exposing fault lines between traditional advocates for the poor and a new coalition of healthy-food activists.

The underlying premise of the modern food stamp program, shaped in the Kennedy/Johnson years, was that the American poor were starving and in need of calories, any calories at all. But there is now a well-documented overlap between the country's staggering rate of "food insecurity" (the term used by the USDA in lieu of "hunger") and its escalating obesity rates. In 2009, 43 percent of households below the federal poverty line experienced food insecurity. And if you're poor, you're more likely to be obese. Nine of the ten states with the highest poverty levels also rank in the top ten of obesity rates.

That one can be simultaneously food insecure and obese seems like a paradox. But consider that many low-income neighborhoods have few full-service supermarkets. Grocery shopping in the neighborhood likely means buying at corner stores with limited options for healthy choices. Even if those options do exist, they are not necessarily the rational economic choice for someone on a tight budget. The cost per calorie for foods containing fats and oils, sugars and refined grains are extremely low, but these are precisely the foods linked to high obesity rates. Healthy choices like fruits and vegetables are as much as several thousand times more expensive per calorie.

In a California Department of Public Health survey of eating habits, low-income people said they knew the importance of healthy eating. But they still eat fewer fruits and vegetables than the government recommends, less than the American population as a whole. "People said they couldn't afford it," says George Manalo-LeClair, legislation director with the California Food Policy Advocates. "It's cost."

At the heart of this whole mess—poverty, hunger and declining health—is the food stamp program. Nationwide, the average SNAP beneficiary received $125.31 per month in fiscal year 2009. If food stamps constitute a person's entire food budget—as often happens, even though the program is intended to supplement recipients' own money—that translates to just under $1.40 per meal. If you're looking to buy something that will satiate you for $1.40, you probably won't be buying broccoli.

Researchers have long studied whether food stamps contribute to obesity. Previously the conclusion was, probably not. But in an Ohio State University study released in the summer of 2009 the finding was, quite possibly yes. The study found that the body mass index (BMI) of program participants is more than one point higher than nonparticipants at the same income level. The longer one is on food stamps, the higher the BMI rises.

If the link exists—and it is exceedingly difficult to prove a causal relationship between food stamps and any one physical condition—it exposes a weakness in the program. The food stamp program has certainly evolved since the "war on poverty," but fundamentally it is still operating as though the only health threat facing the poor is insufficient calories.

The roots of the City Heights farmers' market date back thirty years, to an incident in 1980 Gus Schumacher calls "the case of the broken pear box." Schumacher was helping his brother, a farmer outside Boston, load a truck after the Dorchester farmers' market closed when he dropped a box of Bosc pears in the gutter. A woman passing by bent down and retrieved the damaged fruit, explaining that she was on food stamps but still couldn't afford fresh fruits and vegetables for her children. Schumacher ended up giving her an additional ten pounds of apples and pears. "People should not be picking fruit out of a gutter," he says.

A former under secretary in the USDA, Schumacher is now vice president of policy at Wholesome Wave, a Connecticut-based nonprofit that helped City Heights and similar programs get off the ground. For him, the broken pear box was a revelation: people on food assistance desperately want the products that small farmers like his brother were selling. If those pricey pears could be made affordable for these new shoppers, it could be a win-win for buyer and seller.

City Heights was an ideal community to put Schumacher's theory to the test. The average income in the neighborhood is around $26,000, as opposed to $63,000 in the county as a whole. The types of fruits and vegetables on offer are tailored to fit the cultural preferences of shoppers, mostly Latino, Vietnamese and Somali. The market's operators say more than 1,800 customers, 250 of whom are regulars, participate in their double voucher program, dubbed "Fresh Fund." In a survey of marketgoers, 90 percent said that they include more fresh fruits and vegetables in their daily diet, thanks to Fresh Fund. The market's small farmers have reaped benefits too. Bernardino Loera, Gebere's orange vendor, says Fresh Fund dollars account for three-quarters of his sales.

City Heights customers say they love the quality of the market's produce—"the food is so fresh," "it's natural," "it's organic." But it is also surprisingly economical, given the reputation farmers' markets have for designer produce. Lemons run six for $1 here; at the Albertson's down the street, lemons were selling two for $1. Other items, like kale and onions, were pretty much equal to Albertson's offerings. Loera says he adjusts his prices to match what customers can afford. The wares are made even cheaper by the Fresh Fund. Each time shoppers visit the market, their SNAP electronic benefits transfer (EBT) card is swiped, and they receive wooden tokens in $1 denominations they use at individual stalls. The Fresh Fund is a true match program. Customers can deduct up to $20 per month from their benefit accounts; they then receive an equal amount in Fresh Fund dollars.

In three years, Wholesome Wave and its affiliated programs have secured funds from major philanthropies, including Newman's Own Foundation and the Kresge Foundation. The group had a $1.4 million operating budget last year, and Schumacher expects $1 million more in 2011. But the real money is federal money—almost $70 billion spent in fiscal year 2010 on SNAP. If just 3 percent went to fruit and vegetable incentives, that would be more than $2 billion to make healthy food affordable at farmers' markets and grocery stores.

Incentives are already on the radar at the USDA. Later this year, a fifteen-month pilot program in Massachusetts will attempt to apply the double-voucher theory—extra money for healthy foods—to the supermarket, where most food stamp purchases are made. Taking advantage of SNAP's EBT card, which functions like a debit card, the program will add 30 cents to select recipients' SNAP balance for every dollar spent on fruits and vegetables—fresh, frozen, canned or dried. The experiment cuts to the heart of nutrition incentives: would a little extra money back change people's shopping behavior—and how much money would it take to make an impact?

Food stamps have long had a vigorous network of advocates in Washington; the healthy-food advocates are the new kids in town, with backgrounds in public health with emphasis on nutrition. The convergence of the two groups has not been particularly graceful. "I have to say we got off to kind of a rocky start," says Manalo-LeClair, whose organization has worked with both types of groups. "People were pleased that the food stamp program has the ability to fight hunger, and we haven't solved that problem. So then they were saying, 'Are we asking too much to have it do more in terms of preventing obesity as well?'"

To some in the anti-hunger lobby, the emphasis on nutrition is a political Trojan horse, a pretext for cuts or restrictions to the program. "Nine times out of ten, the people in these debates who use the term 'reform' use it as a sugarcoated way of just slashing benefits," says Joel Berg, director of the New York City Coalition Against Hunger. Indeed, the link to obesity has been raised in Congress as a reason not to increase funding for the program. Also, critics worry that it's a short road from incentives to disincentives: New York City Mayor Michael Bloomberg recently suggested banning the use of SNAP benefits for sugary soda, and Schumacher once proposed a surcharge for Coke and Twinkies (he has since dropped the idea). To some, this approach smacks of paternalism, implying that low-income people cannot be trusted to make their own decisions. "The right and left said we were being nannies," says Schumacher.

The people who run City Heights argue that their initiative would actually expand choices for low-income people who want to include fruits and vegetables in their everyday diet. Imagine if everyone on food stamps enjoyed the same choice. What if there was a place like City Heights in East Oakland, where Dudley could get $20 more each month to spend on fresh produce? Is that something she'd be interested in?

"If they'd match me? Yeah. . . ." She trails off, imagining how that would work. "Yes!" she says, getting louder now. "Oh, my God—I would love that!"

Maybe she could buy fruit all month long. Maybe fresh vegetables wouldn't just be for holidays. For a moment, Dudley adjusts her battle plan to indulge in this new fantasy.

"Twenty dollars a month," she says. "That would change a lot."

Critical Thinking

1. Explain how double vouchers could be used to increase the fruit and vegetable intake of SNAP participants.

2. What is the average amount of food "vouchers" a SNAP participant will receive per month? How does that break down to cost per meal?

3. Describe the food assistance project that occurred in City Heights, CT.

MELANIE MASON, a journalist in Washington, DC, has been published in the *New York Times, Politico,* the *Dallas Morning News* and *The New Republic.* This article was written with the support of a Kaiser Permanente Institute for Health Policy fellowship.

Fixing the Global Nitrogen Problem

Humanity depends on nitrogen to fertilize croplands, but growing global use is damaging the environment and threatening human health. How can we chart a more sustainable path?

ALAN R. TOWNSEND, AND ROBERT W. HOWARTH

Billions of people today owe their lives to a single discovery now a century old. In 1909 German chemist Fritz Haber of the University of Karlsruhe figured out a way to transform nitrogen gas—which is abundant in the atmosphere but nonreactive and thus unavailable to most living organisms—into ammonia, the active ingredient in synthetic fertilizer. The world's ability to grow food exploded 20 years later, when fellow German scientist Carl Bosch developed a scheme for implementing Haber's idea on an industrial scale.

Over the ensuing decades new factories transformed ton after ton of industrial ammonia into fertilizer, and today the Haber-Bosch invention commands wide respect as one of the most significant boons to public health in human history. As a pillar of the green revolution, synthetic fertilizer enabled farmers to transform infertile lands into fertile fields and to grow crop after crop in the same soil without waiting for nutrients to regenerate naturally. As a result, global population skyrocketed from 1.6 billion to six billion in the 20th century.

But this good news for humanity has come at a high price. Most of the reactive nitrogen we make—on purpose for fertilizer and, to a lesser extent, as a by-product of the fossil-fuel combustion that powers our cars and industries—does not end up in the food we eat. Rather it migrates into the atmosphere, rivers and oceans, where it makes a Jekyll and Hyde style transformation from do-gooder to rampant polluter. Scientists have long cited reactive nitrogen for creating harmful algal blooms, coastal dead zones and ozone pollution. But recent research adds biodiversity loss and global warming to nitrogen's rap sheet, as well as indications that it may elevate the incidence of several nasty human diseases.

Today humans are generating reactive nitrogen and injecting it into the environment at an accelerating pace, in part because more nations are vigorously pursuing such fertilizer-intensive endeavors as biofuel synthesis and meat production (meat-intensive diets depend on massive growth of grain for animal feed). Heavy fertilizer use for food crops and unregulated burning of fossil fuels are also becoming more prevalent in regions such as South America and Asia. Not surprisingly then, dead zones and other nitrogen-related problems that were once confined to North America and Europe are now popping up elsewhere.

At the same time, fertilizer is, and should be, a leading tool for developing a reliable food supply in sub-Saharan Africa and other malnourished regions. But the international community must come together to find ways to better manage its use and mitigate its consequences worldwide. The solutions are not always simple, but nor are they beyond our reach.

The world is capable of growing MORE FOOD with LESS FERTILIZER.

Too Much of a Good Thing

Resolving the nitrogen problem requires an understanding of the chemistry involved and a sense of exactly how nitrogen fosters environmental trouble. The element's ills—and benefits—arise when molecules

---

Nitrogen's Dark Side

Doubled up as N_2 gas, the most abundant component of the earth's atmosphere, nitrogen is harmless. But in its reactive forms, which emanate from farms and fossil-fuel-burning factories and vehicles, nitrogen can have a hand in a wide range of problems for the environment and human health.

1. The nitrogen produced during fossil-fuel combustion can cause severe air pollution . . .
2. Before it then combines with water to create nitric acid in rain . . .
3. And joins with nitrogen leaking from fertilized fields, farm animal excrement, human sewage and leguminous crops.
4. When too much nitrogen enters terrestrial ecosystems, it can contribute to biodiversity decline and perhaps to increased risk for several human illnesses.
5. A single nitrogen atom from a factory, vehicle or farm can acidify soil and contaminate drinking water before entering rivers . . .
6. Where it can travel to the oceans and help fuel toxic algal blooms and coastal dead zones.
7. At any point along this chain, bacteria may transform the rogue atom into nitrous oxide, a potent greenhouse gas that also speeds the loss of protective stratospheric ozone. Only bacteria that convert the atom back to innocuous N_2 gas can halt its ill effects.

of N_2 gas break apart. All life needs nitrogen, but for the vast majority of organisms, the biggest reservoir—the atmosphere—is out of reach. Although 78 percent of the atmosphere consists of N_2, that gas is inert. Nature's way of making nitrogen available for life relies on the action of a small group of bacteria that can break the triple bond between those two nitrogen atoms, a process known as nitrogen fixation. These specialized bacteria exist in free-living states on land and in both freshwater and saltwater and in symbiotic relationships with the roots of legumes, which constitute some the world's most important crops. Another small amount of nitrogen gas is fixed when lightning strikes and volcanic eruptions toast it.

Before humanity began exploiting Haber-Bosch and other nitrogen-fixation techniques, the amount of reactive nitrogen produced in the world was balanced by the activity of another small bacterial group that converts reactive nitrogen back to N_2 gas in a process called denitrification. In only one human generation, though, that delicate balance has been transformed completely. By 2005 humans were creating more than 400 billion pounds of reactive nitrogen each year, an amount at least double that of all natural processes on land combined.

At times labeled nature's most promiscuous element, nitrogen that is liberated from its nonreactive state can cause an array of environmental problems because it can combine with a multitude of chemicals and can spread far and wide. Whether a new atom of reactive nitrogen enters the atmosphere or a river, it may be deposited tens to hundreds of miles from its source, and even some of the most remote corners of our planet now experience elevated nitrogen levels because of human activity. Perhaps most insidious of all: a single new atom of reactive nitrogen can bounce its way around these widespread environments, like a felon on a crime spree.

Reaping the Consequences

When nitrogen is added to a cornfield or to a lawn, the response is simple and predictable: plants grow more. In natural ecosystems, however, the responses are far more intricate and frequently worrisome. As fertilizer-laden river waters enter the ocean, for example, they trigger blooms of microscopic plants that consume oxygen as they decompose, leading later to so-called dead zones. Even on land, not all plants in a complex ecosystem respond equally to nitrogen subsidies, and many are not equipped for a sudden embarrassment of riches. Thus, they lose out to new species that are more competitive in a nutrient-rich world. Often the net effect is a loss of biodiversity. For example, grasslands across much of Europe have lost a quarter or more of their plant species after decades of human-created nitrogen deposition from the atmosphere. This problem is so widespread that a recent scientific assessment ranked nitrogen pollution as one of the top three threats to biodiversity around the globe, and the United Nations Environment Program's Convention on Biological Diversity considers reductions of nitrogen deposition to be a key indicator of conservation success.

The loss of a rare plant typically excites little concern in the general public or among those who forge policy. But excess nitrogen does not just harm other species—it can threaten our own. A National Institutes of Health review suggests that elevated nitrate concentrations in drinking water—often a product of water pollution from the high nitrate levels in common fertilizers—may contribute to multiple health problems, including several cancers. Nitrogen-related air pollution, both particulates and ground-level ozone, affects hundreds of millions of people, elevating the incidence of cardiopulmonary ailments and driving up overall mortality rates.

Ecological feedbacks stemming from excess nitrogen (and another ubiquitous fertilizer chemical, phosphorus) may be poised to hit us with a slew of other health threats as well. How big or varied such

responses will become remains to be seen, but scientists do know that enriching ecosystems with nitrogen changes their ecology in myriad ways. Recent evidence suggests that excess nitrogen may increase risk for Alzheimer's disease and diabetes if ingested in drinking water. It may also elevate the release of airborne allergens and promote the spread of certain infectious diseases. Fertilization of ragweed elevates pollen production from that notorious source, for instance. Malaria, cholera, schistosomiasis and West Nile virus show the potential to infect more people when nitrogen is abundant.

These and many other illnesses are controlled by the actions of other species in the environment, particularly those that carry the infective agent—for example, mosquitoes spread the malaria parasite, and snails release schistosomes into water. Snails offer an example of how nitrogen can unleash a chain reaction: more nitrogen or phosphorus run-off fuels greater plant growth in water bodies, in turn creating more food for the snails and a larger, faster-growing population of these disease-bearing agents. The extra nutrients also fuel an exponentially increasing effect of having each snail produce more parasites. It is too soon to tell if, in general, nutrient pollution will up the risk of disease—in some cases, the resulting ecological changes might lower our health risks. But the potential for change, and thus the need to understand how it will play out, is rising rapidly as greater use of fertilizers spreads to disease-rich tropical latitudes in the coming decades.

Mounting evidence also blames reactive nitrogen for an increasingly important role in climate change. In the atmosphere, reactive nitrogen leads to one of its major unwanted by-products—ground-level ozone—when it occurs as nitric oxide (NO) or as nitrogen dioxide (NO_2), collectively known as NO_X. Such ozone formation is troubling not only because of its threat to human health but also because at ground level, ozone is a significant greenhouse gas. Moreover, it damages plant tissues, resulting in billions of dollars in lost crop production every year. And by inhibiting growth, ozone curtails plants' ability to absorb carbon dioxide (CO_2) and offset global warming.

Reactive nitrogen is an especially worrisome threat to climate change when it occurs as nitrous oxide (N_2O)—among the most powerful of greenhouse gases. One molecule of N_2O has approximately 300 times the greenhouse warming potential of one molecule of CO_2. Although N_2O is far less abundant in the atmosphere than CO_2 is, its current atmospheric concentration is responsible for warming equivalent to 10 percent of CO_2's contribution. It is worth noting that excess nitrogen can at times counteract warming—by combining with other airborne compounds to form aerosols that reflect incoming radiation, for example, and by stimulating plants in nitrogen-limited forests to grow faster and thus scrub more CO_2 out of the atmosphere. But despite uncertainties regarding the balance between nitrogen's heating and cooling effects, most signs indicate that continued human creation of excess nitrogen will speed climate warming.

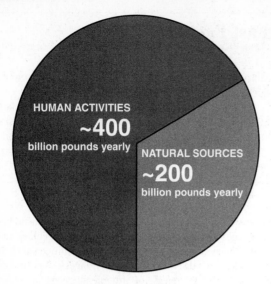

HUMAN ACTIVITIES
~400
billion pounds yearly

NATURAL SOURCES
~200
billion pounds yearly

● Synthetic fertilizer, fossil-fuel combustion, industrial uses of ammonia (plastics, explosives, etc.), cultivation of soybeans and other leguminous crops

● Nitrogen-fixing bacteria on land, lightning, volcanoes

HUMAN ACTIVITIES have tripled the amount of reactive nitrogen released into terrestrial environments and coastal oceans every year.

Global Perspectives
Shifting Hotspots

Regions of greatest nitrogen use were once limited mainly to Europe and North America. But as new economies develop and agricultural trends shift, patterns in the distribution of nitrogen are changing rapidly. Recent growth rates in nitrogen use are now much higher in Asia and in Latin America, whereas other regions—including much of Africa—suffer from fertilizer shortages.

- **Southern Brazil:** Rapid population growth and industrialization around Sao Paulo, poor civic sewage treatment and vibrant sugar cane production all contribute to this new South American nitrogen hotspot.
- **North China Plain:** More vigorous application of fertilizer has produced stunning increases in maize and wheat production, but China now has the highest fertilizer inputs in the world.

What to Do

Although fertilizer production accounts for much of the nitrogen now harming the planet—roughly two thirds of that fixed by humans—abandoning it certainly is not an option. Fertilizer is too important for feeding the world. But an emphasis on efficient use has to be a part of the solution, in both the wealthy and the developing nations.

It's up to You

Making certain personal choices will reduce your carbon and nitrogen footprints simultaneously:

- Support wind power, hybrid cars and other policies designed to reduce fossil-fuel consumption.
- Choose grass-fed beef and eat less meat overall.
- Buy locally grown produce.

Wealthy countries have blazed a path to an agricultural system that is often exceptionally nitrogen-intensive and inefficient in the use of this key resource. Too often their use of nitrogen has resembled a spending spree with poor returns on the investment and little regard for its true costs. Elsewhere, a billion or more people stand trapped in cycles of malnutrition and poverty. Perhaps best exemplified by sub-Saharan Africa, these are regions where agricultural production often fails to meet even basic caloric needs, let alone to provide a source of income. Here an infusion of nitrogen fertilizers would clearly improve the human condition. Recent adoption of policies to supply affordable fertilizer and better seed varieties to poor farmers in Malawi, for example, led to substantial increases in yield and reductions in famine.

But this fertilizer does not need to be slathered on injudiciously. The proof is out there: studies from the corn belt of the U.S. Midwest to the wheat fields of Mexico show that overfertilization has been common practice in the breadbaskets of the world—and that less fertilizer often does not mean fewer crops. The simple fact is that as a whole, the world is capable of growing more food with less fertilizer by changing the farming practices that have become common in an era of cheap, abundant fertilizer and little regard for the long-term consequences of its use. Simply reducing total application to many crops is an excellent starting point; in many cases, fertilizer doses are well above the level needed to ensure maximum yield in most years, resulting in disproportionately large losses to the environment. In the U.S., people consume only a little more than 10 percent of what farmers apply to their fields every year. Sooner or later, the rest ends up in the environment. Estimates vary, but for many of our most common crops, a quarter to half immediately runs off the field with rainwater or works its way into the atmosphere.

Precision farming techniques can also help. Applying fertilizer near plant roots only at times of maximum demand is one example of methods that are already in play in some of the wealthier agricultural regions of the planet. By taking advantage of Global Positioning System technology to map their fields, coupled with remotely sensed estimates of plant nutrient levels, farmers can refine calculations of how much fertilizer a crop needs and when. But the high-tech equipment is costly, prohibitively so for many independent farmers, and so such precision farming is not a panacea.

The solutions are not all high tech. Cheaper but still effective strategies can include planting winter cover crops that retain nitrogen in a field instead of allowing a field to lie bare for months, as well as maintaining some form of plant cover in between the rows of high-value crops such as corn. Simply applying fertilizer just before spring planting, rather than in the fall, can also make a big difference.

The world can also take advantages of changes in meat production. Of the nitrogen that ends up in crop plants, most goes into the mouths of pigs, cows and chickens—and much of that is then expelled as belches, urine and feces. Although a reduction in global meat consumption would be a valuable step, meat protein will remain an important part of most human diets, so efficiencies in its production must also improve. Changing animal diets—say, feeding cows more grass and less corn—can help on a small scale, as can better treatment of animal waste, which, like sewage treatment facilities for human waste, converts more of the reactive nitrogen back into inert gas before releasing it into the environment [see "The Greenhouse Hamburgerr" by Nathan Fiala; *Scientific American,* February 2009].

On the energy side, which represents about 20 percent of the world's excess nitrogen, much reactive nitrogen could be removed from current fossil-fuel emissions by better deployment of NO_x-scrubbing technologies in smokestacks and other sources of industrial pollution. Beyond that, a sustained global effort to improve energy efficiency and move toward cleaner, renewable sources will drop nitrogen emissions right alongside those for carbon. Removing the oldest and least-efficient power plants from production, increasing vehicle emission standards and, where possible, switching power generation from traditional combustion to fuel cells would all make a meaningful difference.

Of course, one source of renewable energy—biofuel made from corn—is generating a new demand for fertilizer. The incredible increase in the production of ethanol from corn in the U.S.—a nearly fourfold rise since 2000—has already had a demonstrable effect on increased nitrogen flows down the Mississippi River, which carries excess fertilizer to the Gulf of Mexico, where it fuels algal blooms and creates dead zones. According to a report last April by the Scientific Committee on Problems of the Environment (then part of the International Council for Science), a business-as-usual approach to biofuel production could exacerbate global warming, food security threats and human respiratory ailments in addition to these familiar ecological problems.

How to Get It Done

Society already has a variety of technical tools to manage nitrogen far more effectively, retaining many of its benefits while greatly reducing the risk. As for our energy challenges, a switch to more sustainable nitrogen use will not come easily, nor is there a silver bullet. Furthermore, technological know-how is not enough: without economic incentives and other policy shifts, none of these solutions will likely solve the problem.

The speed at which nitrogen pollution is rising throughout the world suggests the need for some regulatory control. Implementing or strengthening environmental standards, such as setting total maximum daily loads that can enter surface waters and determining the reactive nitrogen concentrations allowable in fossil-fuel emissions, is probably

Solutions Are within Reach

- Industry can install more NO_x-scrubbing technologies in smokestacks and other sources of pollution.
- Farmers can use less fertilizer. For many crops, applying less fertilizer would not sacrifice yield.
- Community officials can ensure that crop fields are fringed by wetlands that can absorb nitrogen-laden runoff before it enters streams or lakes.
- Nations can institute farm subsidies that reward environmental stewardship.

essential. In the U.S. and other nations, regulatory policies are being pursued at both national and regional scales, with some success [see "Reviving Dead Zones," by Laurence Mee; *Scientific American,* November 2006]. And as much needed policy changes bring fertilizer to those parts of the world largely bypassed by the green revolution, those areas should employ sustainable solutions from the outset—to avoid repeating mistakes made in the U.S. and elsewhere.

Promising improvements could occur even without the regulatory threat of monetary fines for exceeding emissions standards. Market-based instruments, such as tradable permits, may also be useful. This approach proved remarkably successful for factory emissions of sulfur dioxide. Adoption of similar approaches to NO_x pollution are already under way, including the U.S. Environmental Protection Agency's NO_x Budget Trading Program, which began in 2003. Such policies could be extended to fertilizer runoff and livestock emissions as well—although the latter are more difficult to monitor than the smokestacks of a coal-burning power plant.

Other approaches to the problem are also beginning to take hold, including better use of landscape design in agricultural areas, especially ensuring that crop fields near bodies of water are fringed by intervening wetlands that can markedly reduce nitrogen inputs to surface waters and the coastal ocean. Protected riparian areas, such those promoted by the U.S. Conservation Reserve Program, can do double duty: not only will they reduce nitrogen pollution, but they also provide critical habitat for migratory birds and a host of other species.

Substantial progress may also require a rethinking of agricultural subsidies. In particular, subsidies that reward environmental stewardship can bring about rapid changes in standard practice. A recent not-for-profit experiment run by the American Farmland Trust shows promise. Farmers agreed to reduce their fertilizer use and directed a portion of their cost savings from lowered fertilizer purchases to a common fund. They then fertilized the bulk of the crop at reduced rates, while heavily fertilizing small test plots. If such plots exceeded the average yield of the entire field, the fund paid out the difference.

As one of us (Howarth) reported in a Millennium Ecosystem Assessment in 2005, such pay-outs would rarely be required, given the current tendency to overfertilize many crops. The average farmer in the breadbasket of the upper U.S. Midwest (the source of the great majority of nitrogen pollution fueling the Gulf of Mexico dead zones) typically uses 20 to 30 percent more nitrogen fertilizer than agricultural extension agents recommend. As predicted, farmers who participated in this and similar experiments have applied less fertilizer with virtually no decrease in crop yield and have saved money as a result, because what they paid into the fund is less than the amount they saved by buying less fertilizer. As a result, such funds grow with no taxpayer subsidy.

Finally, better public education and personal choice can play critical roles. In much the way that many individuals have begun reducing their own energy consumption, so, too, can people from all walks of life learn how to select a less nitrogen-intensive lifestyle.

One big improvement would be for Americans to eat less meat. If Americans were to switch to a typical Mediterranean diet, in which average meat consumption is one sixth of today's U.S. rates, not only would Americans' health improve, the country's fertilizer use would be cut in half. Such shifts in dietary and agricultural practices could simultaneously lower environmental nitrogen pollution and improve public health: nitrogen-intensive agricultural practices in wealthier nations contribute to overly protein-rich, often unbalanced diets that link to health concerns from heart disease and diabetes to childhood obesity.

Making personal choices designed to reduce an individual's carbon footprint can help—not just on the industrial side, as in supporting wind power and hybrid cars, but on the agricultural side as well. Eating less meat, eating locally grown food and eating grass-fed rather

Where Fertilizer *Shortage* Is the Problem

Synthetic fertilizer has been, and will continue to be, critical to meeting world food demands, particularly in malnourished regions, such as sub-Saharan Africa, where increased fertilizer use is one of the leading strategies for developing a reliable food supply.

Humans already produce more than enough fertilizer to feed the world, but inequitable and inefficient distribution means that excessive use is causing problems in some places while poverty-stricken regions are mired in a cycle of malnutrition. Making synthetic fertilizer available to those who typically cannot afford it has clearly played a role in bettering food security and the human condition in parts of rural sub-Saharan Africa, where wide-spread malnutrition stems directly from nutrient depletion and soil erosion.

Fertilizer subsidies are one pillar of the African Millennium Villages Project, an ambitious proof-of-concept project in which coordinated efforts to improve health, education and agricultural productivity are now under way in a series of rural villages across Africa. Launched in 2004, the project was implemented on a national scale in Malawi. After a decade of repeated food shortages and famine, Malawi created subsidies that provided poor farmers with synthetic fertilizer and improved seed varieties. Although better climate conditions played a role, the approach clearly worked: Malawi went from a 43 percent food deficit in 2005 to a 53 percent surplus in 2007.

—A.R.T. and R.W.H.

More to Explore

Nutrient Management. R. W. Howarth et al. in *Ecosystems and Human Well-Being: Policy Responses.* Millennium Ecosystem Assessment. Island Press, 2005.
Transformation of the Nitrogen Cycle: Recent Trends, Questions, and Potential Solutions. James N. Galloway et al. in *Science,* Vol. 320, pages 889–892; May 16, 2008.
Biofuels: Environmental Consequences and Interactions with Changing Land Use. Edited by R. W. Howarth and S. Bringezu. *Proceedings of the SCOPE International Biofuels Project Rapid Assessment,* Cornell University, April 2009. http://cip.cornell.edu/biofuels.
Nutrient Imbalances in Agricultural Development. P. M. Vitousek et al. in *Science,* Vol. 324, pages 1519–1520; June 19, 2009.

nitrogen production continuing to rise, we will face a future in which the enormous benefits of Fritz Haber's discovery become ever more shrouded by its drawbacks.

Still, as we have argued here, nitrogen cycle problems could be significantly reduced with current technology at relatively affordable costs. We can and must do better. It will take immediate and ongoing effort, but a sustainable nitrogen future is entirely achievable.

Critical Thinking

1. How did the creation of nitrogen-based synthetic fertilizers change agricultural production?

2. How do synthetic fertilizers affect the atmosphere, rivers, and oceans?

3. Why does raising animals for consumption require more fertilizer than raising vegetable, fruit, legumes, and grain crops for consumption?

ALAN R. TOWNSEND is incoming director of the Environmental Studies Program at the University of Colorado at Boulder and is a professor in the university's Institute of Arctic and Alpine Research and department of ecology and evolutionary biology. He studies how changes in climate, land use and global nutrient cycles affect the basic functioning of terrestrial ecosystems. ROBERT W. HOWARTH, who is David R. Atkinson Professor of Ecology and Environmental Biology at Cornell University, studies how human activities alter ecosystems, with an emphasis on fresh water and marine locales.

than corn-fed beef all tackle the carbon and nitrogen problems simultaneously. Individual choices alone are unlikely to solve the problems, but history shows they can spur societies to move down new paths. The well-known trade-offs between climate and energy production that were long ignored as hypothetical now appear everywhere from presidential speeches to roadside billboards to budding regulatory schemes.

Unfortunately, the nitrogen problem is in one critical way tougher than the carbon problem. In solving the latter, it is reasonable to work toward a future of one day producing energy without CO_2-emitting fossil fuels. But it is not possible to envision a world free of the need to produce substantial amounts of reactive nitrogen. Synthetic fertilizer has been, and will continue to be, critical to meeting world food demands. Yet if we stay on a business-as-usual trajectory, with

Perennial Grains
Food Security for the Future

Developing perennial versions of our major grain crops would address many of the environmental limitations annuals while helping to feed an increasingly hungry planet.

JERRY D. GLOVER, AND JOHN P. REGANOLD

Colorful fruits and vegetables piled to overflowing at a farmer's market or in the produce aisle readily come to mind when we think about farming and food production. Such images run counter to those of environmental destruction and chronic hunger and seem disconnected from the challenges of climate change, energy use, and bio-diversity loss. Agriculture, though, has been identified as the greatest threat to biodiversity and ecosystem function of any human activity. And because of factors including climate change, rising energy costs, and land degradation, the number of "urgently hungry" people, now estimated at roughly 1 billion, is at its highest level ever. More troubling, agriculture-related problems will probably worsen as the human population expands—that is, unless we reshape agriculture.

The disconnect between popular images of farming and its less rosy reality stems from the fact that fruits and vegetables represent only a sliver of farm production. Cereal, oilseed, and legume crops dominate farming, occupying 75% of U.S. and 69% of global croplands. These grains include crops such as wheat, rice, and maize and together provide more than 70% of human food calories. Currently, all are annuals, which means they must be replanted each year from seed, require large amounts of expensive fertilizers and pesticides, poorly protect soil and water, and provide little habitat for wildlife. Their production emits significant greenhouse gases, contributing to climate change that can in turn have adverse effects on agricultural productivity.

These are not the inevitable consequences of farming. Plant breeders can now, for perhaps the first time in history, develop perennial versions of major grain crops. Perennial crops have substantial ecological and economic benefits. Their longer growing seasons and more extensive root systems make them more competitive against weeds and more effective at capturing nutrients and water. Farmers don't have to replant the crop each year, don't have to add as much fertilizer and pesticide, and don't burn as much diesel in their tractors. In addition,

soils are built and conserved, water is filtered, and more area is available for wildlife. Although perennial crops such as alfalfa exist, there are no commercial perennial versions of the grains on which humans rely. An expanding group of plant breeders around the world is working to change that.

Although annual grain crops have been with us for thousands of years and have benefited from many generations of breeding, modern plant breeding techniques provide unprecedented opportunities to develop new crops much more quickly. During the past decade, plant breeders in the United States have been working to develop perennial versions of wheat, sorghum, sunflowers, and legumes. Preliminary work has also been done to develop a perennial maize, and Swedish researchers see potential in domesticating a wild mustard species as a perennial oilseed crop. Relatively new breeding programs in China and Australia include work to develop perennial rice and wheat. These programs could make it possible to develop radically new and sustainable farming systems within the next 10 to 20 years.

Currently, these efforts receive little public funding in marked contrast to the extensive public support for cellulosic ethanol technologies capable of converting perennial biomass crops into liquid fuels. Yet perennial grain crops promise much larger payoffs for the environment and food security and have similar timelines for widespread application. Public research funds distributed through the U.S. Department of Agriculture (USDA) and the National Science Foundation (NSF) could greatly expand and accelerate perennial grain breeding programs. Additionally, the farm bill could include support for the development of perennial breeding programs.

The Rise of Annuals

Since the initial domestication of crops more than 10,000 years ago, annual grains have dominated food production. The agricultural revolution was launched when our Neolithic ancestors began harvesting and sowing wild seed-bearing plants. The earliest cultivators had long collected seed from both annual and perennial plants; however, they found the annuals to be better adapted to the soil disturbance and annual sowing they had adopted in order to maintain a convenient and steady supply of grains harvested from the annual plants.

Although some of the wild annuals first to be domesticated, such as wheat and barley, were favored because they had large seeds, others had seeds comparable in size to those of their wild perennial counterparts. With each year's sowing of the annuals, desirable traits were selected for and carried on to the next generation. Thus, selection pressure was applied, albeit unintentionally, to annual plants but not to perennials. Evidence indicates that selection pressures on wild annuals quickly resulted in domesticated plants with more desirable traits than their wild relatives. The unchanged wild perennials probably would have been ignored in favor of the increasingly large, easily harvested seeds of the modified annual plants.

The conversion of native perennial landscapes to the monocultures of annual crops characteristic of today's agriculture has allowed us to meet our increasing food needs. But it has also resulted in dramatic changes. Fields of maize and wheat require frequent, expensive care to remain productive. Compared to perennials, annuals typically grow for shorter lengths of time each year and have shallower rooting depths and lower root densities, with most of their roots restricted to the surface foot of soil or less. Even with crop management advances such as no-tillage practices, these traits limit their access to nutrients and water, increase their need for nutrients, leave croplands more vulnerable to degradation, and reduce soil carbon inputs and provisions for wildlife. These traits also make annual plants less resilient to the increased environmental stress expected from climate change.

Even in regions best suited for annual crops, such as the Corn Belt, soil carbon and nitrogen levels decreased by 40 to 50% or more after conversion from native plants to annuals. Global data for maize, rice, and wheat indicate that they take up only 20 to 50% of the nitrogen applied in fertilizer; the rest is lost to surrounding environments. Runoff of nitrogen and other chemicals from farm fields into rivers and then coastal waters has triggered the development of more than 400 "dead zones" that are depleted of fish and other sea dwellers.

Annual crops do, however, have some advantages over perennial crops in terms of management flexibility. Because they are short-lived, they offer farmers opportunities to quickly change crops in response to changing market demands as well as environmental factors such as disease outbreaks. Thus, annual grain production will undoubtedly be important far into the future. Still, the expanded use of perennial grain crops on farms would provide greater biological and economic diversity and yield additional environmental benefits.

tripling, and even quadrupling the yields of important annual grains, success that would seem to challenge the notion that a fundamental change in agriculture is needed. Today, however these high yields are being weighed against the negative environmental effects of agriculture that are increasingly seen around the world. And with global grain demand expected to double by 2050, these effects will increase.

The development of perennial crops through breeding would help deal with the multiple issues involving environmental conservation and food security in a world of shrinking resources. We know that perennials such as alfalfa and switchgrass are much more effective than annuals in maintaining topsoil. Soil carbon may also increase 50 to 100% when annual fields are converted to perennials. With their longer growing seasons and deeper roots, perennials can dramatically reduce water and nitrate losses. They require less field attention by the farmer and less pesticide and fertilizer inputs, resulting in lower costs. Wildlife benefit from reduced chemical inputs and from the greater shelter provided by perennial cover.

There are other benefits as well. Greater soil carbon storage and reduced input requirements mean that perennials have the potential to mitigate global warming, whereas annual crops tend to exacerbate the problem. With more of their reserves protected belowground and their greater access to more soil moisture, perennials are also more resilient to temperature increases of the magnitude predicted by some climate change models. Although perennials may not offer farmers the flexibility of changing crops each year, they can be planted on more-marginal lands and can be used to increase the economic and biological diversity of a farm, thereby increasing the flexibility of the farming system. Perhaps most important in a crowded world with limited resources, perennials are more resilient to social, political, health, and environmental disruptions because they don't rely on annual seedbed preparation and planting. A farmer suffering from illness might be unable to harvest her crop one season, but a new crop would be ready the next season when she recovers. Meanwhile, the soil is protected and water has been captured.

The increased use of perennials could also slow, reverse, or prevent the increased planting of annuals on marginal lands, which now support more than half the world's population. Because marginal lands are by their nature fragile and subject to rapid degradation, large areas of these lands now being planted with annuals are already experiencing declining productivity. This will mean that additional marginal lands will be cultivated. This troubling reality makes the development of crops that can be more sustainably produced a matter of necessity. Developing perennial versions of our major grain crops would address many of the environmental limitations of annuals while helping to feed an increasingly hungry planet.

Perennial Advantages

Developing new crop species capable of significantly replacing annuals will require a major effort. During the past four decades, breeders have had tremendous success in doubling,

Perennial Possibilities

Recent advances in plant breeding, such as the use of marker-assisted selection, genomic in situ hybridization, transgenic technologies, and embryo rescue, coupled with traditional breeding techniques, make the development of perennial grain crops possible in the next 10 to 20 years. Two traditional approaches to developing these crops are direct domestication and wide hybridization, which have led to the wide variety of crops on which humans now rely. To directly domesticate a wild perennial, breeders select desirable plants from large populations of wild plants with a range of characteristics. Seeds are collected for replanting in order to increase the frequency of genes for desirable traits, such as large seed size, palatability, strong stems, and high seed yield. In wide hybridization, breeders cross an annual grain such as wheat with one of its wild perennial relatives, such as intermediate wheatgrass. They manage gene flow by making a large number of crosses between the annual and perennial plants, selecting offspring with desirable traits and repeating this cycle of crossing and selection multiple times. Ten of the 13 most widely grown grain and oilseed crops are capable of hybridization with perennial relatives.

The idea that plants can build and maintain perennial root systems and produce sufficient yields of edible grains seems counterintuitive. After all, plant resources, such as carbon captured through photosynthesis, must be allocated to different plant parts, and more resource allocation to roots would seem to mean that less can be allocated to seeds. Fortunately for the breeder, plants are relatively flexible organisms that are responsive to selection pressures, able to change the size of their resource "pies" depending on environmental conditions, and able to change the size of the slices of the resource pie. For example, when plant breeders take the wild plant out of its resource-strapped natural environment and place it into a managed environment with greater resources, the plant's resource pie can suddenly grow bigger, typically resulting in a larger plant.

Many perennial plants, with their larger overall size, offer greater potential for breeders to reallocate vegetative growth to seed production. Additionally, for a perennial grain crop to be successful in meeting our needs, it may need to live for only 5 to 10 years, far less than the lifespan of many wild perennials. In other words, the wild perennial is unnecessarily overbuilt for a managed agricultural setting. Some of the resources allocated to the plant's survival mechanisms, such as those allowing it to survive infrequent droughts or pest attacks, could be reallocated to seed production, and the crop would still persist in normal years.

Breeders see several other opportunities for perennials to achieve high seed yield. Perennials have greater access to resources over a longer growing season. They also have greater ability to maintain, over longer periods of time, the health and fertility of the soils in which they grow. Finally, the unprecedented success of plant breeders in recent decades in selecting for the simultaneous improvement of two or more characteristics that are typically negatively correlated with one another (meaning that as one characteristic increases, the other decreases, as is typical of seed yield and protein content) can be applied to perennial crop development.

Although current breeding efforts focused on developing perennial grain crops have been under way for less than a decade, the idea isn't new. Soviet researchers abandoned their attempts to develop perennial wheat through wide hybridization in the 1960s, in part because of the inherent difficulties of developing new crops at the time. California plant scientists in the 1960s also developed perennial wheat lines with yields similar to the then-lower-yielding annual wheat cultivars. At the time, large yield increases achieved in annuals overshadowed the modest success of these perennial programs, and the widespread environmental problems of annual crop production were not generally acknowledged.

In the late 1970s, Wes Jackson at the Land Institute revisited the possibility of developing perennial grain crops in his book *New Roots for Agriculture*. In the 1990s, plant breeders at the Land Institute initiated breeding programs for perennial wheat, sunflowers, sorghum, and some legumes. Some preliminary genetics work and hybridization research have also focused on perennial maize. Washington State University scientists have initiated a perennial wheat breeding program to address the high rates of erosion resulting from annual wheat production in eastern Washington. In 2001, some of those perennial wheat lines yielded 64% of the of the yield produced by the annual wheat cultivars grown in the region. Scientists at Kansas State University, the Kellogg Biological Station at Michigan State, the University of Manitoba, Texas A&M, and the University of Minnesota are carrying out additional plant breeding, genetics, or agronomic research on perennial grain crops.

The potential for perennial crops to tolerate or prevent adverse environmental conditions such as drought or soil salinity has attracted interest in other parts of the world. The conversion of native forests for annual wheat production in southwest Australia resulted in the rise of subsurface salts to the surface. This salinization threatens large areas of this non-irrigated, semi-arid agricultural region, and scientists there believe perennial crops would use more subsurface water, which would keep salts from rising to the surface and produce high-value crops. During the past decade, Australian scientists have been working to develop perennial wheat through wide hybridization and to domesticate a wild perennial grass for the region. More recently, plant breeders at the Food Crops Research Institute in Kunming, China, initiated programs to develop perennial rice to address the erosion problems associated with upland rice production. It is believed that perennial rice would also be more tolerant of the frequent drought conditions of some lowland areas. Scientists at the institute have also been evaluating perennial sorghum, sunflower, and intermediate wheatgrass for their potential as perennial grain crops.

Vision of a New Agriculture

The successful development of perennial grain crops would have different effects on the environment, on life at the dinner table, and on the farm. Producing grains from perennials rather than from annuals will have large environmental implications, but the consumer will see little if any difference at the dinner table. On the farm, whether mechanically harvested from large fields or hand-harvested in the parts of the world where equipment is prohibitively expensive, perennial grains 20 to 50 years from now will also look much the same to the farmer. The addition, however, of new high-value perennial crops to the farm would increase farmers' flexibility.

Farmers could use currently available management practices, such as no-till or organic approaches, but with a new array of high-value perennial grain crops. These would give farmers more options to have long rotations of perennial crops or rotations in which annuals are grown for several years followed by several years of perennials. Crop rotation aids in managing pests, diseases, and weeds but is often limited by the number of profitable crops from which farmers can choose. There are also opportunities to simultaneously grow annual and perennial grain crops or to grow multiple species of perennials together because of differences in rooting characteristics and growth habits. And because perennial grains regrow after seed harvest, livestock can be integrated into the system, allowing for greater use of the crops and therefore greater profit.

Although the environmental and food-security benefits of growing perennial grain crops are attractive, much work remains to be completed. For the great potential of perennial grain crops to be realized, more resources are needed to accelerate plant breeding programs with more personnel, land, and technological capacity; expand ecological and agronomic research on improved perennial germplasm; coordinate global activities through germplasm and scientist exchanges and conferences; identify global priority crop-lands; and develop training programs for young scientists in ecology, perennial plant breeding, and crop management.

Where, then, should the resources come from to support these objectives? The timeline for widespread production of perennials, given the need for extensive plant breeding work first, discourages private-sector investment at this point. As has occurred with biofuel production R&D, large-scale funding by governments or philanthropic foundations could greatly accelerate perennial grain crop development. As timelines for the release and production of perennial grain crops shorten, public and philanthropic support could increasingly be supplanted by support from companies providing agricultural goods and services. Although perennial grain crops might not initially interest large agribusinesses focused on annual grain crop production, the prospect of developing a suite of new goods and services, including equipment management consulting, and seeds, would be attractive to many entrepreneurial enterprises.

Although public support for additional federal programs is problematic given the current economic conditions, global conditions are changing rapidly. Much of the success of modern intensive agricultural production relies on cheap energy, a relatively stable climate, and the public's willingness to overlook widespread environmental problems. As energy prices increase and the costs of environmental degradation are increasingly appreciated, budgeting public money for long-term projects that will reduce resource consumption and depletion will probably become more politically popular. Rising food and fuel prices, climatic instability that threatens food production, and increased concern about the degradation of global ecological systems should place agriculture at the center of attention for multiple federal agencies and programs.

The USDA has the greatest capability to accelerate perennial grain crop development. Most important would be the use of research funds for the rapid expansion of plant breeding programs. Funds for breeding could be directed through the Agricultural Research Service and the competitive grant programs. Such investments directly support the objectives of the National Institute of Food and Agriculture (NIFA), created by the Food, Conservation and Energy Act of 2008, which will be responsible for awarding peer-reviewed grants for agricultural research. Modeled on the National Institutes of Health, NIFA objectives include enhancing agricultural and environmental sustainability and strengthening national security by improving food security in developing countries.

As varieties of perennial grain crops become available for more extensive testing, additional funds will be needed for agronomic and ecological research at multiple sites in the United States and elsewhere. This would include support for the training of students and scientists in managing perennial farming systems. Currently, less than $1.5 million directly supports perennial grain R&D projects around the world. USDA funds will provide less than $300,000 annually over the next few years through competitive grant awards, primarily for the study and development of perennial wheat and wheatgrass. Much of the rest is provided by the Land Institute.

Once the suitability of a perennial grain crop is well established, support from federal programs for farmers might be needed to encourage the initial adoption of new crops and practices. Farm subsidies, distributed through the USDA and which now primarily support annual cropping systems, could be used to encourage fundamental changes in farming practices, such as those offered by perennial grain crop development. Public funds supporting the Conservation Reserve Program (CRP) could be redirected toward transitioning CRP lands, once the federal contracts have expired, to perennial grain production. The CRR initially established in the 1985 farm bill, pays farmers to remove highly erodible croplands from production and to plant them for 10 years with grasses, trees, and other long-term cover to stabilize the soil. Some 36 million acres are enrolled in the program, and most are unsuitable or marginal for annual grain crop production but would be suitable for the production of perennials.

One obstacle to supporting programs necessary to achieve such long-term goals is the short timeframes of current policy agencies. The farm bill is revisited every five years and focuses primarily on farm exports, commodities, subsidies, food programs, and some soil conservation measures. Thus, it is poorly suited to deal with long-term agendas and larger objectives. The short-term objectives can change with changes in the political fortunes of those in charge of approving the bill. The Land Institute's Jackson has proposed a 50-year farm bill to serve as compass for the five-year bills. This longer-term agenda would focus on the larger environmental issues and on rebuilding and preserving farm communities. In the near term, Jackson proposes that, during an initial buildup phase, the federal government should fund 80 plant breeders and geneticists who would develop perennial grain, legume, and oilseed crops, and 30 agricultural and ecological scientists to develop the necessary agronomic systems. They would work on six to eight major crop species at diverse locations. Budgeting $400,000 per scientist-year for salaries and research costs would add less than $50 million annually to the farm bill, a blip in a bill that will cost taxpayers $288 billion between 2008 and 2012.

Some limited federal money has already been awarded for research related to perennial grain through the USDAs, competitive grants programs. Most recently, researchers at Michigan State University received funding to study the ecosystem services and performance of perennial wheat lines obtained from Washington State University and the Land Institute. The Green Lands Blue Waters Initiative, a multistate network of universities, individual scientists, and nonprofit research organizations, is also advocating the development of perennial grain crops, along with other perennial forage, biofuel, and tree crops.

Although agriculture has traditionally been primarily the concern of the USDA, it now plays an increasingly important role in how we meet challenges—international food security, environmental protection, climate change, energy supply, economic sustainability, and human health—beyond the primary concerns of that agency. Public programs intended to address these challenges should consider the development of perennial grain crops a priority. For example, programs at the NSF, Department of Energy (DOE), Environmental Protection Agency, and the National Oceanic and Atmospheric Administration and U.S. international assistance and development programs could provide additional incentives through research programs or subsidies.

Currently, no government funding agencies, including the USDA, specifically target the development of perennial crops as they do for biofuels. In the 2009 federal economic stimulus package alone, the DOE was appropriated $786.5 million in funds to accelerate biofuels research and commercialization. The displacement of food crops by biofuel crops recently played a significant role in the rise of global food prices and resulted in increased hunger and social unrest in many parts of the world. Although some argue that biofuel crops should be grown only on marginal lands unsuited for annual food crops, perennial crops have the potential to be grown on those same lands and be used for food, feed, and fuel.

Substantial public funding of perennial grain crops need not be permanent. As economically viable crops become widely produced, farmers and businesses will have opportunities to market their own seeds and management inputs just as they do with currently available crops. Although private-sector companies may not profit as much from selling fertilizers and pesticides to farmers producing perennial grains, they will probably adapt to these new crops with new products and services. The ability of farmers to spread the initial planting costs over several seasons rather than meet these costs each year opens up opportunities for more expensive seed with improved characteristics.

Although the timelines for development and widespread production of perennial grain crops may seem long, the potential payoffs stretch far into the future, and the financial costs are low relative to other publicly funded agricultural expenditures. Adding perennial grains to our agricultural arsenal will give farmers more choices in what they can grow and where, while sustainably producing food for the growing population.

Adding perennial grains to our agricultural arsenal will give farmers more choices in what they can grow and where, while sustainably producing food for the growing population.

Recommended Reading

T. S. Cox, J. D. Glover, D. L. Van Tassel, C. M. Cox, and L. R. DeHaan, "Prospects for Developing Perennial Grain Crops," *BioScience* 56 (2006): 649–659.

J. D. Glover, C. M. Cox, and J. P. Reganold, "Future Farming: A Return to Roots?" *Scientfic American* 297 (2007): 66–73.

Green Lands, Blue Waters, *A Vision and Roadmap for the Next Generation of Agricultural Systems* (www.greenlandsbluewaters.org).

W. Jackson, *New Roots for Agriculture* (Lincoln, NE: University of Nebraska, 1980).

W. Jackson, *A 50-year Farm Bill* (www.landinstitute.org/pages/50yrfb-booklet_7-29-09.pdf).

N. Jordan, G. Boody, W. Broussard, J. D. Glover, D. Keeney, B. H. McCown, G. McIsaac, M. Muller, H. Murray, J. Neal, C. Pansing, R. E. Turner, K. Warner, and D. Wyse, "Sustainable Development of the Agricultural Bio-Economy," *Science* 316 (2007): 1570–1571.

Critical Thinking

1. Are the current grains that feed the world annual crops or perennial crops?

2. How do perennial grain crops differ from annual grain crops?

3. What are the advantages and disadvantages of creating perennial grain crops?

4. Identify the three grain crops that provide 70 percent of calories for human consumption worldwide.

JERRY D. GLOVER is an agroecologist with the Land Institute in Salina, Kansas. **JOHN P. REGANOLD** (reganold@wsu.edu) is a Regents professor in the Department of Crop and Soil Sciences at Washington State University in Pullman, Washington.

Reprinted with permission from *Issues in Science and Technology*, Winter 2010, pp. 41–47. Copyright © 2010 by Jerry D. Glover and John P. Reganold.

Test-Your-Knowledge Form

We encourage you to photocopy and use this page as a tool to assess how the articles in *Annual Editions* expand on the information in your textbook. By reflecting on the articles you will gain enhanced text information. You can also access this useful form on a product's book support website at www.mhhe.com/cls.

NAME: DATE:

_____

TITLE AND NUMBER OF ARTICLE:

_____

BRIEFLY STATE THE MAIN IDEA OF THIS ARTICLE:

_____

LIST THREE IMPORTANT FACTS THAT THE AUTHOR USES TO SUPPORT THE MAIN IDEA:

_____

WHAT INFORMATION OR IDEAS DISCUSSED IN THIS ARTICLE ARE ALSO DISCUSSED IN YOUR TEXTBOOK OR OTHER READINGS THAT YOU HAVE DONE? LIST THE TEXTBOOK CHAPTERS AND PAGE NUMBERS:

_____

LIST ANY EXAMPLES OF BIAS OR FAULTY REASONING THAT YOU FOUND IN THE ARTICLE:

_____

LIST ANY NEW TERMS/CONCEPTS THAT WERE DISCUSSED IN THE ARTICLE, AND WRITE A SHORT DEFINITION:

NOTES

NOTES

NOTES

NOTES

NOTES

NOTES

ANNUAL EDITIONS

Nutrition 12/13
Twenty-Fourth Edition

EDITOR

Amy Strickland, MBA, MS, RD
University of North Carolina–Greensboro

Amy Strickland is an Academic Professional Assistant Professor and the Director of the Didactic Program in Dietetics in the Nutrition Department at the University of North Carolina at Greensboro. She currently teaches Nutrition Education, Management Practices in Dietetics, Nutrition Assessment, and Medical Nutrition Therapy. In past semesters she has taught sections of Introductory Nutrition, Advanced Clinical Dietetics, and Food Safety/Sanitation as a certified ServSafe Instructor/Proctor with the National Restaurant Association. Recent emphasis in her work at UNCG includes overseeing service learning projects in which UNCG students create and implement nutrition education programs for elementary-school-aged children, with special emphasis on educating children of low-income families. Prior to working at UNCG, Amy worked six years as a clinical dietitian, one year as a consultant dietitian, and five years in a biomedical laboratory. She is a member of The American Dietetic Association, American Society for Nutrition, and American Society for Parenteral and Enteral Nutrition.

McGraw Hill

Connect Learn Succeed™

ANNUAL EDITIONS: NUTRITION, TWENTY-FOURTH EDITION

MHID: 0-07-351560-4
ISBN: 978-0-07-351560-1
ISSN: 1055-6990 (print)
ISSN: 2158-4117 (online)

Managing Editor: *Larry Loeppke*
Developmental Editor: *David Welsh*
Permissions Coordinator: *DeAnna Dausener*
Senior Marketing Communications Specialist: *Mary Klein*
Project Manager: *Melissa M. Leick*
Design Coordinator: *Margarite Reynolds*
Cover Graphics: *Studio Montage, St. Louis, Missouri*
Buyer: *Susan K. Culbertson*
Media Project Manager: *Sridevi Palani*

Compositor: Laserwords Private Limited
Cover Image Credits: © John Lund/Blend Images LLC (inset); © Image Source/
          PunchStock (background)